This Way Out

A Narrative of Therapy with Psychotic and Sexual Offenders

VOLUME TWO

Joseph Isaac Abrahams

UNIVERSITY PRESS OF AMERICA, ® INC.

Lanham • Boulder • New York • Toronto • Plymouth, UK

Copyright © 2010 by
University Press of America,® Inc.
4501 Forbes Boulevard
Suite 200
Lanham, Maryland 20706
UPA Acquisitions Department (301) 459-3366

Estover Road
Plymouth PL6 7PY
United Kingdom

Library of Congress Control Number: 2009936853
ISBN: 978-0-7618-4636-9 (paperback : alk. paper)
eISBN: 978-0-7618-4637-6

Contents

VOLUME ONE

VOLUME TWO

Chapter Three

The Integrated Group

In forming a group on Howard Hall 10, comprised of the integrated population of Howard Hall, I was employing a group formation that had been developed at Fort Knox during that pioneer work. There we were able to conduct groups as large as 225 psychopathically inclined individuals, notoriously bad actors. We had found that the larger the group, the more suggestible the members, and the easier it was to lead them in groups. Of course, missteps could be highly unfavorable. However, the gain in the large group's capacity to reach the regressed member, and to reach and control the acting out ones, were the countervailing factors.

The Integrated Group was conducted in the Chapel, on the top floor of Howard Hall. There was a view of Capitol Hill, across the Anacostia River. The overtly paranoid patients were quite aware of the "Federal Buildings" there.

FIRST MEETINGS OF THE INTEGRATED GROUP: VERBAL COMPLAINTS, ATTACKS RE THE FOOD, THEN CALLS BY MEMBERS FOR RATIONAL REPRESENTATION

Integrated Group Sessions #1,2,3   July 11,17,18, 1947

After verbal attacks on me, this group of 80 got around to complain about the food, agreeing on the need to make rational representation concerning it. Colored-white tensions were then manifest, in an attack by a colored patient on one who had attacked a white patient in a psychotic fashion. Lauton was almost lucid.

These sessions contained approximately 80 patients, both colored and white approximately equally divided. Disturbed members were in this group, among this number Loren Jones. The sessions were at first marked by verbal attacks on me, in covert and increasingly overt fashion. This was mixed with testimonials by members on my wish to help and group discussion of ways to help individuals.

The session on July 18 was particularly interesting, in that the group utilized about two-thirds of the session to figure out the problem of the food which they objected to, coming to fairly rational conclusions as to how to help themselves in this regard, namely, to "talk sense." They also discussed means of helping individuals, and the objectives of the group. The colored-white tension broke into the open, mainly in the nature of an attack by a colored patient on Thomas, who had attacked a white patient in a psychotic fashion. Goodman, in turn, turned on me and attacked me verbally. The session was marked by increasing openness on the part of various patients. Lauton spoke without hardly any psychotic content today.

Members who were active in the large session are Jefferson, Laurence, James, Warner, and various others. There are approximately 20, out of the 80-some patients, who are vocal at the moment. In asking the group how they liked the sessions, whether they liked to have them, approximately 18 raised their hands with enthusiasm, and two didn't like them. The favorable responses were from both colored and white approximately equally.

COMMENTARY

These large group sessions are proceeding in a manner similar to that of the experience in the Army. The members in the larger group are both freer to express negative material, and more amenable to group persuasion and control. As an illustration, a vociferous member quieted down immediately when members in the group turn to him and ask him to keep quiet. The withdrawn members appear interested in discussions, and participate much more frequently than they would in a small group.

FILM SLIDES ON GROUP THERAPY IN THE INTEGRATED GROUP; GROUP DECIDES TO HEAR MINISTER

Integrated Group Session #4   July 23, 1947

The group today viewed film slides developed at the Fort Knox Rehabilitation Center for Military Prisoners on orientation of its psychopathic population to group therapy, entitled, "Group Therapy, What Is It?" The response was that usually found in the groups at Knox, with open-going, aggressive identification with the characters on the screen in a wide range of reactions. There was also heated discussion on whether James B. Hall, a minister, should address the group, and finally it was decided that he should. The group received his address in good style, and members apparently received a great deal of release from the session.

Again, this group is evidence of the utility of large groups in the treatment of the severe disorders. As noted, at Knox we were able to handle groups of several hundred. In Howard Hall, the group size was 80-110. 87 chronic schizophrenic patients, plus a dozen observers and ward personnel participated meaningfully in a group at an experiment at the Perry Point Veterans Administration Hospital, reported in *Group Psychotherapy*, by Powdermaker and Frank, Harvard Press 1953.

BORDERLINE FISTICUFFS BETWEEN JEFFERSON AND JAMES ON RACE IN THE INTEGRATED GROUP, BENIGN INTERVENTION BY BLACKS

Integrated Group Session #5   July 25, 1947

Group of 80, marked by borderline fisticuffs between James and Jefferson over race relations, discussed by the group as rank rivalry, with equal participation by colored and white, and reconciliative transaction.

This group of 80 plus patients had just previously seen a movie in Howard Hall 10. The windows had been closed, to keep out the light, and the atmosphere extremely warm and humid.

However, there was considerable interest in the set-up of a projector for viewing of the slides to be projected for group psychotherapy. The members were quiet as the slides were shown on the screen and participated rather well and in good order in bringing up their feelings concerning the various figures on the screen. The subject was concerning what makes a man a human being, nature of good and evil, with points about the views that were held concerning what makes a man bad—the evil spirit theory, and theory on the sort of life that one.

Towards the end of the slide series, a discussion suddenly broke forth between Jefferson and James relevant to race relations, in which Warner tried to play a part. James and Jefferson threatened to fight, and others and I intervened, and Jefferson was brought to the front of the room to be near me. An analysis of the interaction was then attempted by the group, under my leadership, and it developed and was agreed on by the two participants

they were fighting about who was able to whip the other. Apparently an out-
break of rivalry had been developing in their small administrative group led
by Dr. Cruvant. Several black patients recognized the nature of the conflict,
and tensions were considerably lowered in relation to the white and black
members of the group.

Further analysis of the nature of the reasons for the fighting and the results
of fighting was pursued, in which I took the stand that expression of one's
views was a good thing, but that one should consider what effect it would
have on the group when fisticuffs were involved. I was attacked for even
bringing up the question of open expression of views by various members
of the group, but toward the end of the hour, in summation of what had happened, most members agreed that it was best to bring up problems as they
were, and not let them smolder.

The group was quite disturbed during the 45 minutes following the out-
break of the conflict, but progressively became quieter. A member stood up
and delivered a tirade against people who had been mistreating him during
his entire stay at the hospital. Various others showed similar behavior. I gave
a short, soothing lecture summarizing the views expressed in the group and
the group broke up in fairly good spirits.

A fascinating influence of the slides upon the bringing up of the basic
feelings of the group was evidenced today. The group mores seems to be
developing further, with general consensus that fisticuffs is not a good idea,
and that problems involving race relations should be settled in the open by
discussion. A number of colored patients had a full chance to express their
views, namely Lauton, Holster, and about five others, and the same with the
whites. At the end of the session, I asked how many thought that they got
things off their chest, and approximately 20 people raised their hands. The
attendance of the group was 80 plus.

COMMENTARY

The session was an extremely difficult and exciting one, and I consider it to
be a natural one for this stage of the group's development. This large group
session may be considered as a landmark one, with participation by black
patients in defusing an open fight—James versus Jefferson—within the ranks
of the white patient population concerning race relations. This had a profound
effect on the politics of therapy, leading to opening of dynamics of the White
Therapy Group comparable to that of the Black Therapy Group. Also, it
paved the way to the joint colored-white editorial board espoused by Cohen
for the Howard Hall Journal.

BACKWARD SWING OF THE INTEGRATED GROUP

Integrated Group Session #6   September 26, 1947

I started the hour with a question about the classes, but was attacked successively by a number of members. There was interaction between myself and single members of the group. Those who came up with positive feelings were downed by others. There was a fair amount of schizophrenic language display, by hebephrenics. But on the whole the attacks were quite pertinent.

COMMENTARY

The group is in a backward swing, no specific cause discernable.

MOVING THROUGH BLACK/WHITE DIVIDE, MEMBERS WORKED THROUGH COHEN'S PARANOIA

Integrated Group Session #7   September 30, 1947

At first, four or five white patients, from Howard Hall 6 angrily asked that they not stay in the Chapel, but that they be allowed to stay in the bathroom. Several colored patients asked for the Howard Hall 2 patients to be brought up, to join the group.

I then asked what the group as a whole wanted to talk about. A member stated that James wanted to talk about why patients did not want treatment. James asked if he could draw on the board, and did so, doing an ostrich with his head in the sand. Another patient suggested—see and speak no evil, which I drew for him.

We then discussed how to get divergent opinions together. James stated that it lay in three words -irritation, agitation, and another word. I asked what the group thought of this, and many nodded their heads. At this, Cohen violently attacked a member for agitating him. The member replied by calling him psychotic. The group helped to quiet them down, and I suggested that, "All together, we figure it out."

A black member stated that in his opinion Cohen got upset when people did not approve of him right away, and that was the trouble he had with him. Cohen stated angrily that the person who agitated him always was looking for sympathy and that was why couldn't stand him, inasmuch as he never asked for it. Under great pressure, he went on to state that even though he was condemned nobody cared for him and everybody hated him.

Jefferson stated that Cohen believed he had many enemies. Cohen turned and stated that Jefferson "hated his guts." Jefferson denied this, stating that at times he got irritated by Cohen. Jefferson stated that Cohen said he hated him to see how much he liked him. He brought up an episode in which he "blew my top to Cohen, when he unnecessarily asked me what time it was."

A member broke in to state that he didn't like Cohen and didn't care who "knowed it." Cohen calmly stated that he should forget it because that was something else. The member showed a great deal of affect. A friend then warmly stated that "Hank seems to be always trying out people, whether they like him, by telling them they hate him, a persecution complex." Several members verbally agreed.

Cohen stated he had a few friends, that everybody wasn't against him.

The hour was almost up by this time and I asked the group it thought had been accomplished during the hour. Thomas stated that it was improving. Others agreed. The group appeared quite warm. A member stated Cohen was hated. Lauton stated the group should thank the doctor.

COMMENTARY

The interaction in this large group at first had to do with the racial divide, then moved to Cohen's paranoid character, and his need for narcissistic supplies, gradually working itself into a state of bonhomie. Lauton, a hebephrenic who usually spoke in vague, hyperbolic manner, speaking clear English, stated that the group should thank me.

INTUITIVE CONNECTEDNESS APPEARS IN THE INTEGRATED GROUP, TALK OF ALONENESS

Integrated Group Session #8   October 7, 1947

After a silence, the members agreed to talk about agitation, which was then exemplified by several members. The first ascribed it to his confinement. The second, on an existential level, related it to aloneness, asking acceptance by the members on a simply human level. The group was euphoric at the end.

COMMENTARY

The silence is of great significance. The members are communing, prior to assumption of a union in the ego ideal, marked by my experience of what

I came to call my intuitometer, a sense of cogency in my chest. After the silence the members are prepared to act autonomously as a group. The first member's thesis is matched here by the second's antithesis, and the members are joining in a mutual messianism that is becoming durable in this large, integrated group.

MEMBERS' PROBLEMS COME CENTER STAGE

Integrated Group Session #9   November 4, 1947

This 70 member group is on the cusp of adoption, alongside the two small groups, of the new therapeutic mores versus the usual "dog eat dog" way. James (for his perversion with his daughter) and Cohen (for his delusions of persecution) came center stage, and I directly countered the attacks on them, as attempts to "harm" them. This was backed up by the members from the White Therapy Group.

COMMENTARY

The integrated group is assuming its place of being somewhat ahead and yet behind the two other groups. In this session James and Cohen frankly opened up re their problems, and were blasted by members who had been kept in check by the idealism of the smaller groups. I spontaneously "stuck up for them." Members from the white group joined me, and the group ended on a good note.

MILLER ACT MEMBER OFFERS SELF
FOR DISCUSSION, COHEN HELPFUL

Integrated Group Session #10   November 18, 1947

Reardon, a Miller Act patient, offered himself for discussion, with Cohen in a helpful role.

COMMENTARY

Cohen is entering into a frankly messianic role, especially in the large group. The psychotic patients are working with the Miller Act patients.

DISCUSSION OF MEMBER'S PROBLEMS
CONTINUED FROM PREVIOUS SESSION,
PRECEDED BY ENTERTAINMENT PHASE

Integrated Group Session #11   November 25, 1947

The group worked on Reardon's problems further with continuation from the
last group and increased affability on the part of the patients.

COMMENTARY

The group is settling into this mode of operation, preceded by an entertainment phase, or exhibition of the slide series.

INTERMITTENT YET SYSTEMATIC INQUIRY
INTO INDIVIDUAL PROBLEM SOLVING

Integrated Group Session #12   November 25, 1947

More consistently than in the White and Black Therapy Groups, this group
settled into a pattern of work, in which a member brought up a problem,
members associated in helpful manner, followed by further elucidation of
genetic data, then exemplification elsewhere in the group, settling on deeper
analysis of another individual . In this, James set forth that he and others in
the Hall suffered from a "hypnotized state." He cited loneliness in his marriage as genetic, and members, empathizing with his felt loneliness, noted
one's need for mutual relationships. Then members reached out to members
of the group: one asked about his dementia praecox, followed by allusion to
Cohen as such. With Cohen's collaboration, the members discussed his sensitivities and impaired sense of manhood.

   Then members reached out to members of the group: one asked about his
dementia praecox, followed by allusion to Cohen as such. With Cohen's
collaboration, the members discussed his sensitivities and impaired sense of
manhood. The negro patients then conducted an entertaining comedic routine,
telling risqué jokes.

COMMENTARY

I might note here that Cohen is the chair of this group, attending to its course,
while subject of its ministrations.

INTEGRATED GROUP OPERATES AUTONOMOUSLY; COHEN YIELDS DELUSION OF IMMINENT DOOM

Integrated Group Session #13   December 9, 1947

Starting with Cohen's query re his delusions of imminent doom, which I responded to as an internal state, and which a member responded to as the production of an overgrown boy, a member asserted his own subjective sense of injustice. Another member noted that their provocative behavior was related. Then there was a generalized discussion of how members "ask for it," in the context of insanity.

A member asked what he had to do to himself, for acceptance of society. James then brought up that attendants were picking on him. I noted that the group was acting as a mirror to itself, with acceptance of this notion by the members. Reardon, with a black eye, was the chairman, and was little called on to render guidance.

COMMENTARY

The group conducted itself on its own, and the members are moving their delusions closer to analysis in reality.

COHEN, CHAIR, IS HUMILIATED, RECOUPS

Integrated Group Session #14   December 12, 1947

The group started to mobilize its regressed members by encouraging them to speak up, with demonstration by them of virulent racist ideology. Cohen responded strongly, and was calmed by a hitherto quiet patient. Cohen finally wrote and recited a plea for harmony on the basis of national allegiance.

COMMENTARY

Cohen as chair had urged its backward members, assembled here by the attendants, to express themselves. They did so, coming out with the prejudices of the attendants. Cohen, Jewish, became combative, but was quickly brought to his new reality as leader by a patient who had not spoken before.

MEMBERS COMPARE THE SENSED HELPLESSNESS OF PATIENTS ELSEWHERE IN THE HOSPITAL, AND THEIR OWN CAPACITY TO HELP THEMSELVES

Integrated Group Session #15   December 21, 1947

A continuation of the last large group session, with general discussion of problems of the patients elsewhere in the hospital, with emphasis on their helplessness, and the advantage of the program in Howard Hall.

COMMENTARY

Howard Hall had been known as the "hellhole" of the hospital, and the members are girding themselves for their next step in the therapy.

JEFFERSON DRAWN INTO ANALYSIS OF HIS MURDER

Integrated Group Session #16   December 29, 1947

The group was slow today in getting started, with Cohen at the helm, its size larger than usual. Cohen was authoritarian and part of the hour was spent in relation to his sensitiveness to criticism, which he enjoyed, following a blow up when a member criticized him for a remark to Jefferson. Then a member brought up the influence of the moon on people and their disturbances of mood. It ended with Jefferson's conflict with a woman, his wife, resulting in murder, and his current concept of a woman as a worthless creature. The group was tolerant. The interaction at the end was chiefly between Jefferson and myself.

COMMENTARY

It is interesting that Jefferson chose this venue to work further on the intimacies of his relationship with his wife. An item at issue is one of worthlessness; here he has her worthless, and his behavior lately has been "low down."

TURNING IN THE INTEGRATED GROUP, RE JEFFERSON'S BULL HEADEDNESS, COHEN'S COMMITMENT TO HELPING SELF

Integrated Group Session #17   December 30, 1947

The group lasted 2 hours. Two visual aids were presented, one on fleeing (from self) and one on fear (especially internal). They were very favorably received by the group. James, quite cooperative, projected the film slides. Chief interaction was in relation to society, its role in the group especially on who should take initiative. Jefferson again emerged, at his instance, as a case in point, on whether he or society should give way and change. I took a vigorous approach in relation to Jefferson's "bullheadedness," and he accepted that he was so. There were small sub-group interactions—Cohen, Certa. Cohen read a letter, written by him, on his intentions to help himself.

COMMENTARY

The film slides had been produced for the program at Fort Knox (see *Turning Lives Around*, Author House, 2006), pitched for psychopaths, but apparently adaptable for this population. They were in color cartoons, which readily evoked reactions. Jefferson continued to be the chief participant, arguing against personal change.

MEMBERS AWARE OF GUILT TOWARDS DR. CRUVANT, AUTHORITY FIGURE

Integrated Group Session #18   January 6, 1948

Members revealed inner guilty feelings towards Dr. Cruvant, not so with me, experienced as one of them.

COMMENTARY

The remarkable thing here is the revelation of guilty feelings toward an authority.

INTEGRATED GROUP RUNS ITSELF

Integrated Group Session #19   January 22, 1948

After the entertainment period, there was further work, significantly in the large group, in contrast to the White Therapy Group, on Cohen's obstinate pride and fear of losing face, this time coupled with similar configuration in Lauton, a black hebephrenic member. Also members reflected on Sullivan's holding back after he blew up, after offering himself for interaction. At the end, Reardon impulsively offered to confess his guilt.

COMMENTARY

The difference here is the large group's capacity for autonomy, running itself. It is remarkable how its size of 70 to 100 does not inhibit its attainment of intimacy. That factor of autonomy, with its accompanying self determination (about going to the adjoining bathroom) may play a part in future difficulty with the attendants.

REARDON RELATES HIS LIFE STORY
IN THE INTEGRATED GROUP

Integrated Group Session #20   January 30, 1948

The group was active during the showing of a filmstrip pertaining to one's life story, especially Reardon. After Reardon badgered the doctor and was told so, with advice to take up his case by relating his life's story, he agreed to do so. James spoke up for the patients, asking for more personnel, lawyers and ministers.

COMMENTARY

The large group, though regressing, is still engaging members productively. In this instance it oriented a member towards work in his small group.

THE INTEGRATED GROUP GETS
TO WORK ON INTERPRETATION

Integrated Group Session #21   February 12, 1948

There was active ambivalence on the part of the members of the group at first. I reflected this to the group and it then voted to keep working with Jordan,

Smith, Reardon, and Cohen. I gave an example of dependency that results from not caring about self, which was applauded.

COMMENTARY

This interpretation was similar to the one I came up with in the previous session, in the Black Therapy Group.

JEFFERSON-COHEN MUTUALITY AGAIN; JEFFERSON: "WONDERFUL WORK"

Integrated Group Session #22   February 19, 1948

Cohen was shown affection by Jefferson on his "wonderful" work with regressed patients.

COMMENTARY

This again is a most significant development, and is reflective of Cohen's new found messianism, apparently developed in the large group. My thesis is that in the union in the ego ideal of this dyad, Jefferson's belief in Cohen is stabilizing Cohen's ego, sufficient to enable him to grieve the loss of his delusions, which are anchored in his relationship with his mother. This man was profoundly alienated from her, believing she was a fraud when she visited him at Mason General Hospital and St. Elizabeths. Jefferson suffers from a comparable alienation from women.

COHEN SHEDS HIS AUTHORITARIANISM AS CHAIRMAN

Integrated Group Session #23   March 18, 1948

Cohen is now an appropriate chairman, having shed his bossiness, and the group is quite acceptant. The entertainment phase has attained a rather high quality. James and a black patient dance together.

COMMENTARY

This is a matter of great moment. The group now has become a fixture in Howard Hall, this group's racial integration an accomplished fact. But the racially prejudiced Southern attendants are still to be heard from.

INTEGRATED GROUP SETTLED
INTO THERAPEUTIC PATTERN

Integrated Group Session #24   March 24, 1948

The group now has settled into a pattern of first entertainment, then interaction on personal problems. The illustrative photograph on the cover shows Jones, a regressed chronic patient asking for help, re "rays" coming from a Federal Building on Capitol Hill.

COMMENTARY

Under Cohen's benevolent chairmanship, other chronic patients will emerge in the interactive phase. Cohen has called on me to run that phase of the session, and in the photograph I am holding forth re Jones' complaint.

THE INTEGRATED GROUP WORKS FURTHER
ON PROBLEMS OF THE CHRONIC PATIENTS

Integrated Group Session #25   April 15, 1948

The group is increasingly taking up personality problems, increasingly of the chronic members. They join in the dancing.

COMMENTARY

The chronic patients are moving towards the front, and joining in the dancing to the orchestra. I join them.

DELUSIONS AND FAMILY DYNAMICS OF CHRONIC
PATIENTS WORKED WITH IN THE INTEGRATED GROUP

Integrated Group Session #26   May 5 1948

There was further work with three cases. This work consisted of report of delusional experience and acceptance by the members and myself of its validity per se, then attention to the affective state of the person. The group intuited into the family dynamics of a member from the Philippines, who complained of peremptory action by authorities in separating him from his wife.

COMMENTARY

The Filipino member became a spectacularly participative member, both of this and the White Therapy Group

INTEGRATED GROUP: MEMBERS NORMALLY RIVALROUS, AS FAMILY

Integrated Group Session #27   June 29, 1948

Members spoke and sang with me. There was open play for me by Jefferson and Cohen.

COMMENTARY

The open play is increasingly taking on a family cast, with the members acting like rivalrous brothers.

HOLDING ONESELF IN THE HOSPITAL; ADMITTING TO ONE'S GUILT AND DELUSION

Integrated Group Session #28   July 2, 1948

Discussion started in relation to the advisability of voluntary admission to the hospital, and how the members were ultimately holding themselves in the hospital. A member then stated his lack of desire to leave. James and others defended their (delusional) ideas and their right to defend themselves against others' antagonistic opinion.

Jordan stated that James, with his offense of incest, was better off in the Hall than in prison. James replied that in the Hall because of his offense--"hundred times worse off than prison." I fostered the interaction between James and Jordan. A member ended the hour speaking about the members not wanting to leave—giving Jefferson as example. The members were quite pleasant to me today.

COMMENTARY

The members have returned to voluntary initiative in their work on themselves, in the context of submitting to Dr. Cruvant's dictum on involuntary group therapy. A member kicked it off by admitting to his hiding out in the hospital. Then James started his inquiry by justifying his right to his hegemonic delusion that included incest. Then Jordan edged up on its relation to reality, and James replied, edging into his subjective state, hinting at what I take to be devastatingly worse than the catastrophe he would have met in prison. Tinsley, dialectically, returned to the issue of what the members were avoiding, through refuge in the hospital.

INTEGRATED GROUP MEMBERS, LED BY TEX, BRIEFLY STATE THEIR PROBLEMS

Integrated Group Session #29   July 6, 1948

Cohen is still chair. Tex sang his message, on "we are trying together." Then Morton, a sex psychopath, brought up his proclivity towards young girls, and members advised abstinence. Then a member revealed his wish to "kill the King of England." He then advised Lauton to quit smirking. Then Tex sang again, requesting that I speak on confidence and fear, and the group then discussed it briefly.

COMMENTARY

The remarkable thing about this group is the readiness of members to stand up and recite their problem as a contribution, then sit down.

TEX AND MEMBERS CONTINUE COLLABORATIVE ACTIVITY

Integrated Group Session #30   July 20, 1948

Tex and others were active in a usual session, marked by music by the black patients, followed by a discussion period led by Cohen.

COMMENTARY

This activity is of a piece with the harmony present in all three groups, and the general growth of the program.

THE MEMBERS OF THE INTEGRATED GROUP EAGER TO BEGIN; REGRESSED PATIENT: THE HOSPITAL IS MY BOSS

Integrated Group Session #31   July 27, 1948

For the first time, the orchestra played before I came. Then members sang and danced spontaneously, with vying for the stage. Then I led the singing, at the group's request. The delusions of Jones and another member were then worked on, Jones citing that the hospital was his boss.

COMMENTARY

Jones was the patient in the photograph who was persecuted by rays from the Federal Buildings. Here he is closer home in his delusional content, by acknowledging a human tie.

JEFFERSON AND OTHER "KNOW-IT-ALLS" EXPOUND ON RAISING CHILDREN AND PARENTAL ALIENATION

Integrated Group Session #32   July 31, 1948

Jefferson and others expound on the treatment of a boy from the National Training School, to the effect that his parents should not have divorced, and he should have been whipped.

COMMENTARY

An inference I draw here is that the members, at Jefferson's instance, are in contact with their deviant oppositional impulses, and join society in calling for compliance. They also relate divorce to psychopathy. The National Training School personnel had visited Howard Hall and at the request for the kinds of problems they treat, cited that of a youth who fought with his parents and set off on a career as a thief.

THE INTEGRATED GROUP REGRESSES; BAND BOYCOTTS SECONDARY TO CULTURAL CRITICISM

Integrated Group Session #33   August 3, 1948

Cohen acted again in an authoritarian manner, borderline asking/telling patients to come up for help. Several singers presented their problems, along with their songs. The band was absent, after criticism by white members of its boogie-woogie style.

COMMENTARY

The group is regressing somewhat, manifested by Cohen's authoritarian way. It is of interest that the singers combined their art with presentation of their problems.

IN INTEGRATED GROUP, COHEN APPROPRIATE LEADER

Integrated Group Session #34   August 10, 1948

Cohen acted in a reserved manner. The band returned, and the singing done by an accomplished singer who was a sex psychopath. Visiting Tuskegee doctors questioned colored patients on how they experienced the group. They answered affirmatively. Tex butted in, in a hebephrenic, borderline abusive manner.

COMMENTARY

The group returned to its benevolent way, and Cohen appropriate as leader.

ATTENDANTS IN INTEGRATED GROUP BRING UP
A THERAPEUTIC ROLE IN A PARANOID MANNER

Integrated Group Session #35   August 17, 1948

At the beginning of the session, three attendants came to the fore, grouped around me, and a spokesman stated that I had made a remark last time about "sitting on lazy asses," "should do some work." I replied that we needed to talk it over elsewhere, and the attendants agreed.

The session then continued, with the entertainment, then a brief discussion of snitching. Then Tex entertained. Then the session broke up after I gave a reassuring speech relative to "putting out" with Certa as a positive example.

COMMENTARY

This was a full scale confrontation with attendants, in which they claimed that I had accused them of sitting on their lazy asses, and which I later noted as a wish for a more ultimate therapeutic role. The group worked well, nevertheless.

WHITE PATIENTS ENVIOUS OF MISS SAWYER'S RELATIONSHIP WITH THE BLACKS

Integrated Group Session #36   August 20, 1948

Black members were resentful of a white patient's attack on them re Miss Sawyer's favoring friendliness, and on a black patient's following her with his eyes. He retorted that he was "trying to find something to do." The members laughed, and tensions were relieved.

COMMENTARY

The racial politics continue, but the members are able to discuss their tensions.

DATA SURFACES IN THE INTEGRATED GROUP ON ABUSE BY ATTENDANTS

Integrated Group Session #37   August 23, 1948

The conflict with the attendants continues, with negro patients complaining of brutality. I counseled cooperative consultation.

COMMENTARY

A central role of the attendants in the racial conflict surfaced, with the negro patients' complaint. I am waiting here for Dr. Cruvant to take both administrative and training initiatives.

LOPEZ AND OTHERS GROW IN CAPACITY FOR SELF REPRESENTATION IN THE INTEGRATED GROUP, TELL THEIR LIFE STORIES

Integrated Group Session #38   August 24, 1948

The group had smaller attendance than previously--because of resistance by the attendants. It started with the music and singing. Chairman Cohen was calmer than he has been for a long while. He began the meeting by denouncing the attendants and patient agitators, and told them group therapy and occupational therapy would continue and grow despite them, "keep your fucking mouths off of us."

Then a member got up and told of his being cut off from communication by authorities and I advised him to keep trying. Then Lopez came up with a letter and we went into it, with Lopez' permission, about his political animus concerning defects in the democracy of the Philippines.

Lopez and Cohen got into an argument over Lopez's letter. Lopez turned to shake my hand and stated his wife would come by to see me. He also mentioned the Jehovah Witness' method of looking at things. I advocated that he describe it for the Howard Hall Journal. Then Bostic made a speech about cooperation and I followed it with suggestions to the patients on the need to keep one's room clean, to cooperate, and try to understand the other fellow's point of view.

COMMENTARY

The conflict with the attendants is still playing itself out, with reduced attendance. Cohen is now a calm chair. There were several paranoid presentations, increasingly coherent, and demonstrating increasing cognitive capacity and intelligence on the part of the presenters.

COHEN NEAR ASSAULTIVE, LOSES CHAIR; GROUP CARRIES ON

Integrated Group Session #39   September 14, 1948

Cohen reported that a member had blown his top on the ward. Cohen was then attacked as a Jew by a member. Cohen became almost assaultive, and lost the chair to a calmer, black member. Several paranoid patients presented their problems. A white member subtly wooed me. The microphone was exceptionally active.

COMMENTARY

What is remarkable about this session was how the members continued the session, despite the disruption occasioned by the long time chairman Cohen.

Another remarkable development was the fact that the black member, himself prone to assault, volunteered.

SIMPLY HUMAN DISCUSSION IN THE INTEGRATED GROUP, INCLUDING THE DOCTOR'S MARRIAGE: WHAT LIFE IS

Integrated Group Session #40   September 15, 1948

During the discussion phase, Bostic told me of the group's surprise at my marriage and how they would like to meet my wife and asked for a photo. I was surprised at the warmth and intimate family feeling, and agreed hesitatingly. I stated that I was flattered. Then I stated to Lauton that I saw something about his brother in the paper, and noted the contrast between Lauton's hiding and defeating his talent against his brother's displaying it. Lauton came up with a vague statement about discussion methods learned in the Army, away from it so long, and in an asylum and away from home.

However, Lauton was more pertinent than ever before. Then I referred to Smith as likewise self-defeating, citing experience with him in this group. Smith answered obliquely, on food and stomach and of his ability to recover without food. I noted Smith's tendency to make a fool of himself and Smith then talked in general re life and living.

Vince Jordan asked Smith what he called living. Thereupon ensued discussion of various ways of living in which Smith told Vince Jordan that he needed to learn to crawl before he walked, solve his problems of having participated in the riot and then go from there. Vince Jordan came back with that Smith couldn't talk for 15 minutes without talking about food. The discussion ended on a friendly note with relation to what life is. A great deal of ad hominem character analysis went on during this session.

COMMENTARY

Remarkable session, in which the group was intimate with me re my recent marriage, and my hesitant acceptance of such. Then I, in a person-to-person way, addressed Lauton's self defeating ways, contrasted with his brother, and on Smith as likewise. Smith stated obliquely that he did not need food, and then in transaction with Vince Jordan, in which advised him to deal with his participation in the riot in the Army, then go on from there, with ending in a friendly discussion on what life is.

AFFECT UNDERLYING DELUSIONS
OF REGRESSED MEMBERS BECOME MORE
EVIDENT IN THE INTEGRATED GROUP

Integrated Group Session #41　　　September 21, 1948

Remarkable entertainment phase. Members then presented problems, Lopez delivering his political speech re Philippines, and Jones in particular on how he felt "hurt" when he was not believed, re the influence by rays of the Federal Buildings across the river.

COMMENTARY

The increasing involvement, with show of affect, of these two chronic, regressed members is a positive sign.

THE INTEGRATED GROUP OPERATES AUTONOMOUSLY,
COHEN ON HIS PROBATION RE OUTBURSTS

Integrated Group Session #42　　　September 28, 1948

There was an active entertainment phase. Cohen pitched for reinstatement, but group was critical of his temper-tantrums, yet positive re his paternal-maternal concern for the members.

COMMENTARY

The group is operating autonomously. The members are asking Cohen for display of his capacity as a regular member.

RACIAL CONFLICT ERUPTS;
GROUP CONTINUES ON COURSE

Integrated Group Session #43　　　October 5, 1948

A black patient volunteered and was elected chairman. However, he became borderline assaultive to a white member, who sang about a nigger stealing. This was followed by an exodus by the psychopathic clique from Howard Hall 2. I took over the session; Miss Sawyer spoke then about the occupational therapy, welcoming members. There was no presentation of individual problems.

COMMENTARY

The racial politics of the group continue turbulent, but it continues operating.

JORDAN BECOMES CHAIR; ATTENDANTS BOYCOTT

Integrated Group Session #44　　October 19, 1948

Two thirds of the members were present, much of the white contingent absent, because attendants did not bring them. Vince Jordan volunteered as chairman, accepted by the group. Withdrawn patients joined the singing and dancing, with cake walk by a member. Several more competent members drew a regressed one into animated conversation. Another member came out of a withdrawn state to play the piano. Lopez tried his political speech, but was rebuffed by the group. It was an especially spirited session.

COMMENTARY

The emergence of the chronic members of the group into its messianic reality continues. Vince Jordan's volunteering as chairman was also a remarkable feature of this session, marked as it was by coexistence with markedly regressed members.

FORSYTH IDENTIFIES AMBIVALENTLY WITH THE MADONNA

Integrated Group Session #45　　October 26, 1948

The flux slide series was projected, having to do with life course issues. There were largely projective comments, with a smattering of positive attributions. Forsyth associated to the hands of a woman as that of the Madonna Savior, and the others that they were malevolent in intent. He became perseverative, interfering with the singing which followed. He was acknowledged to be mocking reality, and protesting the hopelessness of taking up the life course material. He had to be removed by an attendant, and became borderline assaultive. A previously mute catatonic joined a duo of dancers, later intruding into my function. Patients applauded at the end.

COMMENTARY

Tex is pointing the way to a feminine identity, or deep identification with a Madonna mother as a problem. Because of his assaultive manner, he was extruded from the group, in time accepting his removal.

INTEGRATED GROUP AUTONOMOUSLY MADE MUSIC, PROSELYZED REGRESSED MEMBERS, IN DEFIANCE OF THE DOCTOR

Integrated Group Session #46   November 2, 1948

The group was already in progress when I came, with the orchestra playing. The slide series on fear was set up by James, and the chairman, now Cohen, called on the group "to be quiet and to pay attention to the slides, which was for the good of all the patients in the room." The room quieted down somewhat, and the slides was shown, with the usual ascriptions by the members to the material, with Tex playing a more active role than previously, with more hostile associations to the material.

He rejected the material as "medical." Vocal members denied that they had any such thing as fear. After the showing was over, the group did not wish to discuss it, and called for music, Certa prominently. The music began, with the orchestra, consisting of a drum, a saxophone, a trumpet, piano, and two guitars in flexible combination began, with a new member of the group acting as singer. The music was boogy-woogy, sweet swing, and some wild bebop. There was a great deal of dancing, culminating in an exhibition by a white member of an extremely active, graceful, and highly sexual dance, done in apparent coordination with another white member. There was also a great deal of couple dancing between Certa and a catatonic member who stood up and shuffled around, and then with the member who sang, who was previously identified as a new member. The group was rather outgoing during the dancing and music, culminating in a highly charged expressive outburst.

After this was over, I was asked to take over, and commented on the music as being almost more than I could stand, at which point a burst of laughing applause greeted the musicians, who themselves applauded. I also commented on the desirability of participation as one saw fit.

I then asked what the group wanted to talk about, and the members asked for some more music. There was a vote taken on whether the group wanted to speak about problems or hear more music and the musicians won six to three. Thereupon followed a series of spirituals by a quintet composed of the colored patients, which were excellent and were participated in by both white and black members, including myself, plus Mr. Anderson, an attendant, and a number of other people in the room. The performance and grouping was entirely spontaneous during the entire session. The session broke up with the members asking me to close the session, which I did by again emphasizing participation as one wishes, repeating a statement to Tex on this point earlier in the hour.

COMMENTARY

Remarkable during the session were the activities of the lobotomized member and another, in which they went around the room encouraging and speaking about problems with members with problems in assault, plus Tex, and several other catatonics in the back of the room. These two had started the session very negative toward the entire performance. After the session was over members of the group asked if one of them could be allowed to attend the rehearsal for the talent show, stating that they didn't believe he would cause any trouble.

Again, remarkable here was the autonomous action of the group and its subgroup activity, in which members, prior rebelling against me, in grassroots manner proselytized sicker members in self expression, also enunciation of their problems. My rule here was that I as willing to hear from members whatever they had to offer in good faith. Here they, in display of great vitality, were celebrating being alive and simply human.

RESOLUTION OF RACIAL CRISIS AND OF THE REVOLT OF THE ATTENDANTS; FELLATIO CALL REACTED TO BY PATIENT SENSITIVE TO FEDERAL RAYS

Integrated Group Session #47   November 16, 1948

As formerly, the group started with entertainment, spontaneously produced. The problem centered portion of the session was marked by a change where the members of the group who brought up problems fitted it into a more group centered fashion. They asked the members of the group their opinion as to their problems. An interesting sidelight related to a display of homosexual behavior. Mr. Dunn called for fellatio on the part of the chair, who pulled away warmly. Jones, the member who complained of the rays from the Federal Buildings, gave him a quick unhostile smack in the face.

COMMENTARY

There was a visitor, Doctor Stronger from Denmark, who was warmly received by the group. There was also much more conviviality and mixing between colored and white, both in the orchestra and the rest of the group. Several attendants spoke to the doctor concerning their desire to help, and the enjoyment they got out of helping the members of the group.

The resolution of the recent crisis with the attendants has gone on behind the scene. The alienation of white and colored is lessening. Jones is moving further into reality, transacting about homosexual issues.

IN CONTEXT OF DISAVOWAL OF RESPONSIBILITY BY MEMBERS, ONE TIES PERVERSITY TO FEAR OF DEATH, "TO FEEL BETTER"

Integrated Group Session #48   November 30, 1948

This session resulted in a member's loss of his headache, and general release of tension on the part of the group. The Chairman would not let several colored patients speak before the music. One of them stated that he was innocent, wished to leave. James again held the hospital responsible for the patients' insanity. Lopez made a speech, on the Great Depression. A black member then organized an impromptu round table, with Smith, Certa, and James, on racial prejudice as deleterious to both colored and white. This was vaguely related to accusations against him. James related there that he also was put in the Hall by a white man. Certa then reported that he preferred colored people to white ones, as more engaging and lively.

A member then asked another to get up, to report a sexual approach by several others. A member cited that this was related to feeling better about still another's fear of execution by the electric chair. The chair asked me to "put it together," and I cited the pattern of relationships that appeared to be emerging, of an underlying not giving a damn for self and others, showing as predatory and homosexual. This was greeted by laughter and acceptance.

COMMENTARY

Lopez, a profoundly psychotic individual, is moving to talking about his depressive affect. Certa's affiliation with colored people is a big step for him, in accepting his identity as Alaskan Indian, in part genetic to his depressive illness, manifested by perversity and hypomania. The members moved inquiry into the relationship between perversity and fear of death. Finally, when the chairman asked me to interpret, he did so in a respectful manner, leading me to think he was taking it in, and perhaps applying it to his case. This member was one of the original group, later alienated, now reconciling with me.

JAMES REVEALS WIFE WON BATTLE FOR DOMINANCE

Integrated Group Session #49   December 29, 1948

I had been away from this group for some time, and it appeared disjointed. James revealed that his wife and he had been in a battle over dominance, and she won. Patients reported that the attendants were saying that the colored patients were taking over the Hall.

COMMENTARY

James is again using this venue for work on his problems. Today, he is making an advance in conceptualizing his marital relation, but is separate from the devastating impact his loss would have on his world. We shall see Jefferson encountering the same realization in his marriage, of a struggle for dominance, a profound loss of masculine identity, on its loss, and its relationship to the offense.

FILM STRIP ON RUNNING AWAY; TEX: BROUGHT TO THE HOSPITAL BY A WOMAN?

Integrated Group Session #50   January 4, 1949

My film strip on running away was received thoughtfully. The group is more coherent, and asking for discussion again. Tex and I engaged on what had brought him to the hospital, and he ventured, "A woman?"

COMMENTARY

Tex is increasingly pertinent, as differentiated from his former outlandish hebephrenic behavior.

JAMES AND LOPEZ REPORT ON ALIENATION FROM AND WITH THEIR FAMILIES; MEMBERS ABSENT FROM THE INTEGRATED GROUP; GROUP PLOUGHS AHEAD

Integrated Group Session #51   January 11, 1949.

The group was missing many members, with half the number of white patients present that should be present. There were no members of Howard Hall 2 present. The session began spontaneously with the usual patients putting up the sound apparatus. The general mood was as before with a somewhat more relaxed air on the part of the entertainers. They seemed self assured. Mr. Davis showed off his new ability at playing the guitar. The dancers were more expressive and less blocked.

Mr. James approached me to talk about group problems, namely how to reach the members of the group. He slipped in several references to the hopelessness of getting on good terms with his family again, and his plans to live by himself away from his family. He stated sadly that they did not want him any more.

The chairman of the group, after the entertainment had continued for about an hour and a quarter, asked me and the group if we wanted to discuss problems. The group was ambivalent but quite vocal. Mr. Lopez had approached me earlier in the session, asked me how I was and how I was getting along, an unusually expansive greeting on his part. He gave me one sheet that he had written. I searched the sheet for clues and found the statement, "No got home. No family, children." There were several other statements referring to his job, the depression and his loss of his family.

Mr. Lopez then went up to the front of the room, and began his harangue. I interrupted him to bring out what he had written, and asked him what he thought of it. Mr. Lopez began again on his political harangue. I pointed out that he really wanted to talk about this other stuff, inasmuch as he had made a great point of giving the sheet with the new statement about his family on it. Mr. Lopez agreed.

I asked the group if members had anything to suggest on the family problem. A member stated that Mr. Lopez' family hadn't visited him even though they were supposed to live in Brooklyn. Mr. Lopez corroborated this. Mr. Jones made a statement about Mr. Lopez' problems being from without rather than from within, projecting his own attitudes relative to someone in the Hall bothering him, after being persecuted by rays from the Federal Buildings.

Mr. Lopez was ambivalent in his response to this, stating that he had his problems with his family, inasmuch as his wife had killed his son in 1926 in the Philippine Islands, and that the son was reborn again in 1929 in America. I repeated and translated much of what Mr. Lopez said. I noted that he was substituting a political approach to the world for his real concern, his family. Mr. Lopez and the group agreed. The attendants seemed to be quite interested. I pointed out Mr. Lopez' artistic ability in his latest poster political endeavor.

The group was restless at this point and I asked if they wanted to continue. There was no response. I summed up and stated that the group could continue on the problem next week. The chairman asked the group what they wanted to do, in reference to continuing on their problems or continuing with entertainment. The group was hesitant, and he ended the session. The group was dismissed.

During the session, members came up to me to ask on how they could reach one another. An example was a member who had been severely assaultive who asked how he could influence several other members who were having that difficulty. He was concerned about one who had cuffs on him when he slept. I asked him to talk with him about his restlessness. A similar discussion was held with Mr. James. I communicated to Mr. James the need for patience and tolerance and for not imposing his point of view on the other person but trying to understand what the other person was thinking.

COMMENTARY

The session was a fairly adequate one. After the session the attendants approached the doctor on Mr. Lopez' modes of expression, and interest in his artistic work. Remarkable was reversal of the attendants' negativism. Half the white patients were absent, as well as Howard Hall 2. Importantly, James slipped in that his family was hopelessly alienated, and he planned to live by himself. There was ample manifestation of the mutual messianism of the group, members seeking to help others.

BOYCOTT BY WHITE PATIENTS OF BOOGIE-WOOGIE MUSIC; JAMES REVEALS WET BED AS CHILD, LATER INCESTUOUS WITH DAUGHTER

Integrated Group Session #52   January 25, 1949

Exposure of his rear by a member to Miss Shannon, as well as revelation by James of his deviant sexual behavior, in the course of a conflictual session, along racial lines, as well as the usual resistances, marked the course of this session. One third of the white patients were absent again. Harvey set up the projector, with Kiddie Habits shown, reacted to in a free, at the same time bad boy manner.

James revealed that he had wet his bed as a child, which I tried to connect with antagonism towards his father, who he reported had beaten him. He denied this connection, citing that it was an "unconscious automatic reaction." Without making any connection to the rest of the data, he later brought up his deviant sexual behavior towards his daughter.

Miss Shannon spoke in support, when members objected to the boogie-woogie music. A white member then broke with the boycott, joining the band. The ending was amicable.

COMMENTARY

James is reaching into his developmental course as background to his deviance. The group is moving along, despite the deep racial conflict.

JAMES DEMONSTRATES HIS FATHER'S
ANGER TOWARDS PROVOCATIVE MEMBER

Integrated Group Session #53   February 8, 1949

With the showing of a visual aid on relationship by the son to his father, members, particularly James cited their obstinacy and negativity towards theirs, leading to punishment. It moved over to evocation by Jones of James's anger, versus his profession of benevolence.

COMMENTARY

Jones is the chronic member who first complained of the rays from the Federal Building, now is an active member. He may here be taking the part of a son, challenging James, as a father, to emit his rays, in what can be described as a transference enactment.

LOBOTOMIZED PATIENT THREATENS
PHOTOGRAPHER OF GROUP; HOLLISTER REALIZES
RESENTMENT TRANSFERENCE

Integrated Group Session #54   March 8, 1949

A hospital photographer took pictures, with Harvey threatening him for it. Smith was disciplined by members for sexual talk on Miss Sawyer's presence. A visual aid on kid stuff was projected, with free and pertinent associations by members. Hollister stated that he realized that resentment got in the way of work and schooling. The entertainment was spontaneous, with a new patient playing piano.

COMMENTARY

The capacity and initiative of the group in taking up cases is in abeyance, but Hollister, a new member does note his problem with resentment.

INTEGRATED GROUP: PLAYING AROUND WITH DELUSIONS; ATTENDANT DANCES WITH PATIENT

Integrated Group Session #55   March 29, 1949

The group started off as usual with music, with a member playing excellently on the piano, and another singing professional style melodies. The dancing was vigorous with a colored patient whose penis was showing, spending considerable time cavorting around, with homosexual gestures, then gradually beginning to smile and fixing his pants in a more conventional fashion.

The group signaled when they wanted to discuss problems and the first member to get up was a belligerent black patient. Both black and white members took the microphone away from him when he became threatening. Then the group discussed Mr. Jones' problem with him in which he vociferously stated that he did not have delusions, moving over to that delusions came from childhood. He said that would happen to him when he had been wronged actually by somebody else and that was not a delusion. He defended his radio wave experience as reality.

The group then asked for someone else to come up and a member stated he did not know whether he had killed three men. If so, he would be very happy. He was not sure whether it was a dream or otherwise and wanted to find out from the group. He wanted to have someone start him off on it and then he would be able to do the rest himself. The members of the group began questioning him, especially Mr. James, relative to the events of the day he had said he had committed this particular crime and he became quite offensive and started to give nonsensical answers.

I role played the scene with him, and he wished to continue. He added that he became angry when people "went over my head to state that my wife was good stuff."

The members interjected that they wanted to see the visual aid on flux again. Participation was free and much was anti-doctor, projecting me into uncomfortable and derogatory positions. One of the situations involved a man climbing and then falling back from a steep mountain. I then asked the presumably homicidal member to visualize himself in that situation. He did so, grabbing for me, tearfully, in the process.

There was a great deal of side play in which members of the group approached me with their new slants on things. A member showed me a pocket telescope in which he saw a pretty nude girl. Harvey came to me to discuss playing a piano and Mr. Jordan also discussed his problem of holding back from people. He also stated that if Loren Jones had gotten up to state that he owned everything, and was the owner of the hospital, he wanted Loren Jones to let him go because he did not wish to be such an unwilling guest. This brought forth a great deal of laughter from the group because of the tragic comic appearance of host and guest.

Harvey participated with the colored patients in their singing and playing. An attendant danced with the patients after the session was over when people were filing out and the orchestra was playing its last boogie-woogie number. When I asked the group on whether it had noted changes, Mr. Hollister stated that he has seen many changes, all under the surface, which would show eventually. He spent a great deal of time during the session with an assaultive member communicating in what appeared to be a significant manner with this patient.

COMMENTARY

A tumultuous session marked by multilocular participation by members, from Jones on his radio wave delusions which he related to childhood injury to a member asking for feedback on whether a multiple murder was reality or delusion. Active discussion of the visual aid on flux, placing me in it. Jordan held back from people, also tragic-comic re Loren Jones's delusion, with laughter from the group.

MEMBER FORMERLY PERSECUTED BY FEDERAL RAYS BRINGS UP ALIENATION FROM FAMILY; HOLLISTER SUPPORTIVE

Integrated Group Session #56   April 5, 1949

This member now locates persecution in his fellows, but supported by Hollister. Members also noted that a beating a member had suffered was sufficient to account for his problems. An attendant was very positive about improvement of the members, and especially Hollister.

COMMENTARY

Hollister, an intellectual elitist, is increasingly participant in this group, affiliative with the colored population. Jones has ceased complaint of persecution by rays from outside, and is volunteering for discussion of his problems, and engaging in discussion of others.

CONVIVIAL DISCUSSION OF HOMOSEXUAL VULNERABILITY; JAMES AS EXAMPLE

Integrated Group Session #57   April 12, 1949

At today's group meeting there was a discussion between the black musicians and a white member who declared the music stank, and they bristled, but admitted it needed improvement. Then followed a discussion of spontaneity on the part of the group, and of the white member's homosexuality. The latter consideration was brought up by Mr. James who recited an experience of his soon after arrival at the Hall, where he was seduced by a colored fellow named Madison. He then cited an experience where he fought off a homosexual assault on the part of an older man when he was a boy of seventeen in the Army in a guardhouse.

The discussion that followed was on why people are homosexual, with a member stating that the mother is to blame in seducing the boy, and another that the homosexual wants to get his nuts off. I stated that the person was afraid of women, did not care for self, lost feeling for self, giving up on self, and then something else happened. Other members stated that when a person is in prison he has no choice and doesn't give a damn. The discussion went on as to how the thing could be cured and various interpretations were given as to what should be done, including a member's that people should be strung up by their penis.

A Southern member then stated that the Ku Klux Klan is a good idea where they do away with a person when they rape, steal, murder, etc. Another member of the group got up and gallantly stated that there was no use having any law if people took the law into their own hands. Mr. James was then asked how come he brought up the problem so much and felt so strongly about the homosexuality angle. He recited his victimization, and a member asserted that Mr. James wanted to have a homosexual experience at that moment and now. Mr. James bristled, challenged him and tension ran high.

Then both stated that they were merely defending their position, defending the colored man, asserting "they should keep their penis in their pants." A member then stated that people could not be told how to live, they had to learn. I agreed and then Mr. James and his opponent stopped debating over the microphone, and agreed that they wanted to be friends, but did not want the other to threaten them. I stated that the issue had to do with taking advantage, and they agreed to continue the discussion next week.

Mr. Hollister was active in the discussion in a vague sort of way, objecting to it, and stating afterwards that it was nauseating. A member showed a great deal of antagonistic feeling, and distress on being asked how he liked the discussion after the session was over.

COMMENTARY

In their intimate wrangling, the members are desensitizing themselves to homosexual issues and issues of cultural discrepancy. They approached personal change when they experienced their reaction to the actions of others, as re the boogie woogie music, nausea, and distress, as clues to their internal dynamics and alienation from self.

GENERAL PARANOID ORIENTATION TOWARDS THE MILLER ACT; FAMILY DYNAMICS AND VULNERABILITY

Integrated Group Session #58   April 19, 1949

The group had begun before I came, with a number of patients from Howard Hall 2 and Howard Hall 6 present today. The session continued with the clang of the music, a great deal of group singing, with the quartet becoming a sex and a septet with Certa and Foster joining the colored patients in singing spirituals. Mr. Foster asked me to get up and talk about problems. When this was done and I asked what the group wanted to talk about, two patients elected themselves to talk with the group.

One had bent my ear for about three-quarters of an hour about his relationship with his father, his intense hatred for him, with the description in great detail of his father's offensive aspects. His noted the role of homosexuality in his many problems. He stated that he doesn't know why but people always tried to have intercourse with him and he would like to find out. I noted that he seemed to center his whole life on thinking about his father. The patient stated that he had never thought about it that way, but that it was so.

We then discussed his "giving in tendencies" and his fear of femininity in relation to an undescended testicle, and how that was part of his problem with others in the hospital. He then informed us that he stated to patients soon after he came to the hospital that he had never had intercourse with a woman. He stated that they then approached him as a queer. I stated that the patient's way of handling himself may be quite related to people's thinking that he was a queer. Members asked if it was more active than that.

He accepted all of these statements and went on to state that everything was like it had been with his father and that did not help him in his current day living. He stated that he could not stop people from coming after him sexually, and from talking about him in a derogatory way. I pointed out that he was self-derogatory before the other person was that way toward him. He then stated that he certainly got a great deal out of talking with me.

The other member then exhorted the group about the Miller Act and about economics. It developed that he considered that the Miller Act was unconstitutional, unfair, and was something that people who had suspicions of other people imposed on them. A member asked what brought him under the Miller Act, and he told about a girl who had framed him by calling a policeman, stating that he had touched her. He then stated that this girl was nine years old. He stated that this happened or was supposed to have happened in an elevator which he was operating, and which he would not have been operating had he been able to find a job which was better suited to his needs.

Members of the group asked him about that, and he stated that he formerly had a job for $50.00 a week with a construction firm, which when it finished the job discharged him, and in order to stay out of trouble took a job at $20.00 a week even though he had dependents. He stated that the former job was one where he worked only with men, and that on the elevator he came in contact with women, which upset him. This was picked up by another new patient under the Miller Act and this patient asked him what it was about women that upset him so. He was rather reluctant to answer that question, but went back to the inequities of the Miller Act. He was pulled back to the point by Mr. Foster. He then went back to the question of the Miller Act and began whipping up a great deal of sentiment in the group over this inequitable and terrible Act.

There was a great deal of hot discussion at this point by members of the group. The act "didn't allow a man to even walk down the street without someone accusing him of making a pass at a woman." Members of the group gave illustrations of what they had heard happened under the Miller Act: a girl asked a boy if he wanted to have a date and when he appeared for it she called a policeman to state that he had been assaulting her. A member related a case that happened about twenty some odd years ago where a man had put his hand on the head of a little girl, was apprehended by a policeman, but actually he had intended sexual intercourse so everything was all right there.

I asked that the discussion relate to the problems of the members, and Mr. Foster as a demanding individual then surfaced.

Two sex psychopaths presented. The first had bent my ear earlier re his father, and I reflected on his fixation. He agreed, and touted that insight re his susceptility to men's advances. The second then attacked the unconstitutionality and inequity of the Miller Act. On remonstrance by a member, he in time revealed that a nine year old girl had complained that he had assaulted her in an elevator. Another sex psychopath asked about his upset with women, which he resisted answering by turning back to complaint re the Miller Act.

COMMENTARY

This session was the first frank, full session on the problem of the sex psychopath and the Miller Act. I had been relying on the Administrative Group to act in an orientative capacity with these patients, but the sex psychopaths have settled down from their previous oppositional stance, and in general worked productively here. Most important was their entrance into looking into the dynamics of their motivation in their individual offenses.

SEX PSYCHOPATHS ASK FOR TREATMENT, WHILE STREET AND LAUTON MAKE LOVE

Integrated Group Session #59   April 26, 1949

The group session had more than an hour of music with a member playing the drums part of the time and also playing on his harmonica quite well in concert, another at the piano, one at the guitar, still another at a guitar, and a last at the drums. During the musical phase, members of the group gathered around me from time to time to ask me for the sex psychopath law which I had with me, on request of members during last weeks session, and to approach me regarding their problems.

Mr. Foster stated that he was better and did not think he needed any more treatment. A member asked for the $2.60 which Mr. Pyles deposited for him, and gradually came out more with his fear of other people. I asked if fear of what was in the other fellow's eyes as what led him finally to the Hall. A member brought his defenses up and then dropped them in rapid succession. I noted to him that was talking to himself, not to me, which had the effect of bringing his defenses down further.

The discussion part of the session was begun when the orchestra terminated the music and I led a brief discussion on which is to come first, the music or the discussion, and when a vote was taken, music won. Then I was asked to read the sex law which I did carefully. The group listened quite attentively. Street and Lauton started to make love at this point, continuing during the entire session with Lauton as the aggressor and Street as the coy one. The question of what treatment was under the sex law was finally brought up and discussion centered around this point with several new members under the sex law shouting that they were getting no treatment and asking what treatment was.

A new patient stood up and said that he wanted to present his case and put himself in the doctor's hands. He then told of stealing a car eleven times, doing it from the same automobile lot. He stated that he bought a car to prevent his stealing other people's cars but that did not help. He would handcuff himself to the bed and that didn't help. He stated that he was amnesic during these episodes and would wake up driving a Cadillac on Pennsylvania Avenue. He stated that it was driving him to distraction and that he had lost his wife and everything because of it and wanted treatment.

A member broke in to state that the man looked desperate and was at the end of his rope and that he needed to turn to God and get benefaction from a priest. The patient stated that he couldn't attend church enough because he was always in jail. Other members of the group stated that this man could be helped by group therapy just as another member of the group downstairs had profited, by watching him blow his top and call the group a bunch of simple assed mother fuckers and learn how he would look in the same position and decided that he preferred not to get himself in such a condition and would try to learn why he would have tended to blow his top.

Then they advised the patient to sit around and watch and learn from what happened around him. One member was especially active in advising the patient on this point of listening and learning. Another stated that the patient didn't really care or else he would learn by himself. The hour wound up, as I delineated the patient's passive state, which a member defined as "Let George do it." This was defined as an impediment to therapy, where the patient felt he and some person had nothing to do with it. The concept of change from his present state was also introduced in the discussion. This was done, however, in rather general terms.

COMMENTARY

Looking back, I would have inserted the enactment in the present of a homosexual act by Street and Lauton into the group discussion, despite the pressure by the sex psychopaths for treatment.

FOSTER ADVOCATES GOING
INTO PROBLEM "IN ITS TOTALITY"

Integrated Group Session #60   May 3, 1949

A member volunteered that the Masons were threatening him. Dialectic arose in the group, on how to discuss his problem, with Forster asserting that one needed to go into his problem "in its totality," versus on how the members reacted to him. There was earlier dancing by colored and white. The member who complained of the Masons at one point hissed at me.

COMMENTARY

Foster here is plumping for systematic discussion of the problem of a member.

INTEGRATED GROUP: MUSIC AND PATIENTS
CITING THEIR PROBLEMS TO ME

Integrated Group Session #61   May 24, 1949

An hour and a half on music, with Mr. Forsyth keeping his back to the group, singing with the chorus. Numbers of patients came up to me during this to cite their problems. A member asked the singer to repeat his blues song, so he could continue talking with me. Mr. Howard, the attendant, commented that it was the heat that accounted for the patients' deviant behavior.

COMMENTARY

Members are plugging through, despite discrepancy and contradictions.

FORSYTH AND LOPEZ COLLABORATE
LOOSELY IN INTEGRATED GROUP

Integrated Group Session #62   June 9, 1949

The group was assembled with Wards 7 and 8 largely lacking. The orchestra was playing in a rather desultory fashion and continued playing for half an hour. Colored members of the group sang into the microphone in competition with the orchestra. After 35 minutes was up I asked the chairman if they would like to continue with discussion. The pianist-organizer packed up his piano and left.

I asked who wanted to speak today. The chairman asked if anyone had a problem and I stated that I had one. The group was silent and Mr. Forsyth raised his hand and said that he would like to take up a problem that he had. He thereupon began to talk in a hypomanic, word-salad fashion about what has bested him, giving details about his mother, calling her vile names and talking about his offers to her of sexual intercourse and her refusal. He then called himself a series of vile names, including "Sister Raping." This was interspersed with songs which he had composed, plus a great deal of neologistic material.

There were a number of responses to his monolog, namely calls for him to sing, statements that he was crazy, and rather serious contemplative listening by members of the group such as Donald Street and others. I got up and stated that Mr. Forsyth apparently wanted the group to tell him how it felt, since he had mentioned the group many times in his talk. Mr. Forsyth agreed and I outlined what the reactions to the members of the group were and the group illustrated by asking for songs, and calling him crazy.

A member walked up in a serious manner to the front of the room to make a statement to Mr. Forsyth, whereupon Mr. Forsyth continued his self-derogatory statements. I interrupted Mr. Forsyth to point this out and he agreed. I asked if anyone else had anything to say after what had happened and Mr. Lopez raised his hand and came up to the front of the room. He began gesticulating and shouting and giving his usual harangue. I interrupted to state that here were two members who wanted to say something to the group and who found that they were received by derogatory comments and requests for performance. I stated that perhaps they could both help one another to express themselves clearly.

Mr. Certa asked Mr. Forsyth to read Mr. Lopez's prepared statement. I asked Mr. Lopez if this were all right and Mr. Lopez agreed. Mr. Forsyth read the statement, slightly mocking Mr. Lopez, with about one third of the group in hilarious laughter by the end of the reading, including Mr. Lopez, himself. Mr. Forsyth did this for some time on another bit of material of Mr. Lopez'. Then Mr. Lopez began his harangue again, saying that all of the people in the group, including he and Mr. Forsyth were ordinary working people in trouble, and he started to give his dates in 1922 and 1942, with members of the group listening to him with increased interest. He then stated that he was through and sat down.

Mr. Forsyth continued with a gibberish talk, aping Mr. Lopez, and then went into material about his father and about his homosexual experiences.

He continued and about this time the group became restless and a musical member asked if he could continue playing. He tried to get the microphone from Mr. Forsyth who stated that he wanted to keep it. After a bit of shuffling, I came up and asked for a vote on who was to continue. The vote was ten for music and two for Forsyth. Mr. Forsyth at this point said he wouldn't accept the vote. An attendant came up and was beginning to lead Mr. Forsyth out when the members of the group and me asked that he stay.

Mr. Forsyth sat down and was quite serious and attentive to the music. Later he got up and danced and clapped and sang with the music in imitation of the colored patients' behavior, along the way doing a strip tease while balancing a chair on his nose. There was some wild dancing between a member and one of the chronic exhibitionistic patients. The session was ended by the chairman with a great deal of singing and shouting by members of the group.

COMMENTARY

In the midst of this Alice in Wonderland session, there was the transaction with Mr. Forsyth and Lopez. I was mobilizing Forsyth's capacity to live in reality, recognize the reality of a fellow regressed patient-with-a-cause, Mr. Lopez. In taking up Lopez's cause and historical data, he gained a modicum of perspective on his own, and through perception of Lopez's alienation from himself, he gained some perspective on his own. He did give up the microphone, and sat down like a good patient, without authoritarian intervention. Along the way, he unburdened himself of some painful data, as did Lopez.

JORDAN AND HARVEY IN DESPAIR ABOUT SELF

Integrated Group Session #63   June 28, 1949

Harvey's dumbness and smartness and ability to change was discussed, then V. Jordan cited that he was in despair about getting anywhere, was still the same person. Foster stated that he was all right. Then I stated that Jordan and Harvey had difficulty being themselves, with the latter trying to convince people that he was dumb, and Jordan that he was popular. Jordan went into how the lack of colored attendants in the Hall made it difficult for him to change.

COMMENTARY

The despair underlying the self abandonment of late is surfacing, cross-racially.

WHITES BOYCOTT; JAMES'S INVENTION
OF UNIQUE LOOM

Integrated Group Session 64   July 19, 1949

Most of the white population boycotted this session. The time was spent in paranoid, anti-psychiatrist ruminations, with James touting his new method of looming.

COMMENTARY

James's loom employed a shuttlecock propelled by gravity, through sideways rocking of the loom. This was an original invention of this man, given to claiming those of others. I cannot account for the regression of the group.

FIGHT IN THE LARGE GROUP, OVER THERAPY, CERTA PRO

Integrated Group Session #65   August 2, 1949.

The group gathered rather slowly and about half the group was present today. Mr. Forsyth left after the group was ten minutes going. At about twenty minutes after nine I got up and started the group since the chairman was absent, by asking what the group wanted to do with the time. Mr. Certa gave his usual remark about nothing to be done and a patient who sits on the right and is usually rather silent spoke up and at length declaimed against his unnecessary incarceration in the Hall for no good reason and the conditions of life on the Hall being quite bad for him.

At this is point a member in the back of the room raised his hand and called out. He was encouraged to come up to the front by the attendants, especially Mr. Howard. He came up and stated that the group couldn't help him. He addressed the group and me on his resentment on being held in Howard Hall beyond his prison term which expired last spring and about his fear of being killed by the wolves, hyenas, donkeys, and other animals resident in the ward with him and his great shame at something he couldn't reveal to the group.

I reflected his statements and members joined in to explain what he was trying to say, to the effect that he was quite resentful about being held in the Hall and that the agitators in the Hall were harming him. A usually silent member burst forth upon the scene to state that what was harming him was all the noise made by other people, especially noise made in group therapy by the orchestra.

The members of the orchestra came to their defense and the subject became music or no music, and what kind of music was to be played. Eventually there was a vote in which the group decided to continue with the music. The musicians became angry at the group for their rejection of the musicians for the while and at the doctor for the continuation of the discussion, beyond the time when the music usually starts. A member asked me to sit down and Mr. Certa came to my defense.

After the discussion was finished, in which Mr. Certa had asked for a vote, I sat down and the member who had asked me to sit down asked me if I were a doctor. He then asked me why I did not exert authority. In a loud voice he stated that what was needed was a strong authority to tell people what to do. I then reflected this statement. Mr. Certa shouted that if he were a doctor he would punch him in the nose.

Following this there was a brief fight between Mr. Certa and the complainer, which Mr. Certa defined later on as a fight over whether the group and the doctor was worth while. Ostensibly Mr. Certa defended the group. The musicians then played particularly loudly and in a boisterous fashion until the end of the session. Afterwards there was a discussion between the attendant, the nurse and myself on whether the attendants should exercise more initiative in telling patients to work their problems in the group, with the nurse taking the position that if the patient spoke against him in the group then his authority would be lost.

COMMENTARY

Very interesting session, with conference with the attendants and a nurse on their role in the group, chiefly relative to taking initiative. They were drawn into it through the action following a complaint by a member on the need for authority. A member from the rear cited his low morale on retention beyond his "term," and sensitivity towards his animal like peers, with particular reference to the noise of the group orchestra. There was a pointed discussion of this, which centered about my identity in the group as a doctor and authority. Certa and a member came to blows briefly, with Certa defending the doctor. An attendant held to the position that without assertion of authority, control was lost and he became impotent.

MEMBERS VOTE FOR INTEGRATED GROUP ADMINISTRATIVE THERAPY SESSION; MEMBER'S IMPOTENCE IN HANDLING SELF AS MAN

Integrated Group Session #66   August 11, 1949

The group voted for an administrative group, four to one. Vituperative conflict on the validity of the vote erupted, with battlers versus peacemakers emerging as the issue, at James's instance. A member who was impotent in handling himself as a man became the centerpiece of discussion in the group. I followed through on his problems with manly self assertion, having given up on it and doing for himself. The group agreed on his doing so, asserting himself, at the moment.

COMMENTARY

Meeting with Dr. Cruvant as an administrative group would be a responsible step forward, and it is not by chance that the discussion following centered on responsible self assertion, versus alienating impotence.

SERIAL REVELATION OF REGRESSED FUGUE STATES, EXEMPLIFYING UNDERLYING ISSUES OF INITIAL COMPLAINER

Integrated Group Session #67   August 18, 1949

The group was operating when I came, with music and dancing, going on for about 45 minutes, much of it single instrumental and singing, quite toned down from previous jive sessions, and in which the dancing was of a more organized variety, with the previously wooden figure dancing replaced by rather able tap dancing on the part of several patients.

The member who has been playing the piano and organizing the orchestra, and has also been taking over the role of chairman in the large group, stated to me that he just wanted to play two pieces and then would give it to me for therapy. After about four pieces, I stood and asked the group what it wanted to talk about, with replies of going home, this is some shit, settling on the question of the malevolence of authority.

The latter was brought up by Mr. Dormer who stated that he was resentful of Dr. Cruvant asking him to state that he wanted to go back to prison before he sent him back. I took this up and there was fairly generalized discussion of authority as non-giving and the world in general and fellow patients as being disinterested in the man who was down.

Mr. Dormer brought out his problem of feeling lost when he left the service, without a pension, and with the advice of a Navy doctor to take a six months' rest. Members of the group asserted that the only doctors who care for them are Dr. Cruvant, Dr. Tartaglino and Dr. Abrahams, with all the rest of society being judges and hostile people. There was generalized discussion of this.

In the middle of it all, when Mr. Dormer was bringing out his hostility and lost feeling when he left the Navy, a member asked to speak, stating that he wanted to says something about politics. He got up and made a long rambling rather incoherent speech which the group laughed at because of his peculiarly comical nature about himself as a George Raft, traveling around the country doing powerful and dangerous things. The identification with entertainment and desperado figures was prominent in his speech as was a certain amount of coherent resentment toward white folks limiting his opportunity. He guardedly mentioned civil rights in his talk.

This was the first time he had spoken. He had previously just danced and sung in a rather wild and impassioned fashion. The next speaker was a member who got up and told of wandering around without any help from society before he was hospitalized, and of his lack of help in other parts of Saint Elizabeths, before he came to Howard Hall. He did this in a rather vague manner. The group discussion continued with the group interested and controlling of its members who shouted for attention and vocalized about malevolent authority.

The pianist worked his way into chairmanship. He played 4 pieces, two more than contracted for. The group then complained that authority was non giving, starting with Dormer' complaint against Dr.Cruvant re wanting him to go to prison. Fellow patients cited that authority was disinterested in the man who was down.

Dormer then cited his feeling of loss on leaving the service. Then a member, who had done some wild dancing and singing, broke in to speak about politics, instead talked like the movie actor, George Raft, drawing laughter. Another member then spoke of wandering without help from society, hospitalized without help elsewhere at St. Elizabeths. Green shouted for attention, was controlled by members.

COMMENTARY

One can infer that the members who followed Dormer, in their disorganized manner, were furnishing the group with a window into Dormer's post-service state, leading medical authority to recommend a "rest." It is apparent he needed treatment.

THE INTEGRATED THERAPY AND
ADMINISTRATIVE GROUP APPEARS REGRESSED;
FOSTER CARRIES ON, HELP TO NEW MEMBER

Integrated Group Session #68   August 25, 1949

At Forster's instance, I worked with a member on why he broke down and heard voices in Lorton, after a fight over cigarettes. Scarce attendance, with buzz of voices, Dr. Cruvant stated that his order curtailing psychopaths' grafting activity in the kitchen may be operative, causing resistance.

COMMENTARY

The group appeared distracted and regressed, yet Foster pushes on, in favor of another patient.

INTEGRATED GROUP: ORCHESTRA ABSENT, MEMBERS CITE PROBLEMS WITH INTIMACY

Integrated Group Session #69   September 1, 1949

The chairman went down to round up the orchestra. On my inquiry, the group gradually volunteered their problems. A member was chosen to speak. He complained of assault by another member during a baseball game, after he insulted him.

Both were identified as agitators by members, and I noted that the members' problems were similar. A member complained of policy limitations on the duration of his family's visit. A member stated when he come too close, a friend becomes an enemy. He gave an illustration of boxing with a fellow prisoner, ending up having to defend himself with a knife. He then asked for the punishment cell block for 2 years, because he had done so much wrong.

A member asked if he was afraid of assault while asleep, and he agreed. A member described him as slow in the past in comprehending things, recommending that he seek help in his ward group. He admitted that he had trouble with men.

COMMENTARY

The subject for discussion turned out to be the representative member, turning against the one was intimate with, then suffering deep guilt.

A MEMBER'S AUTISTIC STANDARDS RESULT IN ASSAULT

Integrated Group Session #70   September 7, 1949

Drs. Meza and Greenberg, Mrs. Sheridan, and Mrs. Williams were visiting. Mrs. Sheridan was cheered, with one boo, asked for cooperation with the talent show. James touted the improvement in the Hall, and quoted a letter from a previous member who had been transferred to Pine Ward, Bolster, asking for return to the Hall and its advantages. The chair asked for a baseball game with the doctors or theology students. I declined, citing we were not in good enough physical shape.

The member who had stated he was "forced" to defend himself with a knife in a fight in prison, asked to discuss his problems, on how he had been forced to cut "Coal yard" in the prison. I asked why he had asked for so much consequent punishment. A member stated it was because he had fallen from a position of being in the good graces of the big shots, and was in danger. He replied that had been in the punishment block for a considerable time, and had heard voices.

COMMENTARY

The chair stated that he did not have any sense, and he replied angrily. Then he called on Dr. Greenberg, concerning Harvey's prospects when transferred to Male Receiving Ward 7, was answered affirmatively, then that patient stated his doubts. He was approaching exposition of his autistic standards, by which he judged self and others.

INTEGRATED GROUP APATHETIC, NEGATIVE

Integrated Group Session #71   September 15, 1949

A new patient was particularly strong and effective as a singer. Members vociferously complained about the food situation, shouting down Foster and others who wanted to discuss their problems. I noted the apathy of the other members. Members acknowledged their switch to the negative. A member was gleeful on seeing me, shaking Forsyth's shoulders.

COMMENTARY

The members are regressing, did respond to my reflection of that development.

FOSTER SPEAKS OF HIS DUAL PERSONALITIES

Integrated Group Session #72   September 22, 1949

Forster brought up the issue of his dual personalities, settling on his orneriness, which he ascribed to maltreatment and isolation from others. He left, after the group criticized his inadequate personality. I compared the personalities of s member who had engaged in a hunger strike, with that of a member who had one foot in the punishment block and the other in a crap game. A member cited his improvement.

COMMENTARY

Foster is taking depth counsel with himself, on possessing dual personalities, secondary to alienating experience when younger.

MUSIC ALMOST OUT OF CONTROL; MEMBER CITES DEPRESSION AT NOT TAKING CARE OF WIFE AS BASIC TO HIS PERVERSE BEHAVIOR

Integrated Group Session #73   September 29, 1949

The music lasted an hour and a half today and my attempts to abate it were to no avail. When the discussion began it centered at first on the separateness of the Hall with desire by the members for participation in activities in other parts of the hospital, and for women to come to the Hall to dance with them. A member stated that the group meeting was just to drive people crazy, bringing up ideas such as that.

Then the pianist came out with his problems with his wife in which he stated that he was droopy and felt very low down for not taking care of his wife. I brought up the other side of the question and the behavior which kept him from approaching the discussion of his problems with his wife in the group on Monday, namely attempting to get people to hurt him by agitating and insulting them. He intimated that he could not bring up disappointment by his wife. Another member and he spoke simultaneously to their disappointment in the doctor, saying that the group session was rather bad. There was a great deal of individual reaching out to me afterwards.

COMMENTARY

The music lasted for an hour and a half, in overt resistance to discussion. A member came out with his depression on not taking care of his wife, hampered in this by his occupation of antagonizing people, also by his disappointment in her. Members showed their disappointment in the group discussion. The phenomenon of disappointment is most likely a transference phenomenon.

FORSYTH OPENS UP IN THE LARGE
GROUP ON HIS SELF ALIENATION

Integrated Group Session #74   October 27, 1949

The group began in its usual way but there was more singing today, with Tex at first acting as the leader, singing in modified music today. Before the session began he sat next to me and was markedly productive. He asked "if the people" in a querulous voice, and I replied that apparently he was quite upset, and asked if the ward had done this to him. He then became extremely angry at me and told me to mind my own business.

When I was asked to get up to talk, I brought up the problem and the session revolved around minding other people's business or not, with Mr. Jones bringing out a poem on not minding other people's business and Murphy, Foster, Jones, and a number of others coming in with their comments on it, to and fro.

Mr. Forsyth brought out feelings of despondency, of himself as a homosexual, of the need to kill, repeating that he was a cruel Caucasian. He was extremely provocative toward all in his vicinity, including Miss Williams and Dr. Bluff. He became more and more appropriate as the session went on and during the final discussion of whether he should be permitted to stay in the group with the usual argument brought out, he joined in with his despondent data, sadly speaking of the fact that he couldn't be helped in a hundred million years.

During the session, I used Mr. Forsyth's panic and the other person's intentions, drawing close to the other person, resulting in dragging the other person into the discussion. He stated that he was being helpful to Miss Williams. Utilizing Forsyth as the representative member, I brought him, after he led the group in singing and bringing up the topic of minding one's own business, to open up about his despondency, homosexuality, homicidal impulses, and alienation. He did state his helpfulness to Miss Williams.

COMMENTARY

In the midst of extreme resistance, the representative member of the chronic members, Forsyth, with affect communicates his self alienation and awareness of alienating others.

FORSYTH REVEALS FEAR OF SPEAKING

Integrated Group Session #75   November 3, 1949

Forsyth again was central, after leading in singing, and after revealing to Miss Williams his fear of speaking. He eventually demanded I tell him what was on his mind. Along the way, Harvey brought out that the members' actions kept them in the Hall. On encouragement by Harvey, a regressed member gestured concerning a female form and a machine gun, A member referred to himself as a Christ sacrifice, and one reported his experience of lacking the courage to speak.

COMMENTARY

Forsyth disclosed a fear, this time of speaking. A member later noted his lack of courage to speak.

DR. MEZA IS GUEST THERAPIST: GROUP IN IMPASSE OVER FORSYTH, WHO OFFERED THE MICROPHONE TO CONTENDING MEMBERS

Integrated Group Session #76   November 17, 1949

Dictated by Dr. Cesar Meza

The group today was centered on the problems of Mr. Forsyth and Mr. Jordan. When I came in Mr. Vince Jordan was tinkering with the piano, playing some sort of a tune with his right hand. He was greeted by Mr. Forsyth in Mr. Forsyth's usual manner. The session began with the music being played and Mr. Forsyth singing. Mr. Murphy and Forster came to the session. I spoke to Mr. Forsyth about my intention to lead the group and he ignored me.

Then he sang, louder and louder, about not giving a damn. Then when the time came to speak, a new patient started to play the piano, and I asked the group to continue and the group didn't want to. Mr. Forsyth then conceded, as Mr. Jordan came in to state that something should be done about Mr. Forsyth, that although he was doing things for the good of other people, Mr. Forsyth seemed to make it impossible for him to hear himself, much less other people hear him, and that Mr. Forsyth should be voted downstairs.

Members joined in discussion of this. Mr. Murphy stated that Mr. Jordan was upset by Mr. Forsyth because of Mr. Jordan's disturbance and that Mr. Forsyth was completely happy and that Mr. Jordan needed to work on his problem. There was a great deal of discussion on the purpose of the group and how it was denied by Mr. Forsyth.

A member saw both sides of the question. Mr. Jordan was careful to note that it wasn't the color line which had to have anything to do with his statement. Mr. Forsyth became increasingly open and vituperative toward Mr. Jordan. The session became quite heated as the thing went along and Mr. Forsyth listened quite curiously to most of the discussion, imitating the doctor and offering the microphone to each who came along, stating that he didn't give a damn what the other person said, but encouraging the other person to say it. A member picked up Mr. Forsyth's manner and began to talk about breaking up the insides of a room if a person were locked up there. The session ended with the question of voting deferred on a member's motion.

COMMENTARY

This is an example of a group in a therapeutic impasse, yet with members, like Forsyth, attempting to be therapeutic. The issue that arose was the expulsion of Forsyth.

BOOTH AS REPRESENTATIVE MEMBER, REPORTS EXPERIENCE "WHEN GROUP LEAVES" HIM, A TRANSFERENCE REPRESENTATION OF THE INCEPTION OF PSYCHOSIS

Integrated Group Session #77   December 8, 1949

Today's session was extremely interesting. Harvey began to speak in an agitated manner, ascribing hostile motivations to others. Another asked me to tell the members of the group what their problems were, and also stated that he realized that the doctor couldn't tell him those things. This led to a call for a show of hands on how many people want to find out what their condition is, and eventually a member told how he was not able to hear; that he was in the newspapers of 12 years ago; that he had given up ever attaining any pride in himself; that he had remorse at having hurt his family, and guilt at having murdered.

There was fairly active interchange between this member and Dormer, Mr. Sullivan, Mr. Murphy, Mr. James, and Mr. Foster, over a period of an hour and a quarter. The group bore with his drawn out repetitious statements of his feelings, and brought it right back to him on the whole. His anticipation and fear of rejection, and refusal to try any other way came out fairly clearly in the discussion. It was shown when Mr. Booth got very upset when I took Mr. James's sympathetic remark on the world's lack of sympathy; Mr. Booth felt that he was being rejected. A black member stated that he didn't know whether the doctor and the group felt the same way about him, after they left him as they did while they were talking to him, and that therefore he had to stick to his guns and stay in his "dream talk."

He stated that if he left the Hall he would then be able to get some pride back and wouldn't have to stay with his dream talk. A member concluded that he didn't care to find out anything about himself.

A member began, by asking Dr. Meza to tell him what his problems were, while acknowledging that he couldn't, and Dr. Meza asked who wanted to find out similarly. A strong show of hands eventuated in a member's volunteering his story, of giving up on any pride in self, and remorse on having hurt his family, and guilt on having murdered. The group was empathetic during his long and repetitious statements, and the member illustrated his difficulty with isolation, with feeling rejected when James stated that society lacked sympathy. He referred to his dream talk in the process, entered into on the experience of being left by the doctor and the group.

COMMENTARY

I take this to be a representation of his prior experience of alienation from himself, the seminal experience in the members.

FORSYTH ENGAGES WITH MEMBERS
ON THEIR INDIRECTION

Integrated Group Session #78   December 22, 1949

Forsyth commented on Murphy's wish for direct reflection by others, in context of his agitating them.

COMMENTARY

My inference is that Forsyth, a master of indirection, is moving closer to direct statements from self.

REMARKABLE SESSION REVOLVING ABOUT
TROUBLE OF THE MEMBERS WITH THEIR FAMILIES

Integrated Group Session #79   December 29, 1949

The group was fairly slow in starting with the usual members plus Mr. Foster, Mr. Murphy and Mr. Harvey present. The music was made by a member on the harmonica, which was well played and applauded, and also on the piano. Mr. Foster played a piece with one hand, picked out on the piano. There was a fair amount of tension as to who should play. I suggested that Mr. Street play. Mr. Foster attempted to get Mr. Street to play and Mr. Street stated that his wrist was bothering him and he couldn't play.

I noted that people hid their talent and asked what it was that kept people doing so to their own detriment. A member stated that he hid whatever talents he had because people never say anything to him. He then brought out that his brother just didn't speak to him and that he hasn't heard anybody say anything for a long time. He went on at great length complaining about his brother's prerogatives in life, his car, looking at the sun, etc, and his own unfortunate position where he was unjustly put away.

A member got up in the middle of this and shouted that another member should try not to be a man and woman at the same time and that that was his problem. The group laughed at this and then a member who had been trying to get to talk came closer to the microphone. He then presented his problem in coming to the Hall again, to the effect that he got into another argument with his father and refused to do as he wanted, not steal cars and get drunk, and in going to the hospital refused to eat or to obey people as per the instruction of his father, breaking out windows and being so wild that people had to tie him down for twenty some odd days.

Members of the group scoffed at this presentation. Then Mr. Foster started a discussion of the OT Shop and how his talent for working mimeograph machines wasn't utilized. A member brought up Mr. Foster's agitated qualities in the OT Shop, illustrating them vividly from an incident where when he was punching the bag, Mr. Foster hit him on the jaw while he was putting the gloves on and how he had exercised grand forbearance in his relationship with Mr. Foster.

Then the discussion between Mr. Foster and the group became fairly generalized with members of the group all declaiming on Mr. Foster's superb agitative qualities and Mr. Harvey stating that Mr. Foster was condemning himself. Mr. Foster stated that the group discussion wasn't getting anybody anywhere and I reflected this statement and then stated that he knew he was agitating people, and wanted to tell why he did it. He stated that he had to have the machine run exactly the way he wanted it at the time he wanted it or else he would try to blow the entire shop up by getting everybody excited and that he had about succeeded in doing so and in doing that he was condemning himself and that he knew that and that he was sorry he had to be doing that sort of thing.

A member got up about this time to state that he believed in civilization, and everybody being civilized. I asked him what it was that was happening between himself and his family to result in his meaning to hang on to civilized ideas that way. In a stumbling, vague way he brought out that he had been in the Hall twenty years already and that he was discouraged about his family when he first came in, but there wasn't much else brought out about his problems in his discussion. I attempted to have him come clear as possible and reconstituted what other members had said about getting into arguments with their family in one way or another.

Mr. Foster asked what it was that he can do to solve his problems. I pointed out that it was important for Mr. Foster to make peace with his family at some time or other just the way he was learning to make peace with these people in the Hall. Mr. Foster stated that he never had any trouble with his family, and then when the doctor reminded him of what he had said in the past, and he stated that he knew he had.

A member called out from the back that perhaps he had talked too much and not allowed his brother to say anything during the time his brother had visited him, and stated that it was necessary for him in solving his problems to come to some understanding with his brother. The hour was up about this time. Many members had been listening actively. Mr. Murphy was in a distant, snappish mood today, taking the doctor up and stating that he shouldn't swear when in the group at the point where I stated that I swear such and such. Mrs. Sheridan was present today and gave a generalized statement early in the session on her delight at the Christmas cards she had received. Mr. Foster held his tongue about Mrs. Sheridan leaving at her request even though he had brought it up to her that attendants had told him that she was leaving.

The group again went into Foster's agitative ways, punching a member in the jaw while he was putting on gloves. On my query, he explained that things had to be running right, condemning himself in his adversive actions. He apologized for that.

A member answered for Jefferson, stating that he did have self respect. I questioned on why then did he not have it for others. He went on, citing that that we Southerners had our form of self respect. At the end, James referred to Jefferson as dominating and loud-mouthing it. I referred to my earlier statement on force and the conniving techniques of dog-eat-dog. I noted that when Forthright fantasized killing all the negroes, he was expressing this point. Jefferson then cautioned Forthright about going too far. The member who had joined with Jefferson asked what was happening between the group and the doctor and stated that the doctor was doing this not because he was interested in the patients but in his own self.

COMMENTARY

This was an active, relatively coherent session, with an earnest struggle between myself and my allies and Jefferson and his, about the group's purpose, and its relationship to the self respect of the members. I rode the "dog-eat-dog, kill all the negroes position" of Forthright. I entered the fray to draw the members out. A member ended the session, asserting that I was there solely for my self interest, to my mind ascribing his motives to me.

Along the way, a member cited his 20 year tenure in the Hall, secondary to an underlying argument with his family. After Foster asked what he could do to solve his problems, I noted that he needed to make peace with his family, as was now beginning with the patients. Booth called out that he needed to reach an understanding with his brother. Mrs. Sheridan's leaving was broached, after she thanked members for their many Christmas cards.

"BIG SHOT" VERSUS "BEST MOPPER" IN THE INTEGRATED GROUP: MEMBERS YIELDED THEIR OMNIPOTENCE

Integrated Group Session #80   January 5, 1950

The session began in a desultory, fashion with desultory kind of music. Mr. Jefferson bent my ear about the radio work that he has been doing around the Hall, and hinted that he wanted to study books on the subject. He noted that he was accomplished about cows and automobile salesmanship. I stood up to start the discussion and, at the suggestion of a member, took my coat off. Another asked if I wanted to fight, and then went into a diatribe against doctors imposing on people and being big shots. Mr. Murphy picked this up and began to rave about big shots and so did a potentially violent member. I took this up as the subject for discussion.

A member marched up to the front and demanded that his charges be dropped, moving on to his experience in the District Jail and the fact that he didn't eat when put into solitary for two weeks. Mr. Dormer and several others supported this stance, "They take your ass if you don't eat every scrap of food when you are thrown into solitary at Lorton."

A patient stated that you needed a strong back and a weak mind to get along in jail. The member who allegedly was in Howard Hall for 20 years for an argument with his family and had sung with the one who had reported he had not eaten for two weeks in the District Jail, stated that it would be better to sit down and quit jabbering, because it wouldn't do any good the way he was doing it. This was one of the clearest statements that he made during his entire course. Mr. Dormer laughed at the humor of this. Later on when a patient in the back came out with some sarcastic statement, Mr. Dormer again laughed. Mr. Street and Mr. Lauton both made unintelligible comments.

I noted that I agreed with them, adding that people behave in the group in the big shot way they object to, pushing people around in the group. A member stated that he was unreliable in what he said, changing his story every time he told it, and therefore it was useless to continue working with him. I noted that the members were that people be straightforward in the group, and asked "who could be reached in a straightforward way." The group was silent with a strained, depressed appearance.

A hitherto silent member then got up and told of his problem with his father and with the hospital and pleaded with the patients not to get him upset, admitting that he needed to have things done exactly as he wanted then done, and asserted proudly that he was "the best mopper in Howard Hall." The member who allegedly acted as a big shot, from the rear, then told about the mopper's atomic bomb he wanted to give to the hospital and how it was recognized by the doctor. I then asked him what his power dreams were before he came to the hospital. He stated that he had considered himself to be a big shot, like the doctor had said. He stated that "the doctor made a great deal of sense to him, and that he would try to behave and get along, and eventually leave the hospital."

A member defiantly told how he would kill people if they got in his way about leaving the hospital, no matter how big they were. The group laughed at this. During the session Mr. Forsyth sat with his back to the group except when the alleged big shot asked about singing a song, he stated that he was interested in hearing a song. He said this in a rather clear language. Sporting a new mustache, a chronic member appeared quite interested during the session. The patient who usually gesticulates about his face was rather serious and interested during the session. Mr. Murphy was rather aggressive, antagonistic toward me and other people during the session.

COMMENTARY

I reinforced the members critical of the alleged big shot member, in reflecting on his intransigence while in solitary in the District Jail, asking who could be reached in a clear forward way. Other members were critical of his unreliability, when a hitherto silent member related a problem with his father, asserting that he had chosen humility here, that he was the best mopper in the Hall, letting go of having to have things exactly as he wanted. Then, yielding, the big shot revealed his omnipotence, admitting he needed to be a big shot, as noted by me. He would try now to behave, and eventually leave the hospital. A member dialectically stated he would kill those who got in his way, responded to by the group with laughter.

INTEGRATED GROUP SURMOUNTS REGRESSION

Integrated Group Session #81   January 19, 1950

The session was already begun when I came, with a member playing the harmonica in sprightly fashion and another on the drums. After about 10 minutes of this, I was asked to begin the session. I started in the usual fashion, by asking what the group wanted to talk about. A member gesticulated in a rather open, childlike fashion about the radio speaker over his head which he felt was controlling him. Mr. Certa wise-cracked that the group had a lot of problems

Mr. Reston opened with a complaint about his not getting attention, and that the authorities really didn't care what happened to him, and that he was beginning to lose control of himself. He didn't know how far he would go, and that he felt like he was going to be something like the gesticulator in a couple of months.

A new patient sitting close by stated he had a head injury and that was what made him insane. Mr. James stated in loud voice that what bothered him was the way an attendant was giving him orders, and belittling him. The attendant's name was Anderson. Then Mr. Foster broke in with a vitriolic statement about being treated like an animal and locked in a room, "for what?"

The discussion continued with a member joining Mr. Reston, and in turn being joined by another on the doctor's being against the patients and not caring. I went into Mr. Reston's medical course, and it turned out that the hospital had taken action on Mr. Reston's arm on the second week of his stay here, but that Mr. Reston's reluctance to let his family know resulted in a delay in getting operative permission. Then he became sick and he just couldn't be operated on. In the face of this Mr. Reston still denied that the doctors were paying any attention to him.

The member who had joined Reston in complaining sat back, silent. Mr. Foster impulsively came in again with his ideation about how he was treated, and a member from behind me, let go with a blast at Mr. Foster to the effect that he needed to learn to let the people around him help him instead of fighting them off all the time. Members joined in on this. The previous big shot also made some statement on this point. Mr. Foster turned on Mr. James to the effect that the group meetings weren't worth a damn, and it didn't do Mr. James any good to bring out his problems with Mr. Anderson, the attendant, that this doctor wouldn't do anything about it.

Mr. James stated that it was good to have other people in the group hear about this, so that then they could take action or think about it. Mr. Foster stated that maybe they could get together and hit Mr. Anderson over the head someday and teach him a lesson. At this point a member talked about a lesson that Mr. Foster needed, and Mr. Reston came out with a statement that what Mr. Foster needed was a good whipping.

I asked what the group thought about this question of people punishing other people to teach them other ways, and there was a great deal of positive assent to this in relation to Mr. Foster. I reviewed what had been said about how people resented being treated like pieces of furniture, treated like animals, and being belittled, and brought it back to Mr. Foster and Mr. Reston with a member stating that Mr. Foster downs the other person and also himself. Mr. Foster at this point got up and walked out of the room.

Mr. Murphy got up and stated that he had a problem which he wanted to talk over, and that after listening to the group and it seemed to him that members of the group were missing the point, and that was to the effect that just as you get benefit from medicine which is given to you, like aspirin or penicillin, and you take it because you believe in the person who is giving it to you and in the medicine, so in the group it was necessary for people to believe in the group and in the doctor and to learn to take the medicine that was given to them there, and then they would be able to help them. Members and Mr. James agreed with this. There was a great deal of noise in the back and I stopped the process until the noise quieted down.

Mr. Foster, who had come back by this time, stated that the ones making noise were listening only to themselves. I stated that one of them must have been listening to him, because he turned to me and pointed, shouting "big shots." Mr. Murphy continued. The member who had stated "big shot" listened seriously, as did Mr. Forsyth and others. Mr. Murphy stated that he had learned that much, that it was necessary to believe in something before you could hear it. Mr. Foster stated that the group was good for some things, but not for him at this point. Mr. Reston stated that he believed in the group for people who didn't know how to get along with other people and going to dances or parties, but for his arm it wasn't any good. He asked me whether the group would cure his arm. I didn't answer.

Mr. Foster stated that the group had done him a great deal of good about himself and the kind of mistakes he makes. Mr. Reston asked if the doctors get the patients and tell them what their mistakes were since they could do something about it. I summed up by stating that I did that with each person in the group at one time or another, but that as the members had stated, when a person feels against authority, they can't be reached by whatever is being said to them. Members agreed with this. I pointed out that it was necessary for a man to go through things before he could learn, and that he needed to talk about it just as he was going through it. At this point Mr. Foster was walking out, and turned to the group and stated that he had learned a great deal and one of them was that people were against him and that he was going to look out for himself, from now on and not bother with other people.

A member stated that Mr. Foster's trouble was that he was an agitator, and gave as an instance how he was bending over in the yard, and Mr. Foster hit him some where or other. Mr. Foster stated that he had something to do with that, and that since he brought it up it should be gone into. The member stated that Mr. Foster was an agitator and that that was all there was to that. The time was up by this time and I notified the group I had been asked to discontinue the group a few minutes early so that music could be played.

COMMENTARY

An important session, illustrating the surmounting of regression. A severely regressed member complained at first of control by the radio speaker above his head. Reston reported that he was regressing to his state, under the neglect by authority. A new patient stated his head injury had caused his insanity. James and Foster voiced increasing paranoid ideas of willful neglect by the doctors. Reston joined the chorus, and I set forth the medical care he had been given. A member blasted Foster on his denial of help, and James then rebutted Foster in his negativism, by a prosocial stance. The members then turned on Foster, citing that he needed a whipping to set him straight.

I then led the group in a discussion of claiming the other from denigrative and denigrated alienated states. Members noted that Foster downs others and himself in the process. Murphy, joined by James and others advocated trust in the group and doctors, and taking their medicine. At this point members made noise, and one shouted, "Big shots!" Murphy reiterated his prosocial beliefs and Foster allowed that the group was good for others, not him, at this point. Reston voiced similar sentiments.

Foster then brought up that he had been helped with his mistakes. Reston asked me to tell the patients in the group their mistakes. I noted that when people were anti-authority, they could not listen, that one needed to go through things, and talk about it while so doing. Foster related that he had learned that people were against him. Gregory gave an instance of being hit while bent over, in the yard. Foster noted that Gregory had asked for it. The group was ended, so music could be played.

VERBAL WRESTLING IN THE INTEGRATED
GROUP; CERTA ASKS FOR HELP

Integrated Group Session #82   January 25, 1950

Foster complained that he had not had real treatment, since he had no doctor assigned to him. Dr. Cruvant, present at that point, noted that Foster was not ready to receive it. Foster fought this and eventually, on his request for data on his problems, was informed by a member that he was an agitator. At this point, a member, physically confronting me, called me a filthy Jew, and that neither Foster nor anyone else was "going down" on him. I noted to him that I couldn't talk while being threatened physically. Smiling, he moved away. It turned out that Foster had agitated him, who in turn held that Foster was a cock-sucker. Foster blushed, appeared unable to speak, and then stated that he would demonstrate how he agitated Baum.

Certa then wanted to go into his problems and a new patient burst forth with that Dr. Cruvant was a Nazi. I noted that the Nazis held that all people were inferior and needed extermination or slavery, and that this problem was present in each person. Certa agreed, stating that he was down on Indians. A colored patient noted the antagonism between light and dark Negroes.

There was real community feeling at this point, with a patient asking me to read a piece by Dr. Blain on 6 million Americans as sick.

A member stated that I was a nut for thinking nuts could help one another. I answered that a person who heard voices could check with another person. I then stated that people were upset when they felt inferior, giving an example of the member who had threatened me, who was on edge about his homosexuality. At the end of the session, that member thanked me. I felt exhausted at the end of the session

COMMENTARY

This session is an example of a deep transaction with Foster concerning the inner state which resulted in the agitator role, an obsessive impulsion to degrade the other, resulting in reciprocal action of that sort, eventuating in alienation and degradation of status, where he did not have to try anymore. This was the converse of his life course prior to his psychosis. In this session, there was exemplification, on the part of a member obsessed with homosexuality, who attempted to agitate me (succeeding, as evidenced by my exhaustion at the end of the session, an unusual phenomenon, since I generally felt better at the end than the beginning of a session, secondary to the exercise of my messianism).

I held my ground in a manner that resulted in his smiling accession to limitation. This transaction appears similar to those I experienced with the psychopathic alcoholics at Ft. Knox, in which my messianism resulted in a messianic response from them. Then Certa took center stage, asking for help, with an impulsive patient intruding with a paranoid ascription to Dr. Cruvant. Again, I intervened benignly yet incisively, designating all humanity as with fault. Certa, an Indian, noted that he had Nazi-like anti-Indian sentiments. A colored patient then extended the observation to his own kind.

I perceived a feeling of community at that point, and a patient spoke psychoeducationally, asking me to read a statement concerning the prevalence of mental illness. Another commented negatively on helpfulness in the group, and I countered on how members could aid themselves to stay in reality. I then returned to the member's problem with his gender identity. He thanked me. Were the group to return to Foster's problems with his ego integrity, this session would be paradigmatic.

MEMBERS DISCUSS HOMOSEXUAL PROPOSITIONING

Integrated Group Session #83   February 1, 1950

The group today was assembled in its usual composition, and was presented with the visual aid on "What makes a man good, what makes a man bad, and the flux film strips. Association to the material was of a far different order than that of a year ago. Here I showed a greater tendency to explain the material as I would with non-hospitalized people, and the patients' now brought in anamnestic data. Prominent in this latter process was Harvey, who identified with the bad child, brought out his feeling that he couldn't do anything about things, that when things upset him he had to let go and show his total reaction.

Another member prone to violence identified with the ideal characters and also with the deviant ones, stating that the man with his hands in his pockets was walking around in a circle, was thinking of feeling something. Members kidded him on this point. This was to the effect that he did a great deal of stealing on the ward, and that he was speaking of himself. There was a great deal of projection on to the flogging scene with Mr. Harvey as the person who gets himself flogged and is chained. Harvey and the members agreed to that characterization.

After the pictures were over, the members seemed to be in a daze and then the alleged thief got up and asked why the attendants write him down as a German, Nazi, etc. A member critical of him replied that it was absurd, that they didn't do any such thing. He went on to cite that the offender propositioned people for homosexual relationship.

The offender then stated that he did it "only because of your face and that of my mother!" I asked what could be the influence there. The critical member objected to an intrusion on his own rights by standing next to him and making propositions to sell him his shoes, etc.

Mr. James interjected that Mr. Certa was victimizing another member with homosexual activity. I asked whether there might be some invitation there. Mr. James agreed to this as did Mr. Street. The latter agreement came as a surprise. During the representation about being called a Nazi, a member shoved a neighbor, with obvious red-faced anger. I attempted to get communication from the shover on this, but unsuccessfully.

The session ended on the note of defining the alleged thief and propositioner's problem as objecting to the thing that he apparently felt himself called upon to do, which appeared to other people as being his own volition.

COMMENTARY

The reaction to the film strips was different from that of a year ago, with more whole person identification with the characters, and acceptance by the members of my explanatory data. Harvey identified with the bad child and the flogging scenes. Stanton identified with the ideal and alienated characters, also "thinking of feeling something." There was rambling, increasingly pointed discussion of objection to behavior ascribed to the other, that originated on one's part.

MEMBERS DISCUSS THE RAISING OF CHILDREN WITH LOVE; FORSYTH BRINGING DOMESTIC ORDER TO WINDOW SHADES

Integrated Group Session #84   February 10, 1950

The group began with an election of a new chairman, the problem being brought up by a member who expected to leave the Hall the next day. A number of people were suggested at random by an apathetic group, among who were Foster and Harvey. Harvey ran a strong second to a dark horse candidate. I congratulated the winner, and reminded him that despite the backhand way of the group the position was realized by all to be a responsible one.

The winner stated that he would do his best in office. The group was then turned over to me for the presentation of the visual aids. The visual aid on flux was shown first, with vivid response by Harvey. He identified the doctor as me in most slides, and himself as falling backwards on the hill of life. During the slides on "What makes kids act like kids" the group entered a rather tense discussion of child-raising problems. The theme was personalized by one of the newer patients who brought out the problem of living with parents who taught him to write, then having to work for a living, then getting exposed to people who were always getting into trouble, and having confusion as to which way he wanted to go, especially after he came out of the Service, and was on his own.

The chairman plunged then into this problem, stating that he had analogous problems in getting in trouble with people. A member who was prone to assault grew quite interested at this point. Mr. Forsyth had to be taken down earlier in the session, when he began objecting to the way the window shades were blowing in the wind, and began replacing chairs around the room in a rather agitated fashion. A member almost attacked Mr. Forsyth when Mr. Forsyth took a chair in the darkness away from him exposing his books and throwing them on the floor. Mr. Forsyth showed passionate anger as he straightened the window shades.

The themes about raising of children were that children shouldn't be beaten, except justly, and that Harvey was in the Hall because he was beaten but not loved. Harvey came out with some statement on somebody needing the milk bottle when they were young and the whiskey bottle when they we were older when they didn't get the proper love.

COMMENTARY

A paradigmatic session, in which the visual aids were exemplified, then carried on further. Forsyth exemplified a fanatically proper parent, in regards to the window shades. The group arrived at a position regarding discipline, relating it to addiction to alcohol later in life.

JAMES'S DELUSION OF PLAGIARISM, THE GROUP'S CONFRONTATION, AND HIS SUBSEQUENT SELF DOUBT

Integrated Group Session #85   February 23, 1950

The group "stayed with" James's problem of claiming ownership of popular songs, and his stout defense of such. A new patient kept up a parallel commentary on the harm he was doing to self and others. James then brought up the issue of his self doubt and doubt of others.

COMMENTARY

James's false self assurance is giving way to self doubt.

JAMES: THE HALL IS UNDER "THE HYPNOSIS OF HATE"

Integrated Group Session #86   March 3, 1950

The chairman informed me that my slides kept people from discussing their problems. The group then discussed a member who derogated the "dummies" in the group. Foster cited he had succeeded in getting a reclusive member to talk by joking with him, but that when the joking wore off, so did the conversation.

A member voiced anger at me and the other doctors for trying to pin things on him. He had acceded to the approaches of perverts along the way because had been hearing voices which told him to do things, and could not say no. Dormer broke in to report how difficult it was for him to report his hallucinations of fire in the group. The member who felt things were pinned on him by the doctors agreed, and asserted that Dormer was sick, not a sex psychopath. Departing from his usual fragmented way, a member reported coherently that a previous bad actor had behaved well in the room with him. He then asked if I understood the bad actor, and I answered in the affirmative. James then diagnosed the Hall as under hypnosis of hate. The member agreed, and that he had turned hate to like, as when he didn't shoot the whites who had beat a colored fellow in Louisiana.

James cited that the hatred came from ignorance, and not accepting him as he was. A member agreed. Members who had been characteristically silent showed animation at this point. He went on to report that, though he had little education, he had a great deal of learning, and saw himself as a leader in turning "hate into like." I asked him whether he had originally turned love into hate.

A member, who had been previously silent jumped up to state that he was hated, though he had given the world the atomic bomb 7 times, and was not paid, had pipe tobacco, no cigarettes. I wondered whether another patient refused to sing without pay, out of feeling he was not appreciated Also he felt hated when not appreciated for what he had done to help. Another patient then continued with his hatred of me for not understanding him. James then attacked me for holding him without reason. I answered that he had a great deal to learn about himself, having in mind his plagiarism and incestuous past. Green and Dormer joined in the chorus of hatred, when the session ended.

COMMENTARY

In this remarkable session, the members are engaged messianically in helping one another, as did Foster in dialoging with an equally vociferous member, and disgorging their wells of hatred, while inquiring into them, then revealing their ways around it through sublimation. Chronic and regressed patients exposed their delusions and deprived states. All this was done in the course of a session in which the members respected each other's right to represent themselves. It is of interest that the members are valuing their discussion period to the exclusion of my visual aids.

Chapter Three

SUMMARY

From the first, the Integrated Group was remarkable for both its turbulence and productivity. It was the arena of conflict between black and white, acute and chronic, and the doctor and attendants. It was sought after by psychiatrists from Europe, Canada, South America, and Asia, to experience an ambience that pro tem did away with alienation, in the formation of a simply human encounter. I had developed the courage and experience sufficient to the task in success with groups twice its size at Fort Knox. There I had learned that secure leadership could bring the advantages of large groups in reaching and controlling its psychopathic members, through inducing guided regression. But could that regression and guidance work with the severely psychotic?

It did not take us long to find out that it could, that the larger the group, the easier it was to bring about its groupness, its feeling for itself as an entity. We soon found that it eagerly elected its own chairman, and listened to him, unless he became too bossy, as did Cohen. And Cohen tended to listen to the members re his behavior, more readily than in the much smaller and ostensibly more intimate White Therapy Group.

It soon assembled a band of amateur musicians, from the talent of the Black Therapy Group, and the white members, including personnel, participated in song and dance. The greater emotional availability and dramatic capacity of the black population induced its members to tell their stories more readily than in the separate groups. I found the group quite receptive to the visual aids I had developed at Fort Knox, with ready exemplification of its characters and theses, leading to fruitful discussion, adoption of the "Figure It Out" approach to problem solving, and training in that in free association to the life situations presented on the screen.

Chapter Four

Courses of Individual Patients in the Groups

We shall present the stories of the individual patients in the order of their appearance in the sessions. The data stem from the sessions and my memory, much of that quite vivid. Lacking their case histories, I confine the data to that of dynamic significance: life course issues, alienation from self and others, and the therapeutic alliance. Basic to the search is the "had to" underlying compulsiveness I encountered in Rampa in the work at Fort Knox.

The names of 60 of the 125 patients in Howard Hall appear in the original record. While the devil is in the details, and we ultimately need them to render these accounts most meaningful, I shall cull the names down to 23. The 23 are representative of the issues that emerged in the sessions, and of the two populations in the study, psychotic and psychopathic. I cite those less dynamically significant as simply members, with qualifiers pertaining to their group role. I continue my practice of guidance of the reader through headlining and running commentary. Of course, I have altered the names.

We were able to convert the 23 from their alienation and train them to be leaders in the establishment of what amounted to a school for living, in which they helped others by helping themselves. In this chapter I shall attempt to trace that drama in their individual lives. In that course, I draw inferences of intrapsychic nature. I present them in order of appearance in the record.

VINCE JORDAN

Mr. Jordan was a 27 year old very dark skinned black patient who had been sent to Howard Hall from Leavenworth Penitentiary several years previously for treatment of a paranoid psychosis with psychopathic features. During his

515

relatively brief service during the war, he had been absent without leave, impersonated an officer, and participated in a dangerous racial riot. During his sentence, while in solitary confinement, he was found to be floridly psychotic and extremely dangerous. The depth of his alienation eventually called for the specialized care afforded by St. Elizabeths. Here, he was found to be imminently assaultive and seclusive. He continued to be housed on the admitting unit, because only there could he receive the necessary close supervision called for by the danger when he was out of seclusion. He would rove about the day room, panther like. He vividly displayed his delusions—Christ, President, Nat King Cole, Inspector General, by his conversation and costumes he was able to create from scraps of cloth. His fellow patients gave him a wide berth because of his dangerousness.

I have already cited my initial, frightening encounter with this man. It was dramatically reminiscent of those I had at Fort Knox, but there, despite the tumult, I never feared for my life. In his fulminating alienation and readiness to kill or be killed, he closely resembled Rampa, the leader of the riot we had experienced at the end of the war. My continuing interest in underlying violence led me to pay both special attention.

I have already hypothesized that in yielding to reality by not assaulting me in our initial encounter, this man had found a place within his ego, as had Rampa in my Army experience, for a possibly constructive relationship with me. I have elsewhere characterized it as an alliance in the ego ideal of messianic sort.

Following our introductory skirmish, he began attending the meetings, and the first notation of such is that he did not speak, and I have no record of his attendance.

Jordan Asks for His War Pay; Begins Systematic Therapy

In B 17, after Loren Jones asked for discussion of the Songs of Solomon, Jordan asked for the pay that was due him from the government.

COMMENTARY

Jordan here begins systematic therapy, in a manner characteristic for the group at the time. He couched it in his concern of the moment; the money owed him by the government, in the form of his payroll. Instead, the members chose to discuss another patient's currently "baby messiah" behavior.

Again, Asks for Money Due Him for War Service; the Story Continues

Again, in B 20, B 21, and B 22 he asked for the money owed him now identified as for his war services. In that course, he cited a delusion of being president. The paradoxical outcome of these transactions was alliance with me; he volunteered to take notes for the group, as I had taken to doing.

COMMENTARY

I infer that this alliance had actually begun in our initial encounter. He yielded his kingship for a contemporaneous student/collaborator capacity.

Dreams of Sex with White Actress Who Transmutes to Man; Group Invests in Work with Jordan

In B 23, after the members chose to continue with Jordan's problem with his delusion re pay for war services, he reported vivid dreams of sexual visits by a white movie actress, who hated him, and who turned out to be a man. Members inferred that he had some lack of masculine capacity developmentally.

COMMENTARY

In this crucial session Jordan relates his problem with reality, through revelation of his autistic nighttime's experience, and the members infer his need for masculine understanding of a defective ego, and hypothesize re a developmental defect, and point out a way for him to obtain centeredness in his masculine identity and present reality, abjuring his psychotic ways. He and the group are setting the stage for his struggles intrapsychically and with them.

Jordan Disavows His Hallucinations and Autistic Identity; Leader of the Pack

In B 26, counseling Jones re his delusions, Jordan related the course of his own "nervous" condition, and his inner conflict re autism versus reality, acting as exemplar of progress for the members.

COMMENTARY

He has begun confiding in me, alongside of the group and establishing himself as a leader of the pro-therapeutic faction in the group, alongside Holden.

Agrees to be "Just Plain Vince"

In B 28, in the context of discussion by the members of their autistic escapes from pain and anxiety, plays a leading role in enunciating his desire to be his normal self.

COMMENTARY

Again, Jordan leads in the inquiry into his intrapsychic life.

Jordan's Delusion Free Letter to Dr. Abrahams: Anticipates Matters of Deep Worry   February 15, 1947

Here Jordan relates the small amount of understanding he had derived from the therapy so far, positing that a meeting with his family would produce matters of deep worry.

COMMENTARY

This letter is delusion free, and hopeful of release through the therapeutic process.

Jordan At Once Identifies with Dr. Abrahams and Jones: "I've Got to Stop Fooling Myself"

In B 30, he identified with Jones on his hegemonic delusions, at the same time, again in alliance with me, interpreting that Jones was "hurting so bad, did it for love." Jordan went further into how, depressed, he had been fooling himself.

COMMENTARY

In interpreting Jones's pain, he is taking a step towards report of his own underlying affect.

Jordan Assumes Role as Librarian and Secretary

In B 31, Jordan appears as keeper of the books and secretary to the group.

COMMENTARY

These roles serve to anchor this man further in reality.

Critical of Jones's Delusions, Counsels "Be Honest with Yourself"

By B 34, he was critical of Jones's delusions, urging him to be honest with himself, which would result in Jordan's support.

COMMENTARY

I would infer that Jordan has engaged intrapsychically with what is called one's executive functions, the capacity for self observation and self evaluation, related in turn to the ego ideal and super ego. His ego is reconstituting itself, and he is widening his interpersonal investments.

Jordan Gives Thanks; Other Step towards Reality

In B 35, he passionately thanked me for my service to the group, also to the Red Cross.

COMMENTARY

I take this passion to be largely messianic in nature, but also in the case of the Red Cross, a governmentally relevant organization, a step towards reality.

In Reorganization of the Group, Follows Holden's Lead

In B 36, Jordan cited what he had learned from the group.

COMMENTARY

Jordan is following Holden's enthusiastic lead.

Letter to Dr. Abrahams: Cites Confidence in Possible Family Therapy

In letter to Dr. Abrahams, of February 15, 1947 he notes his new sense of hope and posits that meeting with his family could be of help.

COMMENTARY

This significant letter is in its entirety in the section on the Black Therapy Group.

Begins Self Analysis through Analysis of Holden: Seeking Seclusion

In B 37, he identified with Holden for his past irrationality in seeking seclusion, citing his own experience in seclusion at Leavenworth.

COMMENTARY

He is now engaging in survey of his life course, reliving its crises internally.

Members Empathize with Mute Catatonic Bostic and "Mortally Pained" Jordan

In B 38, he identified with Bostic, a mute catatonic, citing his own episode in the Army Disciplinary Barracks. He then read the group his poem on suicide, "because of mortal pain, no, eternal pain." He then led a discussion of being feeling alone, unwanted, and subjected to "hard knocks," leading members to empathize with him. He cited a loss of belief in connectedness with others.

COMMENTARY

In this important session, Jordan significantly communicated the "mortal, eternal pain" of the poem. I now infer that it resulted from loss of connectedness with others, involving death of self and an eschatological outcome, involving eternity. I further inferred that he had developed that connectedness somewhere early in his development, the loss of which resulted in the deathly pain. At that point, I had not understood the role of psychic death in the genesis of psychotic and psychopathic disorder, and took this poem to be an expression of depression.

It was later in my psychoanalytic career that I conceived a relationship between psychic death, psychotic and psychopathic disorder, and messianism. Both the messianism and the delusions would stem from a resurrective transcendence. In his account, Jordan cited that he learned to surmount deathly states during isolation at Leavenworth Penitentiary through singing, dancing, and fantasying.

Identifies With Army Rehabilitee; Complains That Army Gave "No Love or Consideration"

In B 39 he identified with an Army rehabilitee in a recording I presented, who after resisting the group's overtures, complained that "the Army gave no love or consideration."

COMMENTARY

This issue of "consideration" played a large part in Jordan's verbal and emotional productions. It was evident that it involved special consideration, as in the possession of an elitist car, a Cadillac, but grew to have meaning relative to his soul's yearnings for recognition in regard to God's design, as was Job.

Volunteers as Judge in Sociodrama; Plays Role Reversal

In B 41 he volunteered as the judge in a mock court, asking the defendant, myself , why I was confined in Howard Hall "hurting." He asked me to prove my hegemonic delusions. He decided I would be "all right" once I was freed.

COMMENTARY

Remarkable here was how Jordan lent himself and appeared to enjoy the psychoanalytic aspect of this psychodramatic exercise. The group would soon be asking him to prove the validity of his delusions. The levity here undoubtedly lightened the bitter life and death aspects of his dilemmas.

Bostic/Jordan Honor Fight; "You're Going to Have to Kill Me!"

In B 46 he evidenced disappointment over not being my favorite in the distribution of model airplane kits. The day before, he had physically fought Bostic, who was defending his honor against Jordan's jealous attack in which he in effect claimed hegemony over Bostic's fiancée. Bostic cited his depth of feeling in the encounter by stating, "You are going to have to kill me."

COMMENTARY

The "kill or be killed" imperative of Rampa of Fort Knox is here expressed by Bostic, indicative of the depth of feeling in this conflict situation. In their rivalry, Bostic is assuming the position of Abel, and Jordan of Cain. This is a manifestation of coupling important to the therapy, to occur with Street later ("he can help me more than I can help him"), with me ("we look alike, eat alike"). This coupling serves as pathway of this Little Prince from commitment to his delusory reality.

Open Hatred of Dr. Abrahams; Analysis Proceeds

In B 47, breaking temporarily from what I considered a messianic mutuality with me, and into analysis of the psychotic aspects of his personality, he showed open hatred of me as his persecutor.

COMMENTARY

Here he reaches the opposite to his messianism, to the delusions he had displayed in our first encounter. In future sessions, he cites an underlying killer mentality. This regression is still in the context of the therapeutic alliance, in which a portion of his personality is leading the group and the rest of his personality in analyzing his situation and motivations.

Letter to Dr. Abrahams: The Low Status of a Big Shot; Flirts with Realization of Mental Illness   April 2, 1947

In this missive Jordan denies he is ill, that I cannot help with that which worried him, thinks he is a Big Shot because of his low status.

COMMENTARY

In denying awareness of his illness, he may be approaching its realization.

Members Address His Need for Superiority, Itself Secondary to a Past Which Haunts

In B 48, members, now accustomed to transaction about troubled aspects of each other's personalities, commented on his need for superiority, itself in the context of the subject of the past haunting them. That haunt came up in B 49 in the form of Jordan's dishonorable discharge from the Army, discussion of which he averted by stating, "let's take someone else's case, maybe I can help somebody else out."

COMMENTARY

I have since learned of the appearance of haunts or ghosts as signals of oncoming mourning, as was Hamlet's father's apparition on the parapet. Here he is beginning to mourn the failure of his military career.

Joins Members in Review of His Incarceration; Exemplifies Street's Haunting Tie to The Past

In B 51, brings up a letter from a Veterans Administration official, and the group reviewed his reality status following courts martial in the Army and dishonorable discharge.

COMMENTARY

Jordan sought and appeared to accept the group's judgment on his reality status re his trial in the Army, dishonorable discharge, and need to accept his task of self rehabilitation.

Becoming a Soldier in the Ranks of the Group

He showed further initiative as a patient among others in joining morning calisthenics prior to session B 52. In B 61 he reflected on the sense of entitlement of Street, a hebephrenic patient, as Jordan moved to open reconciliation with the group and its therapeutic purposes.

"Crying When You Want To Laugh": Jordan, Street, and Bostic Exchange Experience

In B 64 he for the first time openly and frankly asked what members thought of him, avowing that he was hated by whites and despised by colored people. In the course of comments on Bostic's make believe world, he related his own, concerning Hollywood. He affiliated with Bostic, after having fought him, though was disaffiliated from others, asserting he was "in Hollywood." Again, this was further evidence of a wish to become a "regular" member of the group, and in doing so, accept his black man's status.

In B 66 he noted that Street wanted to cry when he laughed (in his hebephrenic manner). In B 68, acting as a counselor, he asked Bostic concerning his furlough, then stated that Bostic must have shot his girlfriend after coming from the Army on furlough. He then tracked through some of his own Army career.

COMMENTARY

Jordan is reaching through to his underlying feelings, through detecting them in others, as re Street's sadness, and Bostic's alienation from his girlfriend.

Letter by Jordan: Unrealistic, but Delusion-Free   April 14, 1947

This was a business like letter to the Commandant of the Leavenworth Disciplinary Barracks, requesting his discharge. While it was in essence unrealistic, it lacked his delusional identities.

Sits Close: "What the Voices Told Me"; Frank Counsel by Members: "Relinquish It All"

In B 70 he sat close to me, in a particularly trusting manner. The members for the first time frankly counseled him to relinquish his delusions and hallucinatory voices. He responded that he "had to" believe what the voices told him.

COMMENTARY

It appeared to me that disbelief in the voices would involve betrayal of a psychotic/psychopathic compact formed during his psychotic break while in seclusion at Leavenworth. His loyalty to them became quite touching, as well as frustrating.

Tells Story of Early Alienation from Self, Ready Access to Women; Still Has to Believe the Voices

This was followed in B 71 by his report on his alienation from himself and others, his inner struggle with the voices, and a claim of sexual intimacy from infancy that followed a most likely fantasized ready sexual access to women as a child. Bostic set himself forth as a role model for Jordan regarding facing reality.

COMMENTARY

The little boy self from which he is alienated can only be inferred by one's intuition, but the members of the group demonstrated it by their patience and ready affiliation.

Simply Human, With Bostic Explores His Alienation from Self and Alienated Worlds, Tearful

In B 72 he reported the natural history of his "feeling bad," a religious experience in the Leavenworth Penitentiary, in the course of solitary confinement. There he hallucinated conjunction with an Eve and exaltation, with singing and dancing. Bostic interpreted that as a "make-believe world," experienced at Jordan's lowest point. Jordan responded that he wished to get drunk, and also that they could help each other. He then cited his alienation at that time, of feeling despised, "a long way from home," and his current fear of making friends. He was tearful in this account.

COMMENTARY

The self from which he is alienated is showing through in his longing for home and wish for friends, above all in his tears.

Aware that Derogates Others When is "King"; Acknowledges Alienation from Self

In B 73 he reported that he would be "making fun" of whites and colored people were he to say he was king, edging into exploration of motivation behind his delusions. Members replied that he would be doing so to himself, addressing the intrapsychic. He agreed. In B 80 he asserted that Street, a severely hebephrenic patient, could help him more than he could help Street, since "he is so knowledgeable."

COMMENTARY

Here he may be edging towards awareness of Street's braininess and his own conscience, and towards a final internal struggle for mastery of his delusions, based on what he sensed was Street's powerful intellect.

Acknowledges Street as Knowing

In B 80 Jordan stated that Street could help him more than he could help Street.

COMMENTARY

This is an indirect reference to the cognitive defect brought about by his illness, and which is gradually yielding, as he lives more in reality. He sees Street's brilliance, hidden to view by others, by his hebephrenic self alienation.

In Tears, Confesses to a Criminal Career

In B 82 he initiated interaction, implicitly asking the group to claim him from his delusions and hallucinations. This he did in the context of his recorder role in the group, announcing his problem of the moment. He accompanied this with a report on his past stealing and lying. A member identified with him in his criminal aloneness. This was followed by tears concerning his criminal career, culminating in his life sentence.

COMMENTARY

I would infer that the tears attest to guilt and also mourning.

Letter to His Family, Reaches Out   June 3, 1947

In correspondence to his brother and sister, he further reached out to his relatives in correspondence to his brother and his sister, both convivial towards them in a mundane manner, yet still indicative of his autistic identity.

COMMENTARY

This act of reconciliation is of great moment, an interpersonal manifestation of his intrapsychic changes.

Sets Self Forth as Model for a Hebephrenic Member

In B 89 he held forth as a model for Lauton, a hebephrenic patient.

COMMENTARY

As a leader of the group, Jordan is currently secretary to the group, taking notes. Having attained a degree of self confidence, here he is encouraging a better educated member to "figure it out"

Jordan Regresses, Fistic with Bostic, Then Reaches Out

He began to fail in his secretarial role, and in B 106 displayed himself in robes made from old bed-sheets, declared himself as Christ. In B 109 he again fought Bostic in the group, citing that was "left out," as a Negro and hated the doctor.

COMMENTARY

After regressing to a frankly messianic role, he recoups his manhood by dueling with Bostic, the current leader of the group.

After Absence, Returns Somber and Reflective,
Asks Member His View of Him

After a long absence, in B 158 he asked a member his view of him, with the reply that he was working against his own will. In B 159, he shared stories of themselves with another patient. In B181, in the context of Bostic's surfacing in a problem solving mode, this time about a member's marital relationship, Jordan appears somber and reflective.

COMMENTARY

Jordan has absented himself from the group, and shall do so, each time relinquishing his initial messianic identification with me. He is now reaching out to members on the same level.

Resumes Work in the Black Therapy Group, as Chair

In B 162, he was elected chair again, encouraging members to present their problems, holding to his transcendent uniqueness, and that pussy was the answer to his problems.

COMMENTARY

Encouraging others was most likely in identification with me. He is also acting from his Don Juan narcissism, an advance from his delusional ways.

In the Integrated Group, Asks Member What He Called "Living"

In I 40 he asked Frank Forster what he called "living." After discussion by members of the ways members dealt with their lives, Smith replied to Jordan that he needed to learn to crawl before he walked, solve his problems in having participated in the riot in the Army, and go on from there.

COMMENTARY

Frank Forster was a hebephrenic member who spoke in parables, but here he gave it to Jordan straight from the hip, pointing out he needed to come off his arrogant stance, in a manner analogous to that of Holden, and, then living in reality, deal with the reality to him of his dishonorable discharge, his low status, crawling before he walked.

Joins with Sex Psychopaths on Man's Inherent Need for Woman

In B 164 he joined two sex psychopaths, following the lead of one of them, in a general discussion on man's need for woman, also on "how to take" psychotic and criminal material.

COMMENTARY

My inference is that here he is seeking further objectivity.

Jordan and Group Begin a Passionate Struggle Over his Past and Current Ties

In B 186 Jordan and the group began a passionate dialog over the validity and reason for his delusions and hallucinations. He held that they were caused by the white man, "Uncle Tomming" and the members remonstrated with him, and he yielded, perplexed.

COMMENTARY

The passion of both is highly significant, also his tentative acceptance of their reason as authentic and not "Uncle Tomming."

Jordan Edges towards Facing and Accepting his Role in Wartime Riot

In B187, he accepted that he had participated in the riot, disavowing being like them, though.

COMMENTARY

He had not quite accepted his criminal status, just as he is still resisting being like the humans in the group.

Asserts That Is To Be Defensive "To the End"

In B 188, comparing himself to an equally resistive member of the group, he noted that he was going to be that way "to the end." In contrast, Bostic identified with me.

COMMENTARY

This "to the end" obdurate way is consonant with that of Rampa, in my long term inquiry.

Jordan Cites and Disavows Servitude to his Delusions

In B 189 he announced that the members would not accept him as all power-ful, followed by his wish to end his servitude to his delusions, including that of being Christ.

COMMENTARY

Again, here he is evidencing his inner struggle.

Jordan's Fear of Contemporaneity, and his Imperishable Ties to the Past

In B 192 he cited that acceptance in the present meant that he was "no good."

COMMENTARY

He had often stated that the members of the group are criminals and no good. He would not be a member of a group that would accept him, also that ac-ceptance of reality meant acceptance of an intolerable, malevolent state.

Becomes Chair of Integrated Group; Withdrawn Members Join in Singing and Dancing

In I 44 he volunteered for and was accepted as chair. Withdrawn members join in singing and dancing; one does the cake-walk.

COMMENTARY

The inference I drew is that he identified with the least among them, and so doing, was able to draw them out.

From Position in Reality, Cites Vulnerability, "Helpless and Hopeless," to the Voices

In B 194, he accepted that he needs to acknowledge his part in the riot, and his real relationship with Nat King Cole, then protests his vulnerability when alone to the torture of the voices.

COMMENTARY

His internal struggle is exemplified clearly in this session.

Together with Psychopathic Member, Jordan Asserts that "Not to Take It from Anyone"

In B214 he joined with a psychopathic member in asserting he was going to stand up for himself, but would do so by being one of his autistic roles. Members and I remonstrated with this as fantasy, and he agreed to relinquish it.

COMMENTARY

Again, he is renegotiating intrapsychically, along with interpersonally.

Reports Delusional and Hallucinatory Preoccupation Keep Him from His Fellows

In B 221 he broke into discussion of dreams by members to report his struggle with his delusions and hallucinations that keep him from relating to his fellow patients.

COMMENTARY

Again, in reporting his internal struggles, he is gaining in ego strength.

Group Deeply Emotional with Jordan As He Cites His Exasperation with His Life

In B 216 in a deeply emotional scene with the members, he cited his exasperation with his life, and that he turns to prayer.

COMMENTARY

I take this to be a step forward in his ego development, of restitutional nature.

Jordan Is Angry at His Voices, Dreams, Veers towards Reality

In B 217, he dreamed that he had hawked and spit on the ground, as pitcher, when someone had stated to him that he was a 2nd Lieutenant. I noted that he was considering entering the game of life, versus his tortured past. He repeated the word "tortured," going on to introduce a recitation of his educational attainments in the past and present, by citing a dream in which the occupational therapist was holding a white box.

COMMENTARY

Jordan's capacity to dream, versus his delusional functioning is a good sign.

Alienated and Alienating, in a "Jiving Fit," Cries re his Birth and Nadir Status

In B 218, in a hypomanic manner, he admitted he was "jiving" in asserting his delusions. He then grew angry and depressed, reporting hatred of women, his own degradation, stemming from birth, and antagonism to affection from others.

COMMENTARY

He is here moving into position to explore developmental and life course issues, relating them to a mother ostensibly in a nadir and self rejecting position, which he then reflected.

Jordan Envisions Leaving the Hall as a Man

In B219 he defended me from criticism by others, and then asserted that he was going to leave the Hall as a man, versus as a god, or child.

COMMENTARY

In criticizing others who had attacked me, he turned to assertion that he was going to attain his own manly identity and grown up status. In going through this exercise, he catches a glimpse of a former infantile and crippled status.

Members Report Feeling of Loss When Give In to the Other Person's Delusions

In B 220, starting with discussion of Jordan's retention of his delusions, the members moved to their affect of loss when they give into the other's delusion. They evidenced close attention and attunement to my feelings, in that regard.

COMMENTARY

I take it that they were attuned to Jordan's loss of his autistic identity, speaking for him.

Jordan Dresses in Ordinary Clothes

In B 221 he came dressed in ordinary clothes, different from the Christ, soldier, prophet vestments he usually displayed. The context was a session devoted to Jones's delusions.

COMMENTARY

This changed of costume to that worn by the other patients is another sign of progress, in this exquisitely expressive and dramatic man.

Jordan Defensive of His Authoritarian Way in Teaching Guitar, Borderline Assaultive

In B 224 he reacted defensively concerning his authoritarian way of teaching guitar, in the context of a one of the members, a minister' having to have it his own way. Jordan then turned his ire onto me, threatening assault, and asserting his alienation from us.

COMMENTARY

Earlier I have noted a centrality of an artistic identity in this man, and it is no surprise that the members are able to get to a core self, through his teaching of the guitar.

Insists on Reality on His Terms, in Contradistinction to Constructive Member

In B 226 insisted that he would only accept reality on his terms, in opposition to a member who avowed constructiveness.

COMMENTARY

Assumed a position dialectical to the other, in a generally convivial debate.

Denies Purpose to His Life

In B 228, in the course of association to a visual aid on growth and the life course, Jordan aggressively denied that his life had purpose. He took on the group in this discussion, the members holding that his position stemmed from him.

COMMENTARY

Jordan is becoming aware of the depth and underlying motivation of his alienation, through debate with the members.

Inner "Torture" As Envisions Being Like Others

In B 230 he cited his insistence that Miss Sawyer take the initiative at mutuality, also his state of torture (by his voices) when envisions being conforming like others.

COMMENTARY

It is significant that he is now citing his experience with himself, interpersonally and intrapsychically, from that of membership in the group.

Reports That Is "Half Man, Half Woman," Needing a Woman's Love Initiative for Restitution

In B 232, in transacting with a hebephrenic member, revealed that he was half man and half woman, need a woman's love to become his own man.

COMMENTARY

This is a seminal revelation, leading to conceptualization as to the genesis of this condition, in his relationship with his mother.

States That Is "Sick, Cannot Get Well"

In B 233 he reported his need for a woman to free him from his hopelessly "sick" state, despairing of recovery.

COMMENTARY

He is edging closer to this intrapsychic conundrum.

In Prospective Court Visit, Would Hold Back on His Delusions, Pending the Judge's Initiative

In B 235 he would yield his aggressive stance, not mention his delusions, unless the judge brought it up, then would fight him.

COMMENTARY

Again, Jordan is trying conformity on for size, holding in reserve his alienated integrity.

If Interested, Could Learn, Like the Members

In B 236, in the context of the members' interest in learning, he cited he could, if interested.

COMMENTARY

He is here reporting his lack of interest in reality, most likely lacking the color. Intensity, and drama of his delusions.

Jordan Asks For Help with His Fear of Ridicule by Others

B 238 he asked for transfer to another ward, to leave the context of ridicule by members for his delusions of grandeur.

COMMENTARY

Here he is reporting his reality ties to others, his susceptibility, and need for help.

Closer to Reality, Realizes Dreams as Delusions; Slept Soundly for the First Time

In B 239 he was voted in again as chair, reported slept soundly for the first time in the Hall. He told a dream of attaining a gold watch from the head nurse, Mr. Broderick, realizing he had none, on awakening. Also, to apologize to another nurse for accusing him of taking his money. He then turned, to counsel a member in solving his problems.

COMMENTARY

These are significant steps, towards reality, intrapsychically and in the group.

Jordan as Chair, Members Take up Evil, Mooning by Member

In B 243 he guided the group through a discussion of evil and the exposure of his buttocks by a member.

COMMENTARY

As chair, is situated in reality.

Lack of Belief in Self, in Context of Concern with Faith

In B 248 he guided the group through a discussion of faith and evil and the exposure of his buttocks by a member. Jordan noted his problem of lack of belief in himself.

COMMENTARY

Again, my inference is that his chairmanship is a stabilizing factor here.

"I'll Never Get Anywhere"; Difficult to Change Due to Lack of Colored Attendants

In I 63 he cited his despair of getting anywhere, in part ascribed to lack of colored attendant personnel.

COMMENTARY

In both lack of belief in himself and despair of progress, he is speaking from his soul. The white attendants are fomenting an anti black move, and Jordan is one of the few who address the issue directly, an act of relative sanity.

Jordan Envisions Self, Post Discharge, as a Formerly Crazy Person, With Dishonorable Discharge

In B 257 he tackled the issue of shame on the part of his family, for his insanity and offense. Members urged that he compensate by having him go into business for himself.

COMMENTARY

He is taking another step towards reality, by acceptance of empathic counsel by his fellows re these crucial issues. He is also leading the group in these regards.

Members in Heart-to-Heart Report Affection towards Jordan But Would Kill Him if He Harmed Mrs. Sheridan, the OT Leader; Could Not Report What Happens at Night; Member Reports My Favorable Look

In B 284 there was affectionate communication between Jordan and the members, but also it's opposite.

COMMENTARY

I consider this closeness to be highly significant, also the look on my face, indicating an identity indicative of what I call a union in the ego ideal.

Jordan in Despair about Getting Anywhere

In I 63 together with others, he stated his despair of getting anywhere. Reassured by members, he stated that lack of colored attendants made if difficult to change.

COMMENTARY

Again, he is empathic with the others.

Jordan Asks About Self Hypnosis through Staring, Volunteers to Bring Paretic Patient to the Group

In B 265 Jordan, who stares a great deal, brings up the issue of hypnosis by staring, in the context of group discussion of mental breakdown and memory loss.

COMMENTARY

I take this to be a further indication of his growing awareness of his sickness.

Tearful Re Being "By Myself"

In B 268 he tearfully reported being by himself.

COMMENTARY

He is allowing others to identify with him.

Reports Graduation from Bible School

In B 269 he displayed a certificate of graduation from mail order bible school.

COMMENTARY

I take it that his messianism is now less autistic in nature, closer to reality role assumption.

Jordan to Give Up on Cadillac and "Search for the Good in Man"

In B 270, in the context of a passionate discussion of living up to an autistic ideal or suffer perversity, Jordan came out with the prospect of giving up on his, but would search for the good in man.

COMMENTARY

He is turning from his autism still further.

Reads His Minutes as Chair, Noting His Lack of a Cadillac

In B 271 he went about his business as chair and secretary, showing his dispassionate way of going about his duties, but leaving out the topic of religion, later brought up by a minister patient, who tearfully reported reconciling with his wife.

COMMENTARY

The reconciliatory event followed Jordan's initial dutiful report.

Striving for Stardom, Achieving One's Ideal: "All or Nothing"; Complains of Not Being in OT, Citing His Delusion of Stardom

In B 272 he edged towards discussion of his delusion of stardom, by complaining he was left out of the OT program. This occurred in the context of a group discussion of having to have one's ideal, or nothing.

COMMENTARY

Jordan is moving towards taking up this delusion, through a paranoid regression.

Star Delusion, Evil Spirits and Assault; Jordan Retreats From Responsibility as Chair

In B 276 he was late, asserting his star delusion, hinting he wanted it discussed, in the context of discussion of evil spirits and assault.

COMMENTARY

It may be held that his regression is in the service of taking up his problem.

Rails Re "No Consideration," Asserts Helps Others

In B 277 he chewed us out re not being given "consideration" then took satisfaction at helping others.

COMMENTARY

This is in conformity with his experience of knowing ahead of time what people say to him.

Be Homosexual or Face the Problem: Jordan and the Group's General Paranoia

In B 283 he at the end noted that I wanted him to be homosexual or face the problem.

COMMENTARY

As a leader of regression in the group, Jordan is settling into his concerns re issues in identity.

Jordan Denied Father Role by Mind Possessing Entity: Working through the Delusions

In B 286, he went through delusions, arriving at wanted a reality role as father of children. This was to be denied to him by an omnipotent entity, reading his mind. He arrived at religious parables and his messianism, in concert with a minister patient.

COMMENTARY

In this session I acted as facilitator to free association, and Jordan is both surfacing in reality and representing his delusional positions.

Has to be Fetched, Wants to Be Trusted, Make Money

In B 287 he had to be called by the members, stated then that he wanted to be respected as somebody, and they responded that they wanted him to act responsibly.

COMMENTARY

Is making deliberate yet reluctant steps towards reality.

Wears Hat and Coat Backwards as Commentary to Group

In B 288 he wore hat and coat on backwards.

COMMENTARY

Action here spoke loudly.

Wishes to be Home, in Reality, Job; When Challenged, Delusional Again

In B 289 he redolently wanted to be back in Michigan, earning money for his Cadillac. Wanted better life, with others not involved in it.

COMMENTARY

He is surfacing, but ready to submerge into delusional world.

Walks Out of the Group, on Discussion of Self and the Godhead

In B 292 he reluctantly acted as chair, asked topic be cleaning of the ward. When challenged on his not participating in that function, and when the group was turned to discussion of the Godhead by Dr. Powell, Jordan walked out of it.

COMMENTARY

I tie Jordan's non participation in cleaning the ward to be due to his Jesus delusion, and his walking out of the group to the challenge implicit in the discussion of spirituality.

He is here envisioning a cure by change of location.

Identifies With Member Who Received Rays from Federal Buildings, Cites His Own Fantasies of Raping and Killing

In B 294 Jordan reentered therapy, through identification with a deeply regressed member, and went on to cite his psychopathic fantasies, centering about violence against women. This was followed by similar expositions by several psychopathic members.

COMMENTARY

It is possible to infer that Jordan was led by the chronic regressed member and in turn led the psychopathic ones in making representations in reality.

Jordan's Lost Childhood Ideal and Delusion of Possession; Christmas Play Trumps It

In B 295 he started the group with increased real feeling, going on to his grieving, and wish to go to the OT Shop. After discussion of Mrs. Sheridan as the ideal woman, his claim to her, and a member's interpretation that she and all were within Jordan, and he was all he loved, he went into how from an early age he never asked for anything. A member cited that he was thereby grieving for his freedom, and he moved over to asking for a part in the Christmas play.

COMMENTARY

Jordan is moving from an autistic concept of freedom from dependence to participating in the reality of relatively humbly seeking stardom in Howard Hall.

Renegotiating With His Stardom Delusion, Lays Hands on Piano, Disciplines Forsyth, the Star of the Show

In I 76 he tinkered with the piano keys, and then later asked for discipline of Forsyth's exuberant singing, entering in the group dialog on the matter. Forsyth was openly vitriolic towards him.

COMMENTARY

Challenging Forsyth's autistic performance is a step towards dealing with his own delusion. He is moving towards volunteering to sing in the Christmas celebration.

Notes his Alienation, Cites Identification with Bird He Had Suffocated

In B 296 he joined with others in noting their alienation, brought up incident where he had held a bird, finding he had suffocated it.

COMMENTARY

A previous allusion to death had to do with suicide and mortal pain, in a poem.

Foray into Reality: Co-Member Criticized For Fighting as a Superman

In B 298 a member had fought with an attendant in West Lodge, been returned to Howard Hall. Jordan criticized him for superman aspiration.

COMMENTARY

Jordan is edging further towards reality.

Reverts to Paranoia, Calls Me a Liar

In B 299, in the context of deep ambivalence on the part of the group, declared that I was a liar.

COMMENTARY

Here he is back to ambivalence.

Jordan Passionately Leads Group from Paranoid Position, Allies Self with Me

In B 302 in the context of contention about antisocial values, citing the golden rule, he vigorously defended me for my troubles in treating the group, and tensions with colored people, like those a colored person would have with whites.

COMMENTARY

In his swings he reaches the point of standing in my shoes.

Continues Defending Me

In B 303 he attacked the members for not facing their problems, in the course of defending me.

COMMENTARY

He is solidifying identification with me, and it is no surprise that in his next swing, he arrives at the essence, the soul as the locus of inquiry.

Asserts Soul is Being Killed by the Doctor, in Non-Recognition of His Entitlement, Alongside Incestuous Possession of His Mother

In B 308, and he held that the doctor sitting and waiting for him to say something was destroying his soul, his spirit, and he had to stand up like a man, take care of himself, and he heard voices on the radio telling him these things. He was entitled to smoke in the dayroom, not be treated like a child.

COMMENTARY

Here he is again a central, representative figure, bringing up his problem with self, soul, and reality. He had been joshed by the group, joining it to cite a radio program, in which Henry Aldridge calls out, "Coming, mother," transmuted by Jordan into a salacious matter.

Members See Jordan and the Doctor as Similar in Features, Jordan Sees Him as Similar in Taste for Foods; Jordan Tearfully Reveals He Is Homesick, Dreamt of Bitten By a Rat

In B 309 he admitted he would have to leave the hospital first, and then get his car. When he stated he would then walk down the street with a brown girl on his arm, members agreed he was improving. Later he tearfully stated he was homesick, like another member of the group. A sentient member of the group cogently asked me to explain insanity, "bit by bit."

COMMENTARY

In this seminal session (see the fuller report in the Black Therapy Group), he and the group members essay into an intimate identity, reaching into his delusions and up into reality. When Dormer asked me to explain insanity, "bit by bit," I infer that the genesis of the psychotic experience going on in himself and Jordan is becoming apparent.

Jordan Cites Desire for "Friendship" With the Doctor, Tearful About "Losing Out on Life"

In B 311, in the context of open ambivalence on the part of members of the group with one another, Jordan opened up about his desire for friendship with the doctor, then was tearful about losing out on his life

COMMENTARY

The salient features here are his tears, evident depression, and awareness of life course issues.

Jordan Cries about Missing His Mother While Reports Prison Psychosis

In B 312, in the context of a discussion of prison psychosis, Jordan wept about missing his mother while in prison.

COMMENTARY

He is capable of reaching his emotions, in the context of the group's initiative in this regard.

Helps Long Term Patient Who Also Had Gone Through Leavenworth

In B 317 Jordan earnestly counseled with and stood up for a long term patient who had gone through an experience with the Army similar to his.

COMMENTARY

This is another step in Jordan's commitment to reality.

Reports That Felt Sick over the Weekend, Hallucinatory Voice Calling Him Jesus; Shocked at Realization Still Here, "Lost"; Writing Book about Himself

In B 324, in context of discussion of god-voices, reported that his voice repeats hegemonic assertions.

COMMENTARY

Jordan is here joining the membership in exchange of the delusions that possessed them, about their possessions.

Mourning Losses, Joins Dormer in Rage at Authority and Missing Family

In B 327 he joined Dormer in rage and disappointment at what they experienced as non giving authority, and then both turned sad at missing home.

COMMENTARY

Here he is in position as a member of the group, identifying with a member who was relatively intact psychically.

Realizes His Suggestibility

In B 328 a member began on his suggestibility when he was examined by Dr. Peretti, saying yes to his questions, on sensing he wanted such an answer. This led to Jordan's statement on how suggestible he had formerly been to the radio. Dormer then revealed that he had been hallucinating the roar of the Navy firefighting school, up to 4 months ago, and it took some time to let go of it.

Then Thomas attacked a member for his evil propensities, in the context of mouthing as a man of God. Then, in a reversal, the member attacked cited that he could not help him, because he was incapable of tears. Jordan reported being troubled all weekend by my noting he needed to find out who he was, with the result that he thought I mean he was a cocksucker. I interpreted it to mean that Jordan, in his suggestibility, desired to make that person happy, in that perverse manner.

COMMENTARY

Dormer and Jordan are testifying to recovering from ego wounds, in which a formerly traumatic situation haunts them. I take it that, in his dialog with Thomas, McClain is identifying the role of mourning in recovery.

SUMMARY

At the end of this therapy Jordan was still vacillating between polar ego positions in his development as a citizen in the group. But it is evident he has come a long way towards yielding his delusions, and reconciling with aspects of a prosocial personality long abandoned prior to his breakdown in prison. He has been reconciling with his family of origin, showing genuine affect about missing them. He has been a central member of the entire therapeutic community at Howard Hall, as evidenced in the Integrated Group, but transacted principally in the black ward group.

As a self styled leader of the psychotic population, "Die Kang," he had challenged me from the first, and then became the group recorder, then chairman during much of its existence, now is partnered with sex psychopathic members of the group in struggles with and grieving the loss of autistic identities.

At the same time, he is moving to reconciling with me, from a position as my executioner, to a simply human one as my friend. He is envisioning graduating from the Hall, to a useful life, starting with reconciliation with his family of origin as the "good boy" they had known, prior to an alienative process early in adolescence.

Systematic individual therapy would have given us more data on his relationship with his mother, father, and siblings for insight into the genesis of his disorder. Cohen, Jones, Bostic, and even Jefferson are to give us more information in this crucial concern.

But this man has taken us through at times poignant inquiry into what was the matter, to his very soul. In doing so, he exemplifies a tie of fealty to the aspect of his ego ideal that keeps him sick. It may be a lead on the negative therapeutic reaction that results in reversion to illness after apparent near recovery.

LOREN JONES

Mr. Loren Jones was a long term District of Columbia patient in Howard Hall. He had been admitted five years previously because of the paranoid psychosis that was noted soon after he had murdered his brother-in-law. Like Vince Jordan, he was kept on the admitting ward because of the manpower called for by his extreme dangerousness. In our work we were able to form what I term messianic mutuality sufficient to open his affective life to transaction about his offense and the attendant marital dynamics. We were able to do preliminary work with his underlying delusions, but when the group was moved to another ward, he could not do so because of continuing dangerousness (intermittent need for manacles). However, he continued efforts to revisit the group, and appears in the record recurrently.

In B 1, in response to my query on how they were getting along, he and another assaultive member in wristlets, asked to have them removed. I suggested that we form a group to discuss it, and they readily did so. Both were then vehement on the injustice of it all. I role played the other member and his problem with ready violence, in the process reaching a mutually messianic stance with the group, Jones was only partially adherent.

It turned out that Jones's assaultiveness had to do with his delusions of ownership of the hospital and everything in it. We discovered that reality when the magazines and games the members had requested came from the Red Cross.

Crisis over Jones's Delusional Ownership of the Red Cross Material; My Inquiry Into its Origin: Death of his Mother When He Was Small

In B 11 the group found itself in a crisis over the custody of Red Cross material, Jones asserted his delusional hegemony over it, going on to his God-identity. I asked for the genesis of it, and he reported it was secondary to the death of his mother when he was very small, also abuse by beating when he was small. He then proclaimed that he was God.

COMMENTARY

I inferred that here he was reporting that he had undergone a psychic death, then a messianic resurrection as the Deity, a transformative experience with the death of his mother. Alongside the messianic it was also satanic in nature. I registered that as a genetic datum in the search for the "had to" compulsiveness of Rampa. I had no data on Rampa's early history.

Use of Intuitometer: Jones's Reason for Murder; Sad Affect Emerges

In B 13 Jones dictated enumeration of his wealth, Holden taking notes. On my query on the when he had become God, and ownership of his wealth, then on what was "eating him," he grew sad, eyes moist, detailing his offense of murder of his brother in law, which stemmed from a long conflict with him.

COMMENTARY

In asking Jones as to what was "eating him," I here initiated what I in time called my intuitometer, reaching for his affect. Again, the sad affect is a departure from the usual picture of schizophrenia. Since this man was generally affectless, displaying an impassive "above it all" demeanor, I would infer that we are making inroads, through a messianic mutuality. In that, he grew coherent and related the narrative of his offense. The members grew hopeful.

Jones's Self Sacrificing Care of His Brother in Law; Derogation of His Sexual Prowess; Alienation of His Wife, and The Need for Love

In B 14 I read a 3 ½ page MS, previously dictated by Jones to Holden, on the self sacrificing care of his brother-in-law, and his provocativeness, especially relating to derogation of Jones's sexual prowess, and alienation of his wife. In I 5, members arrived at agreement that underlying his delusions was a need for love.

COMMENTARY

The depressive affect is now consensualized in the group, an important development, indicating that Jones is in effect leading the members through his self change, into the reality of his forensic situation.

From God Identity to Preacher; Jones and the Song of Solomon "Love the Key Word There"

In B 18 Jones opened his Bible to the Song of Solomon, eventually agreeing with me that love was the key word there. A member cited that his God-ship kept him from that. Jones angrily turned on all with hate for their contradiction.

COMMENTARY

I would infer that Jones's god delusion is closer to operant preacher status than identity as deity. However, the ferocity of his adherence to his deity identity is an indication, similar to that of Jordan, of difficulty to come.

Intrusion into Holden's Self Centeredness: "As God, All Property Is Mine"

In B 19 he broke in on work with Holden and his self centeredness, asserting his right as God, later claiming all property.

COMMENTARY

It turns out that this intrusion into discussion of Holden's self centeredness, exemplifying such, is a step towards asking for help.

Jones Asks for Help: Asks About Homosexual Activity

In B 23 he asked for help, at the same time holding to his delusions. In B25 he asked Holden about homosexual activity on the unit, in the context of Holden's mention of "sodomy, pervert, and degenerate." In B26, concerning the new ward radio, I asked him why he needed it so hard, that had to be God to get it. Members concomitantly challenged and professed their friendship for Jones.

COMMENTARY

This passionate avowal also happened between the members and Jordan, and is of messianic import, reaching him in the arena of his own messianism, and resulting in the emergence of his human concerns.

With Sad Affect, Describes Wife's Alienation

In B 28 he cited his wife's sexual disaffiliation, expressing depressive affect, and joining member's supplying data on their losses. In 30, Jones assumed a peripheral role.

COMMENTARY

An issue here is whether his wife's alienation is not secondary to Jones's split from his sexual self to a religious identity.

In Conversation with His Loneliness, Tears Flow, as Murder Detailed

In B 32 I did role playing, in a role reversal with Jones, with Jordan speaking to Jones's desperate loneliness at root. He again related details of the murder, with tears. He reported hegemonic ideas since 12.

COMMENTARY

As he tells his story, Jones begins to mourn.

Jones Fights with Challenger, Expelled by Decree from Group

In B 34 Jones lost his position in the group, secondary to administrative fiat, after a fistic battle with a member who challenged his hegemonic claims.

The Group Moves to Another Ward, Howard Hall 3

COMMENTARY

Sensitive to issues of safety, Dr. Cruvant and the Chief Nurse moved the group from the Admitting Ward, to another. Jones later sought membership, to continue his dialog with the group.

Individual Interview: Loren Jones, the Doctor, and an Attendant   October 14, 1947

Five minute conversation with Loren Jones, who was brought over from Howard Hall 1, at his request: With an attendant present, I greeted Jones affably and talked over the group's effort to help him leave the hospital. At first, Jones stated that this was his home. I related to the attendant the story of a long time patient who considers the hospital as his home. I then mentioned Vince Jordan, and his difficulties with reality, citing the specifics. Jones appeared increasingly interested, and the attendant and I encouraged Jones to work in the group.

COMMENTARY

This is an instance of the involvement of an attendant in therapy.

Returns to the Group, Cites Loss of Horse, Alienation of Wife, General Resentment re Hegemonic Delusions

In B 221 he returned to the group, at his request. In the course of an account of the loss which lay behind his sense of autistic hegemony, with great feeling he cited his loss of his horse, along with the alienation of his wife. In B 222, as Jones related his residence in his present and past homes, a member surmised that he was "at the bottom of a well." Jones went on to state his resentment of his family, and people in Howard Hall for taking his property.

COMMENTARY

Jones is edging to discussion of relation of his family to the genesis of his delusions. The "bottom of a well" nadirhood designation is of great significance in the group process, bringing to its inquiry the capacity to discern life course and ego estimate issues. Jones has been capable of tears and empathic connection with the members, at the same time, deepest, hard core alienation.

Jordan suffers a similar configuration, in avowing his loyalty to his delusions "to the end."

Individual Interview: A Father's Concern for His Family

Discussion, after preliminary delusional material, of the patient's relations to his wife and children. He stated that he was attached to his wife but did not care to fool with her because she was a drunkard and there were "dangerous people" in their family. He expressed interest in the whereabouts and condition of his children. This interview lasted 15 minutes,

COMMENTARY

This is an instance of how individual therapy needed to be systematic to the program at Howard Hall. He is moving to analysis of his family dynamics and their relation to his breakdown. His interest in his children is a positive sign.

The Problem of Meting Out Justice: Jones Proposes Kangaroo Court

In B 231 he returned, to propose a Kangaroo Court as a means of dealing with problems in the Hall. Members objected, asking him how he would feel if he were the one beaten.

COMMENTARY

Jones has returned voluntarily, to ask for a regressive, authoritarian solution, calling still for autonomous assertion of separate identity, to the sort of untoward behavior that has separated him from the group. There was no mention of the hegemonic delusions that lay behind his assaultive action of the past. The members demurred, asking him to consider that he would be found at fault, punished. But he is still working on the problem of meting out justice.

Returns, To Enunciate Revenge Delusions of Mass Murder

In B 237 he asked for help on the part of the members, citing with great emotion that he had murdered his brother in law, in the role of sheriff, then was hounded as fugitive. He then became floridly delusional, citing an episode of planning to bomb Howard Hall from his 53 airplanes, and vowing life long revenge for his loss of hegemony over vast properties. Members attempted to reach through his delusional state, but the impasse continued. Jordan cited Jones's delusions as cause of the members' alienation.

COMMENTARY

Jones's capacity to enter into his family relevant emotions is increasing, but at a critical point he breaks with reality, into a florid psychotic state. The members are becoming more adept at attuning themselves in the process, comparing it with their own difficulties. Jordan's statement of his alienation resultant to Jones's delusions may be an indication of awareness of the role of delusion in the process of alienation from the other and reality.

Mother as The Real Problem: "My and Everyone's Enemy"

In B 241 Jones passionately related his hatred of his wife, going on to that his mother had been the real problem, "my and everyone's enemy."

COMMENTARY

Jones has progressed from a delusory position that could be characterized as hard core, enforced by a superior capacity at assaultiveness. He has come down from a lonely perch as God and possessor of all, to human status and connectedness with members of the group, sufficient for empathy with him as he relates his situation, including his delusions. They have taken second place in his productions, having to do with family dynamics.

There the picture he draws at the end, of his mother as the enemy, is opposite to that early in the work, in which he, on the edge of grief, cites her death when he was very young as causative of his troubles. Both Bostic and Cohen had delusions that their mothers were dead, and this may been the case with Jones. Again, systematic individual therapy would have been helpful. I would infer that his hegemonic delusion is somehow related to the delusion of death of his mother.

RON HOLDEN

Mr. Ron Holden was a relatively new patient in Howard Hall (hospitalized for several years) at the inception of this study. He was black, light skinned, in his early forties, sent there from the District Jail, having been convicted of a serious assault on a fellow rooming house boarder. He had been diagnosed as paranoid schizophrenic for his pronounced paranoid trends, and delusions of persecution. He was well-known in Howard Hall for sudden assault with minimal provocation.

Mr. Holden first came to my attention as a member of a subgroup that in the session distanced itself from me physically and verbally, attacking me bitterly, then at the end of the session coming up to me to act in an opposite manner, finding good things to say about the therapy.

Holden Seats Self Close to Doctor, During Heated Discussion about Manacles for Assaultive Behavior

In session B 12 Mr. Holden, from the first, sat significantly close to me, during an emotional session dealing with the policy and practice relative to manacles to control assaultive behavior, and the responsibility of the patient in this regard. There are no data in the record on a position he took aside from sitting close to me.

COMMENTARY

This affiliative gesture was displayed by Jordan and others.

Holden Emerges as First Member of Doctor's "Brain Trust"; Supportive of Therapy in Missive He Presents

He presented me with his first missive, an envelope with a letter, dated December 3. In a penciled scrawl, along with supportive advice, he asked for hygienic and other services for the colored patients.

COMMENTARY

It turned out that he became the first member of my Brain Trust, a subgroup that, placing them in harm's way, verbally supported the therapy, against its opponents, patient and staff. Jordan became the group recorder, but did not offer advice and counsel, as did Holden. Another early supporter was a white patient, William Cohen. Both Holden and Cohen used the pen as expression of their sentiments.

In Dyad with Jones, Assumes Position of Patient Advocate

In B 13, he read a 3 ½ page letter that had been dictated to him by Loren Jones.

COMMENTARY

In doing so, he formed a messianically relevant dyad with an even more paranoid member of the group, the "enforcer" of the aberrant mores of this maximum security situation. Jones was even more dangerous than Holden when crossed. The position of patient advocate enabled him to be relatively safely prosocial, at the same time.

In Dual Role, Reflects on Members' Problems

In B 15 Holden wrote on the blackboard concerning the group's task of self-understanding. Then, in concert with others, he associated to Jones's motivations in his delusions of Godhood.

COMMENTARY

Holden is assuming a dual role, one of caretaker and teacher, and the other of student and acolyte. In the latter action, he engaged in a cognitively relevant enactment in which he transacted about another's delusional function, indirectly his own.

Openly Critical of Jones's Delusions

In B 16, he read anew his previous statement on understanding as the aim of the group. Later, he volunteered "Relief Seekers" as a name for the group. He agreed with others on Jones's view of self as all powerful. Then he stated that a five year old would think Jones crazy for thinking he was God.

COMMENTARY

Again, in taking the truth-speaking role, via Jones's delusions, he was placing himself in physical danger. He may have been safeguarded by his previous messianic mutuality with Jones. More important therapeutically, this danger was also of internal nature, inasmuch as he, like Vince Jordan, he was leaving the security of his autistic, alienated world. This opened him to the massive anxiety experienced when he left that autistic reality and attachment to earlier ties. As with Vince Jordan, one could expect that his "devil within" would be mobilized against this danger to its hegemony, and Holden would revert to his former pathology. I had noted this drama at Ft. Knox, where this transitional period of the psychopaths was marked by deep anxiety, confusion, depression, and psychosomatic manifestations.

Holden Suffers Regression

In B 17, apparently anxious, Holden asked to be excused, after finding me chalk for the blackboard.

COMMENTARY

By the following session, Holden resolved his dilemma and emerged as a leader in a march of the members towards analysis by the group.

Asks the Members for Help with Himself; Holden: "Not That Way"

In B 19, he asked members what they thought of him, and on why he was restricted by the personnel. They resisted answering, and I asked if they were afraid. He stated that he was "not that way."

COMMENTARY

This was a seminal development, an open call for help.

An Attendant Joins in the Therapeutic Interaction; Jones Joins Temper with His Godhood State

In B 20 an attendant noted his reaction to Vince Jordan's calling Holden's attention to his violent behavior towards another patient. I asked Holden to describe his appearance when he was angry. He responded with, "flushed face." Then I asked where his temper came from. Before he could reply, Jones exemplified this issue, with a speech on his Godhood. Holden supported Jones's right to his opinion. Jones went on to claim all the property, followed by advice from Holden for him to "stay out of trouble."

COMMENTARY

The participation by an attendant in the doings of the group marked another advance of the group process, in which he departed from the code of the attendants in opposing the treatment, as "mollycoddling which ultimately endangered them." Prior to that I had brought up the internal and external fear the members had in departure from their code of alienation. I believe this opened the way for both the attendant and Holden to proceed with the analytic transaction. This took the form of character analysis, down to his body image when enraged. The dialectical process of the group resulted in the emergence of the delusion genetic to the temper, in the form of Jones's Godhead. At root, Jones was God when angry.

This datum is another element for the puzzle posed by Rampa on his compulsive alienation, relating it to an autistic identity.

Holden Advises Taking Group Member by the Hand, As Parents Failed To Do

Letter from Holden: Holden advised me and the group to take Street in hand, as his parents had failed to do.

COMMENTARY

Holden is now bringing one's family of origin into the equation, at the same time advancing the group as a latter-day family.

Holden on the Offensive, Decries Plot against Him, Promises to Act Friendly, Wishes for Release from Hospital

In B 24, Holden spoke on his wish for release from the hospital, going into a long account of his court experience, and a three year term, following his assault on a fellow boarding room occupant. He held that there was a plot against him. Members held that he was not ready, since he still suffered from the delusions that had rendered him assaultive. He agreed to act friendly, as per advice by H. Jordan, another readily violent patient.

Letter of January 17, Admits Attempts to Overcome His Prejudice through Labor on Behalf of Others, Christ like Ways

In a second letter, on January 17, he admitted his prejudice, which he was attempting to overcome through Christ like thinking and feeling, plus labor for others' welfare. He had cured others in the past.

COMMENTARY

In this missive, he both continues his character analysis, but even more importantly, reveals the messianic aspect of his Dr. Jekyll—Mr. Hyde character diathesis.

Group Works With Holden on His Story: Course in Prison, Homosexual Advances by Others; Group Euphoric at End

In B 25, Holden related his course in prison and subsequently, noting homosexual advances by others. Jordan sighed during the homosexual aspect, asking for explanation of terms like sodomy and degenerate. The members were euphoric at the end of the presentation.

COMMENTARY

Important here were the systematic aspect of Holden's presentation and the sense of gain on the part of the members.

Holden: Put Parental Limits on Jones; Further Analyzes His "Excitable" Character

In B 27, in a crisis with Jones, who claimed he owned the ward radio, Holden urged the members to "handle it like a parent, putting limits on him, and go no further." Beating did not help. He then admitted further to his own excitable nature.

COMMENTARY

Holden here played a central role in formulation of policy and practice with the power struggle about analysis of the pathology of the members of the group.

Holden Accepts Doctor's Formulation re Manic, Assertive Members; Advocates My Group Motif, "Figure It Out"

In B 28, he accepted my formulation that a manic and assaultive member was somehow trying to "figure himself out," coming out of it, and changing himself in the process.

COMMENTARY

The next step was characterization of this policy and practice as an obligation by the members, to "figure it out," in which the member has the lifelong task of figuring self out, leading to adaptive change.

Members Confront Holden's Disruptive and Alienative Character

In B 29 Holden acted in authoritarian manner, after claimed was sleepy, had to drowse.

COMMENTARY

Holden is exemplifying his superioristic character defect, on the way to its analysis.

Holden: "Members Throw Gasoline on the Fire"

In B 31, Holden worked his way back to a positive note, citing the readiness of his fellow patients to an inflammatory way of dealing with psychotic material.

COMMENTARY

Holden's characterization of "throwing gasoline on the fire" was striking, and had a positive effect.

Letter of February 10, 1947: Positive Account of Doctor's Role Playing and Role Reversal Approaches

This was the third letter of his series, featuring a highly positive account of my use of role playing, with role reversal, citing how I "amused the patients with unbelievable surprise." Enacted in role reversal were Loren Jones's delusions of Godhood and hegemony.

COMMENTARY

The positive transference attained here, plus the perspective gained through of role playing most likely facilitated the step he is to take next, that of subjecting himself to inquiry by the members.

Admits to His Mishandling of Self

In B 33 Holden advised the group on how his case had been mishandled by members, in accordance with violation of how much the members could take. He then admitted to contributing to the "mishandling" of his case by previous psychiatrists.

COMMENTARY

Having lessened his superioristic stance and position, Holden is available for therapeutic transaction with the members, in common reality.

Letter of February 11, 1947: Reports Opposition to Therapy by Personnel, Anticipates Its Defeat, Doctor's Martyrdom

This was a relatively brief missive, emphasizing the obtuseness of the attendants, the ignorance of the patients, and that the doctor will land in a position on the outside, despite his efforts for the patients.

Letter of February 12, 1947: Complains of Restraint from Privileges, re Room and Eggnog

Absent in this brief note is the reason, obvious to this very bright man, having to do with the contrariness that led to his restraints.

Holden's Analysis of His Self Righteousness; Similar to Rampa Stance of Fort Knox

Prior to B34, the members experienced a fistic encounter over Jones's delusion of possession, with an impending transfer of the group members, minus Jones, to another housing unit. Ron Holden resisted the transfer, on the basis that he belonged on the unit of most dangerous and alienated patients. In the course of the subsequent discussion, the group took up his self-righteousness and perception of others' malevolence, and their relation to his difficulties in prison and Howard Hall.

COMMENTARY

He is now analyzing his self righteousness, general paranoid positioning, and alienated tough guy identity, a stance I had encountered in Rampa, at Ft. Knox.

Letter of February 13, 1947: Offers to be Custodian of the Group's Property; Act of Courage; Preaches Collaborative Behavior

In a letter of February 13, he briefly offered to be custodian, followed by a lengthy exhortation on collaboration, begun with an allusion to character development, which "begins at home and develops abroad."

COMMENTARY

This offer was an act of great courage and conviction, given the potential for violence in the group.

Becomes Custodian of the Group's Property; Official Recognition

In B35 he was active as custodian of the group's property on Howard Hall 2, recognized officially.

COMMENTARY

Jordan has assumed the position of secretary, and this custodianship on Holden's part is even more important, given Jones's hegemonic delusions.

Letter, February 13, 1947: Lauds Doctor's Efforts, Repeats Philosophical-religious Terms.

This is written for the group, citing its names.

COMMENTARY

Significant is the action behind it, calling for consultation with the members, and their assent.

Holden: Hot Headed, "I Want What I Want When I Want It"

In B 36, he volunteered for the group's scrutiny, citing himself as "hot-headed, want what I want when I want it."

COMMENTARY

This revelation of his inner psychic state and motivational dynamics is of great moment in the group's development.

Letter, February 16, 1947: First Condemning His Unfair Treatment, Admits Nervous Condition

Characterized by lengthy paranoid construction, in this note he cited himself as having a nervous condition, "called a mental illness," which he claimed was brought on by confinement at Dr. Overholser's instance.

COMMENTARY

In the context of this paranoid exposition, he focuses on the "nervous condition" behind his quick temper, bringing it into view, for discussion and analysis.

"Alienated and Self Isolative": Further Analysis of His Deviant Character

In B 37 he resisted the interruption by the members of his positively oriented preachment-lecturing, then accepted the members' reflection of his previous self characterization. He then accepted Vince Jordan's interpretation and assertion of his own motivation and position as alienated and self-isolative. Holden was also characterized as domineering and "crazy," leading to self immolation.

COMMENTARY

Now the character analysis has reached his transcendently relevant position as preacher, an aspect of his "good side," his messianism, which has sustained his capacity to stay in reality. One can speculate that he is furthering his grounding in common reality, without his previous bulwarks of psychopathy and messianism.

Disjunction from Reality and "Eternal Pain": Holden, Jordan, and Bostic Work On It

In B 38 he worked with Bostic on his disjunction from reality, with association by Jordan to his "eternal pain" and loss of consideration by others.

COMMENTARY

Again, in transacting with others on their problems with reality and their depression and loss, he is furthering his own basis in reality and also that of his fellow patients.

Jordan States Holden Wanted Members to "Kiss His Ass," Holden Admits He Was "Acting The Fool, Always Had To Be Right."

In B 39, stemming from a recording of a therapy session at Knox, the group, especially Vince Jordan, came around to identifying that Holden wanted the members to "kiss his ass," as evidence of its consideration. Holden eventually accepted that he was "acting the fool." In B40 there was further playing of recorded Fort Knox sessions and critical discussion by members of Holden's omniscient ways, with his admission that he "had to be right." In B41, the group worked on Holden's continued hospitalization as consequent to his delusions and violence. In B48 Holden cited his pride in his technical ability in road building, though he was uneducated. Then he joined others in citing patients' use of religion as a shield of superiority.

In B 61, he advocated discipline of Street for his high-handed and superiority way. Took the initiative in stating that had been his problem.

COMMENTARY

Holden is engaging in systematic analysis of his ways and state of being, through his reactions to and view of others, but also on his own.

Fistic Confrontation With Alter Ego: Holden's Movement Towards Reconciliation and Regular Membership with Others

In B 64, he reviewed his recent episode of mutual baiting and assaultiveness with another patient who resembled him.

COMMENTARY

Along with Vince Jordan, he is moving towards reconciliation and "regular membership" with the others. His transaction with the members on their interpersonal positioning in reality has reached to point of an *ad hominem* confrontation: a patient may be considered as an alter ego. This would bring in train danger to the previous alienative basis in reality noted earlier, and consequent regression. Vince Jordan had particular difficulty with the fealty involved.

Quits Group, Assert His Rectitude, Fellow Patient "Asked for It"

In B 70 Holden dramatically quit the group, asserting an autistic rectitude regarding his assault on his fellow patient: "he asked for it." Jordan went further into assertion of his hallucinatory experience, and Bostic into his crime. In

B92 Holden returned, to attack me as provocative towards Lauton, in order to prevent him from going to court.

COMMENTARY

This marriage-like quitting of the group, then reconciling, is one of the features of the therapy. The group continued on its course, something Holden was well aware of.

Admits to Rebelliousness towards Parents

In B 141, in the course of discussing the rebelliousness of the group members, admitted to his own towards his parents.

COMMENTARY

Though partially a manifestation of his superiorism, Holden is edging into analysis of his domineering character.

Accepts Members' Feed Back

In B 149 members of the group countered Holden's stance that I was negative towards him and others. In 206 Holden's case was taken up, after Bostic griped about Dr. Overholser's slowness in replying to his letter. Members reflected that he was overanxious and told the doctors "things that made him appear crazy." Holden accepted this, smiling about his own "shenanigans." He then asserted that "each of us has a temper."

COMMENTARY

Holden is increasingly able to accept criticism re his "shenanigans." His previous do-or-die heroic stance for his psychopathic/psychotic integrity exists as a temper that "each of us has," a temper that can be brought under control. Holden is now in position to claim status as a regular patient at St. Elizabeths, worthy of containment outside of Howard Hall.

Holden Leads Group in Analysis of His Superiorism

In B 151, then 152, Holden intervened in a positive manner in an argument between Bostic and a bullying sex psychopath, then engaged in a full fledged inquiry on the part of the members into his own arrogance.

COMMENTARY

The bullying member in question had been the epitome of principled intolerance.

Graduates, Returns, Proselytizes; Group Established
As Therapeutic Instrument

In B 155 Holden informed the group that he was being transferred to West Lodge, and in the subsequent discussion admitted to his superioristic ways. In B 169 Holden visited from West Lodge, enthusiastic about his prospects, and highly supportive of the group therapy, citing that he was trying to get a group started there. He reported that his superiorism is now a work-in-progress.

COMMENTARY

This member played a key role in establishing the group as a therapeutic instrument, one which in turn actively confronted him on his narcissistic character. We do not have data on his organized delusions, nor data having to do with their genesis. An inherent messianism served as the avenue for adherence to the group idea sustaining him through the anxiety and depression that beset him when he abandoned a self-righteous and self-justifying stance.

DONALD STREET

This 20 year old black patient is included in this study of the individual in the group for the representation he affords us of the group's reach into extreme alienation, coupled with a capacity for intellectual clarity and moments of shared reality with the doctor and the patients. His diagnosis was hebephrenic schizophrenia, with psychopathic features. Patients suffering from this disorder are held to be the most difficult to reach. In the groups at both St. Elizabeths and at the Veterans Administration Hospital at Perry Point, Md., I found these individuals to be central figures in the therapy, mock elatedly and agitatedly pointing to the opposite of their evident affectlessness, the depressive states of the paranoid and catatonic members of the group. Donald Street served in that capacity in the groups at Howard Hall. When the members moved towards affect, he became agitated, serving as a group weathervane.

However, when Wilfred Bostic emerged from catatonia into reality, then into mourning over his murder of his girl friend, Donald Street altruistically insisted on staying with him, as a therapeutic agent the full four hours necessary to complete the process. In this account we shall trace Mr. Street's course from inception of his treatment until the end of the project, with particular attention to the development of therapeutic alliance, and transaction about underlying dynamic factors.

Donald Street had assaulted (with attempt to kill) his private psychiatrist, was found guilty, and sentenced to prison. His transfer to Howard Hall was necessitated by agitated hebephrenic behavior. This was characterized by assaultiveness and provocation of assaults by others, a steady monotone of mumbling and meaningless gesticulation. His capacity to care for his hygiene and transact verbally was not impaired, but he needed close watching because of his provocativeness with his peers, and his past assault on a psychiatrist. He was transferred to the therapy ward soon after passing through the admission ward, Howard Hall 1.

Street first appears in the record in an undated note by Holden, in which he recommends discipline as the necessary treatment. Holden complains of Street's presumed "desire of two conductor weeks." One can infer that Street's arrogant and superioristic ways were particularly galling to similarly constituted Holden.

Doctor Role-Plays Street's Arrogance; "I Need Electroshock"

In B 44, In the course of this session, I role played Street's provocative behavior, after which he volunteered that he had been staying away from the group, because of "weakness." After he alienated members though mocking them, uttering nonsense noises, I confronted him on what he was after. He smiled in a superior manner, stating that he needed "electroshock." This evoked reflection from members on Street's dramatic alienation from everybody. At the end of the session, he abstractedly came out with a low muttered monolog.

COMMENTARY

I was struck by an aspect of Street's verbal production, his statement of causality on why he had absented himself, "weakness" and his prescription of electroshock. This was a sophisticated individual whom I could talk with on the most cognizant levels, but for an evident massive alienation. I found his forthrightness in challenging others somewhat appealing. And as weathervane, he helped me with the group dynamics.

Admits That Headaches Related to Disturbed Feelings:
A Step Forward

In B 47, in the context of discussion of members' fights, Street cited a prospective fight with a patient who also made noise. The discussion then turned to his headaches, with Street admitting that they were related to feeling disturbed at others.

COMMENTARY

I took it to be a step forward, Street's admission of a relationship between his hypochondriacal headache and his disturbed interpersonal relations.

Asks For Help, Members Empathize

In B 49, 50 Street asked for help in attaining his objectives, ostensibly having to do with where and how he resided in the Hall, translated by the members to his difficulties with himself and others. Members reflected on his inner state as "feeling bad" and preoccupied with his past, berating himself and others. In the course of the discussion, Street displayed decreased hypochondriasis.

COMMENTARY

Street is establishing a pattern of relating in the group, in which, in rivalry with others (and accepting them as fellow patients), he asks for help, on a subject once removed from his problems with himself. The members are being drawn into reflecting their perception of his underlying emotional state, and alienation from himself.

Admits to Humiliating Self: Character Analysis
Similar to Holden's

In B 51 Street and the group laughed together at the anomaly of the group and Dr. Cruvant referring Street back and forth to one another for his help. The members asked him to address his problems, with Street in frank regression to his hebephrenic and hypochondriacal ways. Members interpreted this as "making fun of himself," leading to Street's explanation of "humiliating myself," following which he left, as Holden had done previously.

COMMENTARY

Having established a give and take in an initial witty man-to-man therapeutic alliance with the members of the group, looking down at anomaly itself as the scapegoat, Street placed himself in position to listen to the members in the act of receiving help. This resulted in frank hebephrenic and hypochondriacal manifestations, eventually to his admission that he had humiliated himself, a bit of character analysis, comparable to that recently undergone by Holden. Thereupon, he fled the group.

Assumes Understanding by Members of His Sensitivity to Noise, Asks for Help to Obtaining Quiet Room

In B 52 he pointed to his ears, assuming members would know what that was about, then asked for help with changing his room. Members felt he was "jiving."

COMMENTARY

At issue was his incapacity and obdurate resistance to exposition of his humiliated state.

"Helpless" In Confronting His Problems; Leaves Group Helpless

In B 55, interpreting the group's silence, Mr. Street cited that it meant the members wanted him to talk. He asked for help with obtaining a quiet room so he would not be upset, then would be symptom free. Members replied that his dissatisfaction was the problem, to which Street responded that the group was "irrelevant." He then denied he had previously cited humiliation as a problem. That led to a discussion of a clown's self humiliation, and Street's facility in having the group laugh at him. Members then cited that he did not take himself seriously. I role played the contrast in how he and Bostic asked for help. Bostic cited that Street was keeping himself from what he really wanted from the group. I noted and Street agreed that he felt helpless in the face of his problems.

COMMENTARY

Street's characterization of himself as helpless may be considered as another step forward.

Cited By Members as Errant and Domineering For Attack on Bostic; Accepts Their Judgment Graciously

In B 56, Street reflected to Bostic on his superioristic position, resulting in Bostic's regression towards anxiety and catatonia. In B 57, Street graciously accepted citation by members as errant and domineering.

COMMENTARY

This may be considered as another step in the analysis of Street's characteristic ways and interpersonal positioning, involving putting his great toe into the waters of the reality of membership in a group he formerly openly despised. The "graciousness" to my memory was tinged with mockery, and extended from an autistic aristocratic height.

Street Acts As Just another Member

In B 58 Street accepted membership in the group as, "Acting as just another member."

COMMENTARY

Again, Street appears to be "trying it on for size."

Group Objects to His Domineering

In B 59 members openly objected to his domineering manner.

COMMENTARY

Identification of his domineering is a step in analysis of his superiorism, a problem it has faced with Holden.

Members Work on His Domineering and Murder Attempt

In B 60 the members worked on Street's domineering and controlling ways, through to his worrying and then speculation on its relation to his murder attempt.

COMMENTARY

From this new intrapersonal and intrapsychic position, he is allowing himself and the group to essay into the past that haunts his present.

"Entitled" Street Brings Group to Impasse

In B 61 members again discussed the issue of disciplining Street for his constant harassment. Jordan commented on Street's sense of entitlement. The members found themselves in impasse with Street, and exhibited depressed affect.

COMMENTARY

Street appears to be retreating to his former defenses, while Jordan works on an underlying dynamic, entitlement, central to his own problems and a link to his personal past.

Members Work on Street and Jordan's Entitlement

In B 62 the members compared Street's and Jordan's entitlement.

COMMENTARY

During this transaction, Street and Jordan formed a temporary dyad in a separate reality, that served, as it turned out, as a way station mainly for Jordan to essay into reality, re his entitlement.

Jordan Sees Street as in Delusionary World

In B 66, after Street cited his frustration, Bostic alleged that it stemmed from problems with his manhood and immaturity, then going into his own world of make believe resulting in murder. Members urged Street to listen to the group, as Bostic was doing. Bostic went on to review his experience, internal and external, in the commission of his crime. Street interrupted him, to complain of headache. Jordan then cited that Street was in a delusionary world.

COMMENTARY

In the dialog, Street, as representative of the complex of vectors and levels of transaction in the group, is complaining that the members are not giving him what he is asking for. He is not asking for a Cadillac, as is Jordan, but to his mind, for simple relief from that which is distressing him, his sensitivity to noise and the headaches which plague him. Bostic ignores the surface manifestations and addresses himself directly to that which is preoccupying him and causing his massive confusion and catatonic state, a world of idealistic obsession which led to murder. Street is in proud, massive denial of that subjectivity. Street refers to his own subjective state, through reference to his headache, and Jordan attempts to bring him to awareness of his delusionary world.

Jordan and a Member Reach into Street's Sad, Lonely, Defective State: "He Wanted to Cry When He Laughed"

In B 67, Jordan, identifying with Street, interpreted that Street wanted to cry when he laughed. This led to Street's statement that he was sad and lonely. I led discussion of it as possibly related to lack of family support of his medical career, and the member cited his experience that Street, though brilliant in High School, was mediocre as a student.

COMMENTARY

Jordan empathically supports Street in transacting about his subjective state of depression and loss, which Street enters briefly, joined by a member, who brings into view his career as a student and whatever internal states and conflict that impeded him in attaining his goals at that point in his development.

Street Briefly Identifies Self as Depressed, Causing Headache

In B 76, Street claimed that depression caused his headaches, then rebuffed Bostic's attempt at mutual identification with him, turning full on the group with derogation.

COMMENTARY

After taking initiative in identification of his internal conflictual states, Street engaged in massive denial of a dependent and mutual relationship with Bostic, presaging a long negative therapeutic reaction.

Stalwart Street Grieves with Bostic as He Struggles through Traversal of Girlfriend's Murder

In B 78, Street insisted on staying through a four hour session, missing lunch, mutely helping Bostic traverse his memory of his murder, and crying with him during the depths of his loss of his lover and their life together.

COMMENTARY

A half century later, I am still impressed by the stalwart, I believe messianic, stance of Street in insisting on staying with me and Bostic, as Bostic struggled through traversal of his murder of his girl friend. Street's alliance with me and Bostic appeared as strong as his later denial of meaning to the group. This alliance surfaced again when he and Thomas seated themselves in the white patients group, in the service of integration of the races.

Street Implores Doctor to Delineate His Depression, Both in Mocking Fashion

In B 79, before the session, Street, in mock serious fashion, asked if I would discuss his depression, its effect on his head and behavior, then failed to follow through in the transaction.

COMMENTARY

In this initiative, it was as if he were clinically discussing someone else's pathology, all done in a mocking fashion.

"Pent Up Inside" Street Portrays State through Identification with Bostic

In B 80, Street jocularly asked the members for help with his painful neck. Jordan responded that Street could be of more help to him than he to Street. Bostic continued tracking through his murder, and when Walker reflected that Bostic was saying that his girlfriend had first killed him, Street replied that he felt, like Bostic, "pent up inside," but that the group was not the place to treat that.

COMMENTARY

Again, Street was able to refer to his inner state through identification with Bostic, but distanced himself from the group as a place to deal with it.

Admits to High Expectations, Murderous Anger towards Others, His Psychiatrist

In B 83 the group and Street discussed his murderous anger towards the attendants and other patients, subsequent to an incident yesterday. Street admitted that he had wanted to murder Dr. Williams when he did not live up to his expectations, later citing subordination as "ass licking."

COMMENTARY

Street here is coming closer to experiencing his internal affective state and intentionality, connecting it with his crime. The connection of murderous anger and high expectation is a step closer to my search for meaning on the part of Rampa and his suicide.

Street Holds Doctor in Violation of "Moral Law"

In B 84 Street held me in violation of "moral law," in not discussing his neck pain.

COMMENTARY

Street is making progress in experiencing me transferentially in a manner analogous to his victim, Dr. Williams. He is the high arbiter of moral law.

Step Towards Reality: Participation In the Instructional Program

In B 86 Street asked that he be allowed to participate as a student in the instructional program initiated at Howard Hall.

COMMENTARY

This is another forward step, in which Street accepts membership in the treatment program, as one among many.

Rival with Bostic for Leadership of the Group

In B 87 Street acted openly rivalrous with Bostic for leadership of the group.

COMMENTARY

Again, another forward step.

Street Opts for Role of Alienated Gadfly

In B 88 Street was subjected to a vote on his exclusion, after a snide remark on Bostic's girl friend. Street opts for role of gadfly

COMMENTARY

From here on out, with the exception of his heroic volunteering to integrate the ward groups, Street compulsively acted the role of the alienated gadfly, who quixotically was pro-therapy when the others were in resistance. He also would become agitated and gesticulating during emotionally charged moments in the group process.

Through Insight into Mourning of Bostic and Jordan, "So Low Down Like A Fool" Street Edges Into Same

In B 90 members commented on Street's martyrdom in being excluded from the group. In B93 Street left his mute state and insisted that the group talk about him, at the point where Bostic broke into tears indicative of mourning. In B104, readmitted, he argued about asking for classes previously. In B 109 during a discussion of Jordan's complaint of not receiving consideration, Street interpreted that he felt "so low down, like a fool, that he did not count for anything."

COMMENTARY

Street, like other hebephrenic members, is peculiarly sensitive to others' affects, and massively resistive to engaging in their own. Again, the clarity of language in his interpretation re Jordan is of moment. It is as if I were speaking, or a normal Donald Street.

Oppositionally Asks for Therapy, Individual and Group

In B 112, in the context of resistance by members—Bostic and Lauton—towards therapy, Street set himself against them, asked for more therapy, individual and group.

COMMENTARY

This stance is reminiscent of his earlier insistence in participation in Bostic's therapy.

Individual Interviews: Shows Greater Tie than in Group

October 7, 1947. Beginning with assertions of envy by others, he went on to his wish to be a medical missionary, as a means of "finding answers to lifelong problems." He went on to his anger at me, for not discussing his problems in living.

October 14, 1947. Donald Street was interviewed on a bench in the ward. He was complaining of his physical symptoms but then went into the question of leaving the hospital and the career he had planned, as a medical missionary, the disappointment he had suffered and his present fear of being disappointed. The patient then went into his stereotyped "disciplinary-patient question." This was skirted and I told of an incident three or four months ago, when Vince Jordan had stated that Donald Street could help him more than he helped Donald Street. I repeated positive statements about Street's ability that had been made by the other patients, and their bafflement on why he didn't use it. Street replied that people did not appreciate his intelligence. I stated I would like to continue the discussion at some further date. On his way to his ward, I asked him about the group. Street stated he could "give no psychiatric opinion." I stated that I was not asking for a psychiatric opinion, but an opinion as a human being. Street stated that "they were hopeless." I denied this. Street stated sarcastically that the doctor was "so good and strong." I asked Street how long he had been pulling peoples' leg that way, and Street answered, "Since so high," showing a child's height.

COMMENTARY

We were here discussing his hebephrenic ambivalence, taking simultaneously extreme positions. It is evident that a systematic course of individual treatment, coincident with therapeutic community would have been of great value with this patient. He appears to have a messianic mutuality with me, a necessary step to therapeutic alliance.

My policy and practice later in my career was to engage in systematic individual therapy, to tolerance, selecting representative members, but potentially with the entire group. This interview with Mr. Street shows their value, inasmuch as Mr. Street exhibited a tie with me here that was much greater than in the group, where he would show a tie by sitting next to me in an affectless manner. He is here confiding his wish to be a doctor and also to understand his problems in living. He had requested the interview.

During Discussion of Insanity by Group, Street is Cited by Bostic as Most Helpful Re His Problems: Intuitive Connectedness and the Intuitometer

In B 191 after a significant silence, members, especially Bostic brought up the nature of insanity—involving worthlessness and loss of motivation towards understanding by others. Bostic cited Street as most helpful to him, and that Street had cried during exposition of his problems.

COMMENTARY

Jordan had earlier cited that he could learn more from Street than vice versa, a straw in the wind re Street's helpful messianism. Street had stayed with Bostic during a four hour session, and here we have testimony to a deep underlying emotional link between the two. Looking backwards, it is apparent to me that the silence and anxiety earlier in the session indicated the intuitive connectedness I have associated with my intuitometer.

Street Stakes Out Claim in Academic Universe While Regressing Further Into Hebephrenic State

In B 258, in the context of discussion of freedom through growth, also alienation from others, Dormer asked Street what he was reading; with the reply that it was a letter from a university.

COMMENTARY

Street lives in another, academic universe, among others, while he regresses further in his hebephrenia, exemplifying the issues discussed in the group.

Street Defends Doctor against Attacks by Group in Its Rage against Authority

In B 285 he defended me against attacks by the group, in its rage against authority. After a lull, a sex psychopath revealed he had molested a young girl.

COMMENTARY

Street is here assuming a position dialectically opposite to that of the members, in his alienation from them, finding himself in my corner, similar to that he enters during our individual sessions. I would infer that the sex psychopath, in his alienation from the masculine position of the members in attacking me, is following the influence of a young female.

Baseball sans Intellectuality: Street Swings towards Simple Membership in Group

In B 291 he brought up his wish to be able to discuss baseball without intellectuality. A member was active in redirecting him towards his problem with reality and his feelings.

COMMENTARY

He is here swinging towards simple membership in the group, eschewing his intellectuality.

Street among Group Leaders Wanting To Make People Over: Homosexual Liason with Lauton in Integrated Group

In B 306 I mentioned Street as a leader, along with Dormer and Thomas, in the context of his wanting to make people over, and representation of aspects of the group. In I 180, in the Integrated Group, Street and Lauton, another hebephrenic patient, made unintelligible comments, in the context of the patient Hall becoming clearer in his expression. Street was cited by members as "conscienceless," like Vince Jordan.

COMMENTARY

This regression eventuated in a homosexual union with Lauton.

Street Mutters in Context of Member's Hearing Voice, Deeply Involved, Sensitive Weathervane

In B 318, in the context of Thomas and Jordan's hearing the voice of God, a member reported hearing the voice of his grandmother since he was 8, Street again muttered and gesticulated. This was interpreted by Thomas as an attempt by Street to "break" him. Thomas had previously assaulted Street for his muttering.

COMMENTARY

I infer that Street, as a sensitive weathervane, is attuned to Thomas's and Jordan's intrapsychic disturbances. Later, Street acts as I would have, asking Jordan what had happened to him, in an assault by Jones. He denied harmful intention with his muttering, claiming that he had been struck by Thomas "in a chance manner." He then amused the members with a demonstration of muttering while reading a newspaper, commenting on it in a schoolmaidish manner.

Street Brings Up Assault on Psychiatrist in Oblique Manner; Doctor Anticipates Street Will Relinquish Psychotic World

In B 319 Street excitedly showed me a picture of a basketball player who had overcome polio at the point where the group was discussing identification of self as God and having elitist possessions, like a Cadillac. He then volunteered that the psychiatrist he had assaulted had retired. In B 140, in the context of discussion as to when one was ready for discharge, I called attention to Street as a member of the group who was "quite sick." In 642, after this session, in which the group had coherently worked on a member's problems, Street, as a co-therapist, asserted it had been "a good session." I replied that he would some day face his "preoccupations and ambitions."

COMMENTARY

Realizing I had failed in helping this member work through to his inner and outer reality, I nevertheless anticipated that he would relinquish his psychotic world and live in reality. The only datum I have to back that up is his ready loquaciousness in the sparse individual sessions.

Street Attempts to Integrate Black and White Ward Groups

In W 216 Street and Thomas came through the open door of the Howard Hall 6 group, and seated themselves. When the members strongly expressed disapproval, Thomas retreated to the bathroom, but Street stoically sat through it, finally leaving when an attendant asked him to.

COMMENTARY

We do not have data on the internal and external factors that kept Street tied to his inner autistic life, but can infer that he was thoroughly invested in it. During the work at Fort Knox with psychopaths, we had seen dramatic evidence of mourning on the part of the rehabilitees of the loss of their superiorism and the safety it afforded them. They manifested depression and psychosomatic disturbances as they relinquished the psychopathic ideal.

So far, in this work, Jordan is giving us a clue on the nature of this internal tie. He tellingly is citing his relation to an inner godhead, experienced as a God-voice, which appears to preempt his capacity to live in reality, and his autonomous will. This aspect of his personality, experienced as an inner and outer voice, obsessively entitles him to an elitist possession, a Cadillac. We can suspect an autistic entitlement on Street's part, especially since he assumed co-therapeutic status with me in regard to Bostic's recovery. In the reality of the group process, though he yielded his superiorism for the humility of a student, he was unable to accomplish what Jordan did, in an excruciating internal struggle with this internal God-voice, relinquishment of his entitlement and its accompanying messianic status. Were he able to do so, he would have succeeded in working out a leadership role in the group, alongside Bostic, a group whose dynamic moved in the direction of reality. Unable to do so, he fell back into his hebephrenic status.

WILFRED BOSTIC

This 24 year old very dark black male, well muscled, medium height, came to Howard Hall in a severely catatonic state marked by absolute mutism punctuated by agitated episodes calling for restraint. On return from service in the Pacific during World War II, in a jealous fit over his girl friend's professed infidelity, he shot and murdered her. His catatonia began immediately subsequent to the deed. His family, especially his mother, maintained close ties during this period and took part in the treatment at one point.

Bostic, Mute Catatonic, Joins Group, Is Able to Express Himself in Writing

In B 38 Thomas introduced Bostic, a new patient in urgent need of help with his catatonic psychosis, characterized by muteness. I helped Bostic to focus and communicate via the written word on the blackboard, resulting in his writing, "I want." Jordan immediately stated that he had gone through a similar episode while in prison, followed by a low period in which he was suicidal. Members associated to it, one reporting that it involved a split from God, then a member exemplified this dilemma in a recent experience, with gradual reconciliation with self and others.

COMMENTARY

The associations of the members were ready and remarkable, Jordan re his crisis while in prison, attended by depression, and the other members, on a break with God.

Bostic Appears Interested, Speaks Responsibly

In B 39-42 Bostic sat through these sessions mute, but appeared interested. In 43 I asked Bostic what he thought of Nelson's feeling of persecution and he whispered, "I don't know, I don't know." This effort galvanized the members, and I led Bostic through making vocal sounds, to clear speech. On his own, he professed that he felt people, including members of the group, were against him. The members reassured him as to their good intentions.

COMMENTARY

In speaking, Bostic revealed a paranoid state.

Bostic Breaks into Discussion, Asks for Help, Evinces Trust in Group

In B 44 Bostic inserted himself into the group's attention to Nelson and Street, asking for help, accepting a rebuke by Nelson. Bostic later joined in discussion of Nelson, citing that he had learned that members were not against him. He then attempted to clarify a misconception, that he had been talking continuously. A member stated that he had been talking, but not understandably.

COMMENTARY

After breaking into the group's discussion of Nelson and Street, Bostic joins in discussion of Nelson, and then adds that he had learned that members were not against him, asserting a reality stance.

Bostic Fights Jordan for His Honor

In B 45 Bostic was restless, grimacing, rubbing his face, then addressed himself to the members who did not help themselves, citing that he did so. This representation was apparently spurred by a fight the previous day between Jordan and Bostic. Bostic showed distress on his reason for fighting, defense of his "honor." The group proceeded to discussion of Jordan's claim of superiority.

COMMENTARY

This fight presages the one Bostic reported having with his victim, over her derogation of his darker color, and a certain specialness of his that became evident in the family therapy, with his mother. He confronts Jordan again, in Black Therapy Group Session 109, when Jordan verbally derogated black people in a manner directly reminiscent of his victim's. That time he exclaimed that Jordan would have to kill him. This seminal encounter will be discussed further in the report of B 109.

Specialness Related by the Members to Not Caring about Self, Having to be Special

In B 48, in a heated discussion of superiority and conflict between the members, Bostic reacted intensely but nevertheless silently to the statements, and agreed with the conclusions of the members on the relation of that specialness to alienation from self and others. In B 52, in the context of the group's discussion of Street's superioristic and destructive behavior, Bostic asked why he had such difficulty expressing himself.

COMMENTARY

Street is the epitome of specialness in the group, and is the most alienated.

Launches Self into Recovery of His Memory

He then launched into recovering his memory for his crime and a consequent revulsion from himself, plus feeling of condemnation by others. In B 53, after a regressed schizophrenic patient cited, "Three ounces of sense, three ounces of sense," Bostic reported he had lost his good sense, and his wish to make sense in the group. Members then engaged with him in traversal of his army career, as an avenue to current reality. Thomas cited worry as a factor, and another member helped him with the military drill, as a means of grounding him in the memory of his military days.

COMMENTARY

The issue of the previous session, alienation from self, is now posed as secondary to commission of his crime.

What Is Wrong With Me? "I Am Sick," Had Aspired To "House on a Hill"

In B 54 Bostic queried the members on what was wrong with him, then, citing his perception of himself as sick, he launched into an associative reverie in which he aspired to a house on a hill, then saw a letter, cringed from an allegation that he had killed a girl, and saw himself on the way to a hospital.

COMMENTARY

At issue is the aspiration re a house on a hill, and the news contained in the letter, ostensibly having to do with the crime.

Regresses to Catatonia on Criticism by Street: The Power of Autistic Superiority

In B 56, in the course of discussion of Street's troubles, Bostic stated that Street had to have his way, in childish fashion. Street reflected back that Bostic was being superioristic. Bostic regressed to a catatonic state.

COMMENTARY

Street touched a chord here, causing anxiety and regression in Bostic from an autistic position of superiority.

"I Cause Trouble": Bostic's Inability to Articulate, Tears and Pain

In B 59 Bostic complained that a quarter was missing from his account, and was reluctant to bring up his other problems, because "I cause trouble." In B 65 Bostic was in tears because of his problems with self expression.

COMMENTARY

This "causing trouble" can be correlated with his mother's orientation to his being a good boy.

Emerging From World of "Make Believe"

In B 66 Bostic cited that Street's frustration stemmed from problems with manhood and immaturity. He then soberly admitted to his murder and emergence from "a world of make-believe." He cited that Street did not want help with that problem. He continued on his course of "waking up" in the group, traversing further his Army time, then to his ultimate fate, with danger of execution, which he would take like a man. Jordan averred his own preference for his delusional state, and the struggle they were engaging in, which at times took a physical form of assault.

COMMENTARY

In this session Bostic forged ahead, emerging from an autistic world. Jordan and Street were still immersed in theirs.

Further Progress from Make Believe World: Bostic and Jordan

In B 68 Bostic continued recapture of his memory. In that course, Jordan exchanged with him their experience with furloughs, and Jordan speculated that Bostic had shot her while on furlough

COMMENTARY

Jordan and Bostic are companions in a journey from their make believe worlds, to reality.

Induces Tears on Jordan's Part re Leaving Make Believe World: Messianic Mutuality

In B 71, as Jordan went into his initial struggle with hallucinatory voices, Bostic set himself forth as a role model in facing reality. In B72 Bostic interacted with Jordan on Jordan's make-believe world. Jordan felt Bostic was turning from him, inducing heartfelt testimony from Bostic, and tears on Jordan's part.

COMMENTARY

Their messianic mutuality played an important part in Bostic's recovery.

Bostic as "The Worst Person in the World"; Killing Mother Figure Following Killing Rejection by His Victim

In B 74 Bostic induced testimony from members, in which they contradicted his feeling that he was "the worst person in the world, as a murderer." In B 75 Bostic centered on his profound disappointment at rejection and derogation by his girl friend.

COMMENTARY

My hypothesis is that she denigrated him as the ego ideal figure he and his mother had developed. She had the same name as his mother, and he thought of her as a mother substitute. He later states that Nancy had killed him.

Family: "Forget It"

Family Therapy: This was marked by efforts on the family to have Bostic disassociate himself from the murder, by "forgetting it."

COMMENTARY

Adherence to the family's way of denial will prove to be a difficulty soon in the treatment, as he enters analysis of his tie with his love objects, his victim and mother.

Bostic: Fiancée Considered Him as "Non-human": Counsels Street to Get Problems off His Chest

In B 76 Bostic attempted to counsel and guide Street to "get it off your chest." Street rejected it. In B 77, lasting 2 hours, Bostic ambivalently went into his fiancée's aggressive derogation of him as "non human."

COMMENTARY

The non-human status is profoundly alienative, and Bostic is peculiarly sensitive to that consideration.

Catatonic in Resistance to Family's "Forget It"

Family Therapy, May 13, 1947

It appeared that these visitors were Bostic's mother, a granddaughter, and his brother. Bostic greeted them in a preoccupied manner, and his mother immediately began exhorting him "not to worry about anything." His brother presented him with a guitar which Bostic had asked for, apparently to test his brother's intentions. His brother threw three packs of cigarettes onto the guitar in a peculiar, aggressive manner.

May 15, 1947

Another episode which occurred on that day was a visit by Bostic's father and brother in which his father urged him to "forget about the whole thing." Apparently contact with his brother resulted in regression and the reappearance of some of his catatonic symptomatology, namely difficulty in phonation, increased preoccupation and profound muscular tension. I attempted to lessen the pressure they were exerting to have him repress, which appeared to paradoxically cause recrudescence of his illness.

COMMENTARY

I would infer that Bostic was sensitive to the aggression displayed in the previous family session, in the manner of throwing cigarettes onto the guitar. Also operative was the inner conflict over revelation versus self continence in accordance with the family myth.

Bostic Relives the Murder, Claims Was the Devil;
Crucial Alienation from Human Status,
As Was Rampa of Fort Knox

In B 78, lasting 4 hours, Bostic inquired into and related an account of the events leading to the murder and then the murder itself, ending with "I'm alive!" Street insisted on staying with him through the lunch period, while the others acceded to my request for them to leave for lunch. In B 79 Bostic again relived the murder. He cried out that he was alive, spared death, to preach.

In B 80 Bostic reported feeling evil, deserving electrocution. His girl friend was in heaven and he was not human. In B81 Bostic held himself responsible for all his actions. I repeated a statement by a member of the group that she had killed his soul first. In B82 Jordan claimed he was Jesus Christ, and Bostic responded that he, Bostic, was the devil.

COMMENTARY

The cry that he was alive was highly significant, leading to the inference that he had been dead before. He later brought up the thought prior to the murder that his mother was dead. His prospect of being a preacher is again significant of a messianic tendency, as is his feeling that he was the devil, as was alienation from human status. All of these spiritual considerations have to do with his soul's vicissitudes. I consider that these soul considerations are crucial, and can be applied to the issue of Rampa's alienation from self.

Brings Up Conviction Prior to the Murder, That His Mother Was Dead

In B 85 Bostic is assimilating loss of his moral self esteem. In B86, it became apparent that Bostic's relations with the group members is increasingly reality oriented. In B91 Bostic brought up a thought he had prior to the murder that his mother was dead. This agitated Lauton, who became violently antagonistic. Bostic responded with agitation and abject apology.

COMMENTARY

This delusion is of seminal importance. My theory centers about a tie by the infant to a mother who is depressed, tied often to a mother similarly constituted, in which the depression is experienced by the infant as death. This psychic death is surmounted by a spiritual resurrection; the infant incorporates this maternal object, and messianically becomes a special savior figure to the mother. This leaves him vulnerable, when the messianic identity is challenged.

Bostic in Tears, re Victim's Contempt for His Color

In B 93 Bostic broke into tears and open mourning, in the context of discussion of color and self respect, eventually revealing Katie's contempt of him for his dark coloration.

COMMENTARY

Other members of the group would be asserting, psychopathically and otherwise, their supremacy as blacks. In Bostic's instance, as mother's good boy, he needed his fiancée to adore him as his mother had.

Bostic Fighting for Leader Position and the Validity of Group Therapy Ideal; Edging on Discussion of Relation to his Mother

In B 99, when challenged by Lauton and another member regarding his pro-social leadership of the group, Bostic walked out, then returned. In B105, there was a power struggle between Bostic and a member, who joined in with Lauton, new hebephrenic patient. In B108 Bostic was reluctant to talk, in context of work with Murphy, another Miller Act patient, who cited his need for his mother.

COMMENTARY

The members are negotiating the validity of the group therapy ideal and ways, on the way to deeper analysis of their familial and intrapsychic ties.

Fist Fight with Jordan in Defense of his Dark Color

In B 109 there was a fistic fight between Bostic and Vince Jordan, over his derogation of darker blacks. The members had been reaching into their dis-advantagement, starting with straight talk about Lauton's verbal disability secondary to his hebephrenia, and then to Jordan's avowal of jealousy as his handicap, Street's low down not counting for anything, moving to Jordan's hatred of his blackness and that of others. Bostic regressed into the encounter with his victim that had edged towards murder-suicide, citing that, as with her, Jordan would "have to kill me."

COMMENTARY

This issue of darker blacks played an important role in his murder of Katie. Here Bostic is standing up for his honor. Katie likewise derogated darker blacks. Further reflection brings to view how I was in an analogous situation with Jordan at the inception of the work, aware of his lethality, and now wondering what I could discern of my motivation in so risking death, an outcome my colleagues would have criticized. What I have learned since is that it was my messianism that led me to that encounter, and what I have learned of its genesis in my relationship to my mother. I have touched on that issue in a study, *A Passionate Psychoanalyst*, Xlibris 2007.

So far, we have scant data on the relationship of the members to their mothers, except for that Jordan was extremely close to his in some undefined way, with massive entitlement resulting. Jones felt victimized by women, and considered his mother as an enemy. I have touched on that issue in a study, *A Passionate Psychoanalyst*, Xlibris 2007.

Bostic, Shirtless and Psychopathic, is Chair Again

In B 110 he appeared preoccupied and on the verge of catatonia, but still led the group, shirtless, a stance highly unusual for this conforming individual.

COMMENTARY

He is reacting profoundly against his previous stance, assuming a psychopathic mode.

Declares Readiness for Discharge, Denying Susceptibility

B 111 as chairman, Bostic led a discussion of his readiness for discharge, and I cited the unfinished business of his susceptibility to women and males who challenge him. In B 112 he continued denial of having any problems.

COMMENTARY

Having fought for his honor and asserted same, he is temporarily on top of the profound anxiety and regression that led to his catatonia.

Skirting Paranoia, Bostic Edges into Analysis of his Vulnerability to His Victim

In B 113 I cited Bostic's evident strong feelings, as related to the events of the murder. In B 114, In the course of his resistance, Bostic admitted that he had killed his girlfriend from his "subconscious," but still felt persecuted by the group. In B 116 Bostic described how he had fallen in love with Katie. She had the same name as his mother. He got terribly upset when she did him dirt. He asked why he had killed her. In B 120 Bostic was actively hostile and paranoid.

COMMENTARY

Bostic is engaged in analysis of the excruciatingly painful subject of loss in his love investment.

Family Interview with Mrs. Bostic and Mr. Bostic's Sister: The Stabilizing Force Family Therapy Could Have Been

October 7, 1947

Mrs. Bostic insisted adamantly that her son leave the hospital. I replied that we wanted her son to be ready to face the world and Courts, etc. We didn't want him to break down, etc. I advised her to tell her son to try to understand self and why he committed the crime. His sister spontaneously stated that her mother tells her son to "forget it all."

Mrs. Bostic agreed that she did that, and reorienting herself, told her daughter to "call off the lawyer deal." She asked how long it would take for Mr. Bostic to attain insight, and was told that it would take as long as she and her son take to cooperate.

COMMENTARY

Mrs. Bostic quickly relinquished her intransigent stance in the family dynamic brought into play by his sister, indicating that family therapy would have had a great stabilizing and analytic factors in this treatment, bringing to light underlying genetic data. In the interview I found her to induce a Don Juan side of my personality, ready to be charmed, a characteristic of her son, and a likely factor in his vulnerability to his victim.

Individual Interview: Through Anger at the Doctor Realizes Anger at Victim

Patient asked for the interview. He started angry at me for telling him he needed further treatment. He then asked if he had slipped, then moved to the subject of his anger. I stated he was now working on why he had killed his fiancée.

COMMENTARY

This is one of the great turning points of this man's treatment, and indicative of the value of individual therapy. I infer that he utilized me here as an oedipal figure, to free him from an alienating tie with his mother.

Bostic Works on Dependent Vulnerability to his Victim

In B 122 Bostic and the group members worked out perspective on his relationship with women, as "dependent on what she thought of you and you thought of her."

Individual Interview: Was It A Search For Mothering?
Doctor's Hypothesis Confirmed

Bostic asked me if he was looking for "mothering" from his girl friend.

COMMENTARY

I take this revelation as confirming my previous hypothesis.

Avowed His Faith in God

In B 129 he passionately avowed his faith in God, in the context of what the members placed their faith in, along with Lauton's citing that he had faith in culture and books.

COMMENTARY

He had announced his wish to preach, right after realizing the fact and enormity of his crime.

Notes on His Schizoid Ways: Withdrawal in Anticipation of Next Revelation

In B 135 he joined with members who were citing how a member withdraws to himself.

COMMENTARY

Bostic is withdrawing to himself, on the way to his next revelation.

Bostic Relinquishes Family's Dictum against Self Revelation, About Faces Re Writ of Habeas Corpus

In B 136 Bostic backed down from a Writ of Habeas Corpus he had submitted, edging towards treatment. He joined in discussion of his stubbornness. In B 147, after Bostic started unburdening, a member broke in re having been beaten by his mother and brother, but asserted that he would commit suicide if he killed a woman.

COMMENTARY

He is in a very vulnerable position at the moment. It was as if the member spoke for Bostic, in this instance, including his self alienation.

Bostic Projects Own Witholding onto Doctor

In B 148, Bostic was angry at me for withholding. In 201 he cited a negative view of the group of personnel and patients.

COMMENTARY

This negative phase can be considered to be transferential, related to the material which is emerging on his problems with the other side of his giving mother's nature, as differentiated from a paranoid one, which would be more generalized.

In Paternal Gesture, Doctor Encourage Bostic to Assume Chair

In B 156, in the context of a struggle of the members over who should be chairman, I found myself encouraging Bostic to do so.

COMMENTARY

I would infer that I sensed his wish to do so, and departed from my abstinence, reaching out in a paternal fashion

Bostic Turns to Cooperation; Discusses Sensitivity to Criticism by a Woman

In B 170 he accepted that he needed to know why he had killed, as insurance for the future. This was experienced as excruciating sensitivity to criticism. He and the members agreed that he was extraordinarily sensitive to criticism by a woman, as he is to criticism in the group, by his fellows.

COMMENTARY

As a member of the group he is no longer protected by his specialness, and is catatonically vulnerable. Jefferson in the White Therapy Group displays a comparable vulnerability, manifesting an ego defect of homosexuality, alongside his hypermasculinity. Acceptance of the sex psychopaths in the group is valuable in detection of that component to his alienation from self that is homosexual.

Asserts in Letter to Overholser That Is "All-right"

In B 173, as leader for the patients' betterment, and anticipating discharge, he read a letter to the authorities that he now was "all-right."

COMMENTARY

Arrogantly going over my head, he swings from denial to admission of his core difficulty. At the same time, he realizes he is in position to deal with it.

Members Detect Homosexuality Component to Bostic's Gender Ambiguity and Vulnerability to Women

In B 175 Bostic asked the members for help, accepting that he needed understanding of why he had killed. He entered character analysis for impetuousness; also, members broached homosexuality as a component of his vulnerability to Katie's denial and his current behavior.

COMMENTARY

The detection by the members of the homosexual component to his gender ambiguity is significant.

Feelings of Loss on Separation

In B 179 he identified with a minister patient re feelings of loss on separation from his woman, and his vulnerability to teasing by her relatives, his intense jealousy and possessiveness.

COMMENTARY

The feeling of loss is not resultant to victimhood, but to his mode of investment in intimacy.

Agrees That Original Member of the Group, Who Fought, Was "Not Tough but Crazy"

In B 181 an original member of the group, Jones, who had remained on Howard Hall 1 because of his dangerousness, and who had challenged me re my statement to his mother on his need for therapy for fighting, returned to the group, to make representation. He softened to agree with me, stating that he was "not tough, but crazy." Bostic stated that he had supported him in his challenge, but that he now agreed that it was not toughness, but insanity, supportive of his new self concept.

COMMENTARY

This is a seminal event in the therapeutic program, as well as indicative of a basic change in Bostic's self concept. First, the member's mother had intervened in favor of her son, conveyed my judgment that he needed therapy for his compulsive combativeness, and finally, that he had relented his obdurateness and admitted that his hitherto proud defiance was crazy. It would point to a Howard Hall wide dynamic on that score, relating ultimately to the stance of the attendants. Re Bostic's analysis, it relates to his honor fight with Jordan, in which, in honor, he stated that Jordan would have to kill him. It is also a datum in the quest for the motivational dynamics of Ramps, of the work at Fort Knox, his psychopathic sense of honor.

Bostic Notes Awareness of Smith's Alienation from Self, Where the Problems of Fish and Insects Take Precedence

In B 184 he drew Smith out on his alienation from his own voice, when Smith claimed he needed to solve the problems of fish and insects before his own.

COMMENTARY

I would infer that Bostic is intellectually discerning his own alienation from himself.

Identifies With Minister Patient, "Street Angel, Home Demon," Who Denies Aggressivity

In B 185 he claimed that his victim was too resentful and afraid of him, denying his own aggressivity, along with a minister patient.

COMMENTARY

I identified the minister patient as a "street angel, home demon." Certainly, the various aspects of Bostic's character are in play in the group's inquiry.

Bostic to Do It the Doctor's Way, Though Ambivalent Still

In B 188 he cited that was "to do it your way," then joined group members in criticism of me as intrusive.

COMMENTARY

His ambivalence is quite manifest, but he tends to identification with me. Doing it my way resembles doing it his family's way, a submissive aspect of his former identity.

Refers to Street's Tears, In Discussion of Low Estate and Insanity

In B 191 centering on Bostic's boredom, impatience, and extreme tension during silence in the group, Bostic joined the others in discussion of insanity, with worthlessness and loss of motivation towards understanding by others. He especially noted Street's tears during his marathon exposition of his problem.

COMMENTARY

It is significant and of great interest that Bostic's mourning was manifested by hebephrenic Street, who was least capable of doing his own. I would observe that he is moving into authenticity, at the moment.

"Must Have Blown Open with Jealousy":
His "Had To" Compulsiveness

In B 193 he volunteered that "must have blown open with jealousy," hinting at an evil state, subject to the woman's influence, where he was susceptible because he loved her "deeply," "worshiped her." Compulsively attempting to master it.

COMMENTARY

In this seminal session Bostic is in touch with issues of transcendence, leading to compulsive behavior. This transcendence is linked in this session with messianism on his and, probably, her part. He is aware of compulsive fixation on this aspect of their linkage.

Bostic Reports Dream Analysis with Dr. Karpman

In B 196 he, very positive re his work with this group, stated he was working productively with Dr. Karpman, at his own instance.

COMMENTARY

True to the tenets of individual psychoanalysis, Dr. Karpman did not share his work with me or the group.

Bostic Able To Take Deep Silences On The Part of the Group, Without Discomfort or Decompensation

In B 197 he was able to take silences on the part of the members, without discomfort or decompensation. The members went on to discussion of the hereafter, and I found myself referring to Jordan's problems in being master of his own fate.

COMMENTARY

Formerly, he had to intervene, because of discomfort. Again, we can only speculate on the effect of Bostic's psychoanalytic commitment to Dr. Karpman.

Bostic Advocates Self Change in the Group; Discharged As Recovered

In B 198 Bostic spoke strongly on the need for the members to change self, avoiding further discussion of his problems.

COMMENTARY

Acting the role of savior in the group I would hold was a way of avoiding further work on his problems. It may be that Dr. Karpman is engaging Bostic in a manner that is hegemonic, keeping him from sharing his material.

I recall the "mother hen" emotions I experienced at this point, feeling as with the others, that they needed more time to become stronger on their feet and pecking around.

Patient was discharged back to D.C. Jail for trial shortly after, as recovered. He was eager to face his charge of first degree murder, somewhat confident of mounting a defense of not guilty by reason of insanity. Street, Jordan and Thomas were in the lead of those who identified with him, in his recovery.

The psychosis appeared to stem from a humiliating rejection by his fiancée, itself of racial nature, related to his dark and her light color. An idealized image vision of her was so closely identified with his very existence that denigration and betrayal on her part was experienced as death by him, and also calling for her death. This configuration was hinted at by Jones, in regard to his mother and wife, and is to be encountered in Cohen and Jefferson. Bostic developed the delusion that his mother was dead early in his psychosis, before the murder.

LAUTON

This 24 year old black male, was one of the first of the Miller Act patients, admitted for homosexual molestation. He was soon noted to be manneristic, and to have an impediment in self expression of near hebephrenic sort, consisting of vague language, filibustering in the group, long diatribes about iniquity. He later mimicked my summaries at the end of sessions; doing brilliantly at times.

Lauton Emerges As Intellectually Pretentious, Rival to Bostic

In B 86 Lauton emerged as rivalrous to Bostic, as he in turn emerged into membership in the group.

COMMENTARY

Lauton here is a mentor and rival.

Unresolved Tie to a Dead Sister, Attempts To Reach Her via Prayer

In B 89, when the members complained of Lauton's vagueness, he related it to a tie to his dead sister, stating that he was attempting to reach her in prayer. At this, Jordan stated that Lauton was improved.

COMMENTARY

Midst the paucity of data on this man's dynamics, the data on a tie to a dead relative stands out. He also took as a fact Bostic's statement at one point that he thought that his mother was dead.

Senses That Bostic Was Provoked by his Victim's Derogation, Inner Conviction of Mother's Death

In B 91 Lauton reacted to Bostic's revelation of his vulnerability to his fiancée, stating that she had provoked Bostic, and that Bostic was affected by his mother's supposed death. Lauton assumed then the role of agitator of a riot, starting with a passionate speech against letting preoccupation with Katie monopolize the group. The group needed restructuring, and moved on to an impending riot. When Bostic became agitated, Lauton attacked him for bringing his girl friend up, for which Bostic apologized. Lauton became openly vituperative re the girlfriend and left the group.

COMMENTARY

My inference is that Lauton was massively defending himself against identifying himself with Bostic, in his vulnerability to his girlfriend, secondary to a developing tie to her. He had previously hinted at such, re his tie to his dead sister.

Along with other hebephrenic patients, Lauton senses the state of Bostic's very soul.

Lauton Filibusters, In an Erudite, Engaging Manner

In B 94 he kept the group from working on its problems, by standing up, as if a legislator, to read an epistle on the improvement of the group.

COMMENTARY

The seminal feature here was the conviviality, the sense he was reaching out. It is to be matched by profound alienation.

Wants to be Normal Boy on the Streets, Had Masturbatory Guilt

In B 97, after filibustering, in which I asked him what was "eating him," he revealed that he wanted to be "a normal boy on the street," and suffered guilt about masturbation. In B103, he complained of past iniquity, but agreed to a patient's feedback that was held here legally.

COMMENTARY

This switch to the dialectical opposite position is a manifestation of his hebephrenic character. He is revealing aspects of his inner life, in fragmentary manner.

Asks For More Organized, Structured Discussion; Resistance to Emergent Material Inferred

In B 98, along with Bostic, he asked for a more authoritarian and structured discussion format.

COMMENTARY

My inference is that both were resisting ordering and managing the material that was emerging.

Members Empathetic, Discuss Lauton's Compulsive Masturbation, Loneliness, Fixation on Mother's Decline

In B 103 the members left the topic of need for authority, to draw Lauton out on his compulsive masturbation, loneliness, and fixation on his mother's decline.

COMMENTARY

He is letting the group into his depressive state, his inner life and tie to his mother.

Elected Chair, Elicits the Concern of the Members for His Regressive Agitation, Pressured Speech

B 107 was elected chairman and central subject, for regressed behavior, mostly consisting of agitation, and excessive speech. In B120 he was discussed at length by the group for his disabled leadership.

COMMENTARY

This man appears to be settling into a therapeutic relationship.

Regresses Further Into Nudity, Hebephrenic Laughter, and Masturbation

In B 112, in paradoxical context of announcement by Bostic that was cured, and generalized group regression, Lauton disrobed, laughed hebephrenically, and openly masturbated.

COMMENTARY

Street has exhibited similar swings. My inference is that Bostic's resistance played a part in this regression. There was open discussion in the Hall on the danger of execution that Bostic envisioned, on discharge to the District Jail, and subsequent court action.

Gave a Masterful Summary

B 139: At the end of the session, Lauton gave a masterful summary of the proceedings.

COMMENTARY

This patient is revealing little about his interior life, but within his limitations he appears to have a good grasp of the group's reality, but is detached, except when he attempts to lead it, to little effect.

Verbal Combat of Believers and Non-Believers; Mobilized, Lauton Emerges Into Reality

In B 223, at the very end of the session, Lauton greeted me effusively, as a fellow member of the group.

COMMENTARY

This reconciliative gesture marks the end of a long, schizoid swing. I inferred that it was evoked by the open emotion of the members.

Joins Discussion of Evil, Stating Was Only Interested in His "Interior Decorating Fantasy Life"

In B 343 he commented, at end of discussion of good and evil, that was only interested in his "interior decorating fantasy life" and would continue such as long as he was hospitalized.

COMMENTARY

He is commenting on reality from the afar of his schizoid retreat.

Integrated Group: Sex Psychopaths Ask Re Treatment; Street and Lauton Make Love Via Masturbation, Mocking Laughter

In I 59 he acted the active agent in masturbatory activity with Street during the entire session. Both were laughing mockingly

COMMENTARY

It appeared that they were defiantly exemplifying the problem presented by the others.

Street and Lauton Make Unintelligible Comments Re "Big Shots"

In I 80, still paired, both made unintelligible comments during a heated discussion of big shots and resistance to authority.

COMMENTARY

Both are still in another reality.

SUMMARY

Inquiry into this man's course and problems gives us some idea of the chasm of pathology that Street was avoiding earlier by his mechanism of total denial.

This brief account of this man's course is an example of the need in a program of this sort for systematic individual therapy. Aside from its putative value to the patient, it would have mobilized him to articulate material useful to the others, relative to his tie to his dead sister, his thoughts re good and evil, and motives towards sexual perversity.

JEFFERSON

This 43 year old white male came 2 ½ years ago from Lorton Prison execution row when he developed a severe catatonia just prior to execution. He had murdered his wife of 17 years, in a rage, by seven blows of a hammer. The immediate and extended family was alienated, and Jefferson remained self justified as to her "asking for it." Since admission, the patient largely recovered his premorbid personality, but his mood instability and tendency to rages left transfer back to Lorton for execution in doubt. In time he worked himself into the role of "Mayor of Howard Hall."

Jefferson Assumes Position as Chair, Exerts Benign Feudal Authority through Devastating Tongue, Brawn

In W 1, the 1st Session of this group, Jefferson, as self appointed chair, mediated a dispute between Cohen and a rival, with the statement that they had "time on their hands."

COMMENTARY

This mediation was done as the Mayor, exercising a semi feudal authority, backed up by brawn and a devastating tongue.

Virulently against Women as Dominant, Feminizing Men: Enters Group's Analysis of His Rigidity

In W 6 he raged against patients who showed womanly traits, asserted he kept his wives in their place.

COMMENTARY

Jefferson is regressing from his Mayor role-taking and his chairman position, into his personal psychology, leading to character analysis. He violently denies dependence on women, through avowal of masculine dominance. This is based in Southern cultural patterns, at its highest, courtly, and basest, brutish rule of the fist. He murdered his second wife, with seven blows of a hammer. When he became vehement in the group, he brandished and banged his fist.

Under their professional role assumption, of benevolently keeping order the attendants held a similar masculine dominant position. Jefferson kept his fellows in order, collaborating. The trend now in therapeutic community will be for people like Cohen, with feminine, hysterical fits, to make representation in the group. Eventually, Jefferson arrived at his homosexual self.

Under Criticism, Quits Chair Position, Returns, Accepting Its Inherent Feedback, Character Analysis

In W 7, Jefferson, under criticism for masculinist, domineering ways, responded angrily, quit, then reassumed chairmanship.

The group has quickly developed the inner workings of the Howard Hall 3 group, with open discussion, a member stating his piece, another opposing, then an attempt at synthesis. In its course, he received "feedback" on his domineering ways. He responded with anger.

COMMENTARY

In leading the group, Jefferson accepts membership, and therefore what is called feedback, with its character analysis. The part of his personality that was capable of asking himself questions re his rulership and gender identity would become manifest to him and would be strengthened. Holden in the Black Group has gone down that path, gradually yielding his authoritarianism.

Jefferson Participates In Resolution of Group Conflict on Homosexuality as a Valid Problem

In W 9, after a deep and vigorous conflict on acceptance of homosexuality as one of a wide range of adaptations on the way to fuller sexuality, Jefferson collaborated in its resolution.

COMMENTARY

This acceptance carried profound implications for the group, and Jefferson, personally.

Jefferson Participates In Acceptance of a Golden Rule, Each Man to His Diverse Own

In W 10, James and Jefferson debated on greasy eggs and reality, arriving at consensus re a golden rule.

COMMENTARY

I would infer that here Jefferson is centered on an Enlightenment view of man's reality, perhaps stemming from colonial and revolutionary times. James was practiced in profound intellectual discourse, perhaps in justification for his crime of incest.

Abandons Chair Position; Members Off On Tacks of Own

In W 18 Jefferson abandoned the position of chair. In choice of a new chairman, the group got into discussion of James's incestuous problem.

COMMENTARY

The members are going off on tacks of their own, beyond Jefferson's controlling ways. Not only that, but they are essaying penetration of problems in increasing depth.

Befriends New Homosexual Member; Significant In Light of Previous Homophobia

In W 19 Jefferson took Reardon, a young homosexual patient, under his wing, defending him from attack by James for taking up his case with the group.

COMMENTARY

This is of great significance, in light of Jefferson's former homophobia.

Defends His Domineering and Amorality, Approves His Father's Chastising Him by Punching

In W 22 the members reflected on Jefferson's domineering stubbornness, as Jefferson engaged in vigorous defense of his amorality re his murder of his wife, "no justice or morality in relation to marriage." He was "the right ruler of his household." Cited approvingly of his father's punching him, hinting an autistic idea of manhood with him.

COMMENTARY

An inference might be that violent punching and murder by hammer blows are possibly related. We have encountered passionate profession of amorality (Karpman's anethnopathy, see Glossary) present also in Rampa, in the work at Fort Knox Rehabilitation Center during World War II.

Jefferson Notes His Father's Strength, yet Submissiveness with His Wife; Members Identify His Domineering and Submissiveness

In W 23 Jefferson admitted that he may have had his father's weakness in expressing his manhood in his own marriage.

COMMENTARY

Jefferson and the members are identifying his domineering as well as submissive character traits and their genesis in his family of origin.

Through Insight into Reardon's Passivity with His Father, Jefferson Edges Into His Impotence and Depression

In W 24 Jefferson identified with Reardon's incapacity for initiative on his own, especially in reference to a fight with his father over the family estate.

COMMENTARY

Jefferson is ostensibly the most potent man in the group, and is edging into awareness of his own impotence and inner depression.

Jefferson Loses Chair; Cohen Alleges Jefferson's Homosexuality; As Member of Group Moves into Inquiry into Jefferson's Crime

In W 27 Jefferson defied me and the group, lost the chair. He then boasted that he had made Certa chair, and protested had held to the "middle" ground.

In W 28, he pushed Cohen into leadership, in context of Cohen's positing homosexuality as Jefferson's problem. In W 29, in context of Cohen's authoritarianism, group discussed American justice, then the question on whether Jefferson should have been condemned to death for his crime. He related fantasy of escape into the Seminole swamp. Less dogmatic.

COMMENTARY

An allegation of Jefferson's homosexuality by Cohen would have earlier resulted in assault. Instead, Jefferson related an escape fantasy, to be enacted in the group in entrance into what was in effect, a swamp of homosexuality itself. He is acting as a member of the group, steadily less dogmatic.

Jefferson Demands that "Society Make the First Move" As He Edges into Awareness of Patient's Responsibility in Therapy

In W 31 he demanded that society make the first move, after Murphy, who had completely identified with me, quit acting as the group secretary, at the group's insistence.

COMMENTARY

Jefferson is here both resisting making the next move in therapy and edging into awareness that he is impelled to make the move in therapy.

Hints at Low Opinion of Women Is Related to his Murder

In W 33, at end of the session, on mood disturbances, and Cohen's sensitiveness to criticism, Jefferson came out with his low opinion of women and hinted at its relation to his murder.

COMMENTARY

Jefferson makes his move here, citing his contempt for women. He is entering systematic analysis of his murder.

Jefferson in Conflict: the Murder of His Wife, Her Worthlessness

In I 16, in the context of discussion of the influence of the moon on mood and crime, Jefferson discussed his conflict and murder of his wife, her worthlessness. In I 17, in the context of discussion of whether he or society needed to change, he accepted that he was bullheaded.

COMMENTARY

He appears to be pursuing a self directed, revelatory course, softening.

Discusses Whether Motive Was Present In Passion Murder Case

In W 34, he presented a published murder case in which the expert discussant denied passion as the motive for it. Jefferson then admitted he had been "that way" for a long time, cited a recurrent dream in which a man with bulging eyes grabbed him by the foot, kicking him in the stomach, citing identification with Daniel Boone.

COMMENTARY

Jefferson is allowing himself to engage in relatively free association, concerning his motivation, related to his life course. In that free association, he came across a dream with a confrontation with a passionate, rageful man, with phallic overtones, is of significance, as well as the identification with a mythic, heroic exceptional character. The recurrent nature of the dream is suggestive of something from the past he is attempting to master, something that is haunting him. At issue was the nature of the long time passion.

Jefferson Cites Cohen's "Wonderful Work with Patients": Their Mutual Messianism

In W 38 they engaged in convivial discussion of Cohen as both agitator and victim. Jefferson then cited Cohen's "wonderful work with patients."

COMMENTARY

This is a critical development, in which these leaders exhibit mutuality I would term mutual messianism. Protected by it, they do not react in paranoid fashion to criticism. They are developing the capacity to view themselves critically, and to conceive and perceive ambivalent ego positions. Cohen had been devoting to socializing mute and otherwise chronic patients.

Jefferson and Reardon Incite Self Derogation, Jefferson Able To "Take It"

In W 42 Reardon badgered members to do good, by helping him, while admitting to it. Jefferson, resistive, stated that all he cared about was making money. Jefferson was laughed at by the group.

COMMENTARY

Here, Reardon, representative of the sex psychopath contingent, slight of build but fearless, is taking on Jefferson, former head of the hard core psychotics. Jefferson "took" being laughed at, a positive step.

Individual Interview

Everything I said was for the good. I was not excited, it was only making progress. I didn't want anything to happen, but what was good. I think you made progress, could have made more. I think eventually the groups and things will turn out all right, providing Dr. Cruvant doesn't get under the influence of certain individual old attendants and routine. The patients find it hard to understand, but they will get better and better.

You can live in this place, there's no getting around it. Nobody knew what group was all about. I never resented the group. You only got out of it what you put into it. Nobody was putting into it, just lost interest at times. I never resented it. It would have got further, if there was more order. I was the first chairman, politician, by holding on to it. I didn't want the chair, but if I could do anything helpful to get the patients understand the doctor and the doctors understand the patients. There is a barrier between the patient and the doctor. The patient wants the doctor to understand him his way. That gap had got to be let down by the doctor, to show he's for him. Not against and not for, that patient is holding himself.

The majority of us are holding ourselves here. You want to get out of your way. An example is Paulson, who raise hell about medications. He knows he can get them, but not his way. He needs understanding with the doctor, and faith.

Being misunderstood upset me the most. They didn't want to understand me, my way. My intentions were good. You need to show me it in my way, that is my intention. Things were going better, and I did not want anything to happen. Got my screwing in the Court. I hit the calendar at the wrong time. About me being wrong mentally, they did not hesitate a bit. It just happened

I got in a bad current. I've made a lot of changes lately; I have more will power, and can put myself in a good current, avoid evil currents. I can handle every situation if I were free. Under some circumstances, like drinking, there is a question. There is a question of marriage, what would be his reaction to another current?

It is a question of acting in an unconscious way, and I would know how to meet it without getting into trouble. My letters home, my people can see a big difference in me, in the last 3-4 years. They make it appear it is my age, that I am more stable now.

Jefferson Becomes a Convert to Therapy, Admires Doctor, Spoke to His Prospect of Death by Execution, on Recovery

In W 45 he admired my directness, as the group worked on Forthright's story. Forthright had asked the group to go "whole hog" with him. In W49, after another patient spoke to the issue of a "spark of decency left," Jefferson reversed himself re his usual position of "not giving a damn." He went on to state that each little thing that happens to people affects him and that he does give a damn. He mentioned the death he faced on recovery.

COMMENTARY

Jefferson is moving into the converse of his former attitudes and orientation.

"Each Little Thing Affects Me; I Do Give a Damn"

In W 50 he feelingly admitted to exquisite sensitivity to others and a caring attitude: "Each little thing affects me; I do give a damn."

COMMENTARY

He is moving into position to identifying his susceptibility to his dead wife's attitude towards him.

A Psychopathic Member Successfully Needles Jefferson and the Doctor

In W 51, during a hot election battle, a psychopathic member successfully needled Jefferson and myself.

COMMENTARY

Being put down by a sex psychopath formerly would have resulted in cold cocking by Jefferson. Evidently his sensitivity is to people's needs, not derogation.

Jefferson: "The Problem Is With Us, the Individual"

In W 52 he held forth that the problem rests with the individual, and his self management.

COMMENTARY

He is here concerned with therapeutic self alteration.

Jefferson and Group Turn Philosemitic: An Approach to Spiritual Aspect of His Crime?

In W 54 he and the group had a long discussion on anti-Semitism, and Jefferson expressed great support for the Jews.

COMMENTARY

Turning to the people of the Book may be a sign of approach to the spiritual aspect of his crime.

"Beating the Bad out of People" and Society's Opinion of Murderers: Attempts to Reconcile Elements of Jefferson's Highly Contradictory Inner Life

In W 55 Jefferson led the group in discussion of society's opinion of murderers. A member hinted that Jefferson may be one. In W 56 Jefferson obliquely approached the difficulty of being one's own person, then to the issue of incest as the extreme of that. In W57, the group took up suicide and homicide, with Jefferson baiting Forthright at the end on whether he had the courage of his convictions. In W 61 I stated that the group seemed to be digging itself into in a rut, and then a member defended Jefferson as having the self respect which goes with striving for his Southern identity. Jefferson then cautioned Forthright as going too far in stating "kill all the Negroes." In W 66, he claimed he would not make the mistake of a choice of mate, like his mother, or of being with a woman again, except a prostitute. In W68, the members noted Jefferson's right to his castle as central to his violence. Tinsley interpreted that as giving Jefferson the right to kill his wife.

COMMENTARY

It seems to me that, in light of the fact that Jefferson was at least in part raised by a colored "mammy," and had evidently positive feelings towards her, it would be a central factor in his highly contradictory inner life. I sensed such an underlying influence in a childlike relationship with me, of transferential nature, when he was in a positive mood. He has been oscillating towards such as we have gone along.

In contrast was his redneck Southern character. He would hold forth on the Southern virtue of beating the bad out of people. In this session he displays a negative view of women, yet he has counseled his fellows on the healing quality of intercourse, re manhood, with black women. For a man who urges people to be up front and courageously state their reality, he has the members talk for him, unlike Bostic, in giving account to his murder.

Smith, Presidential Assassin: Jefferson Is Stubborn, Self Defeating, Related To King of His Castle and To Kill; Jefferson Accepts

In W 68 he yielded to Smith's and members' analysis of his character as stubborn and self defeating, his violence stemming from his right to his castle.

COMMENTARY

As important as Jefferson's yielding to the group was its attainment of comprehension of the relationship of character to crime.

In Convivial Interaction with Jefferson, James, Reveals More of His Inner Life, Hallucinations

In W 70 Jefferson portentously announced he had a statement about me, but was interrupted by James who revealed the had been having auditory hallucinations for 7 years, gradually gaining control over them.

COMMENTARY

Again, somebody else, under some pressure, speaks re an inner concern. My thought is that Jefferson was about to do so about himself, perhaps not about hallucinations.

Following Cohen's Lead, Jefferson Counsels with Chronic Black Patient, Jones

In I 31 Jefferson earnestly talked in the rear of the Integrated Group with Jones, a long term black patient.

COMMENTARY

This is the patient who is reporting the advent of rays from the Federal Buildings across the Anacostia River, in the photograph on the cover. Jefferson has come a long ways from a rigid reactionary position re race. My inference is that he is exercising his messianism and also touching base with early mothering by a colored mammy.

Jefferson "Feels" For Marital Love of Member; Asserts Positive Feeling for Occupational Therapist

In W 73 Jefferson with great feeling, noted that a member who had disavowed such, really needed his wife. A member cited that Jefferson was projecting. Jefferson later brought up the issue of trust, citing his trust for Miss Sawyer, the occupational therapist.

COMMENTARY

I would infer that Jefferson is here edging into the data on his relationship with his deceased wife, a deep trusting love, and paranoid distrust.

"The Heart of the Problem: I Could Have Avoided Killing Her, Lack of Trust

In W 81 citing his expertise in getting to the heart of fixing radios, he stated he could have avoided killing her, and lacked trust.

COMMENTARY

Jefferson is edging up dealing forthrightly with the murder.

Smith Savagely Attacks Jefferson for Belief in Therapy

In W 83 Jefferson is openly and savagely derided by Smith, re Jefferson's hopeful and pro-doctor stance. Jefferson parries the blows in good humor. Then Smith, along with James, voiced despair and hopelessness,

COMMENTARY

Not only that, but the implication is that Jefferson is traitor to his previously devoutly held values. Also f moment is the switch, of comparable significance of Smith from extreme and proud alienation, to admitting to his subjectivity.

Jefferson Attacks Doctor for Supporting Him

In W 87, I praised Jefferson's initiative in electronics, as example to other leaders of the group, especially Captain Bolster. Jefferson then became vituperative towards me and my group idea, particularly regarding its hope, with group attempting to reach him re his bullying.

COMMENTARY

Jefferson is switching back to his previous identity, while the members remain steady in analysis of his authoritarian character. My inference is that he is now seized by the fealty to his previous way of life that Smith accuses him of betraying.

Jefferson States That Cohen's Fear Drove Him towards Unreality

In W 88, he joined a member in denying Cohen had a problem with staying in reality, stating that he was driven by fear.

COMMENTARY

The issue here is how does that apply to Jefferson's inner life. Cohen now transcends the fear, which previously kept him manic and assaultive for days on end, through messianic identification with me. An aspect of that fear may be homosexual panic, another, deeper may be a struggle with conscience exemplified by Jordan in the black therapy group, and already traversed by Bostic, regarding his murder.

Members Bring Up Jefferson's Past That Haunts Him: Sodomized James

In W 89 James reported that Jefferson had sodomized him earlier. Jefferson did not reply to this assertion, and turned convivial when Smith asked what James and Jefferson were about in their mutual attacks. I stated that they were out to break down each others intransigent stubbornness.

COMMENTARY

What I had in mind there was Rampa's "had to," a thrall of imperativeness. He had to reach nadir for some ideal, and sodomy is conceivably such an enactment.

Jefferson's Attachment, Unmourned Loss of Dead Wife

In W 90, members asked Jefferson why he had not sought to marry another woman, venturing that he may be attached to his dead wife. I noted that it appeared that he had not mourned her loss. If so, he would have her in him, her wishes for him torturing him. He would therefore act against his self for not living up to her ideals for him. I went on to note that such a haunting presence would beset him in mourning her and impinge on his daily reality. He noted he got along with everybody but two in the Hall.

COMMENTARY

The members and I are directly confronting Jefferson with the central question of what is "eating him." I have pursued this issue of what was "eating" one from the first, in this work, stemming from leads I developed in the work at Fort Knox, with psychopaths. Though Jefferson confronts everybody else, here he avoided replying.

Jefferson Reveals Love for Black Mother

In W 91, with feeling, he revealed a "deep trust and attachment" to a "colored mammy who raised me."

COMMENTARY

This deeply sentient position is the converse and obverse of his previous character, and is a true breakthrough in his treatment, rendering him vulnerable to the rest of his personality and his fellows. I can still see his glowing face as he arrived at this memory.

Jefferson Swings Pro, Then Anti therapy, Then Back Again

In W 92, Jefferson stated he was pro-OT, in the context of attacks on therapy by new members. In W93, he vigorously attacked therapy, and in W95 was anti authority and anti negro. He stated Colton needed to be a negro to get help. In W 96 he edged towards helping others, and in W97 claimed that the hospital had saved his life, Dr. Cruvant was helping people out of the Hall.

COMMENTARY

In these four sessions, Jefferson swings back and forth, then back again, evidence of the weakness of an ego previously powerful, a situation shown earlier by Cohen.

Jefferson Claims That Trusted His Wife Too Much

In W 98, stated he was not dumb, as smart as anyone, but trusted too much, as had done with his wife.

COMMENTARY

This is an example of vulnerability through a tie based on his ego ideal, similar to that of Bostic. He is settling back to inquiry into his mental and emotional state, addressing his vulnerability to women.

Led by Jefferson, Members Cite their Vulnerability to Dominant Women

In W 100 a member spoke on his own vulnerability to a dominant wife, joined by Jefferson, then James, stating that their wives were entrapping, and they had been slavish towards them.

COMMENTARY

They experience the women as entrapping, and themselves as slaves.

Jefferson Advises Sex Psychopaths to Cure Selves by Intensive Intercourse with a Colored Woman

In W 105 he advised new sex patients to cure self by intensive intercourse with a colored woman. He went on to state he was not interested in anything beyond sex and food and women. In W 106 Jefferson defended James's visual aid of a woman's genitals. He stated that one needed to look at the female genital without fear or anger. Later, a member bluntly called Jefferson a "hammer murderer."

COMMENTARY

Jefferson here resembles Jordan in his swing back and forth towards and from aspects of his dilemmas. The empathic passion of the black therapy group is here replaced by jocular and then blunt confrontation. The bluntness of the last confrontation reflects Jefferson's.

Sex Psychopath Member: Jefferson's Father Playfully Humped, Pawed Him

In W 107 a sex psychopath member, capable of eliciting empathy from the members, from Jefferson's behavior, cited Jefferson's father as playfully pawing and humping him earlier in his life. Jefferson was non-committal, but agreed to speak further on it.

COMMENTARY

Jefferson is well known for such behavior, and we are here confronted with behavior similar to that of his father, direct evidence of what in psychoanalysis is termed an incorporated object.

Jefferson Joins Orgy of Characterization of the other's Perversity

In W 108, several sessions after James provocatively exhibited a graphic drawing of a woman's genitals, the members engaged in an orgy of characterization of the other as perversely destructive, with Jefferson holding and being characterized as agitating to a downfall.

COMMENTARY

Again, the members bring up Jefferson's offenses (in the name of truth) towards them, to haunt him.

Anti-Therapy Again; Called Child Molester, Foster Assaults Jefferson

In W 109 Jefferson, bitterly anti-therapy, lashed out at Foster as child molester, assaulted in turn in defense of a sense of integrity, versus his perversity.

COMMENTARY

Both Foster and Jefferson are dealing with their inner alienation and attain a sense of self in the process. Jefferson is here agitating Foster for perversity that is his own, in this case homosexuality of puerile sort. Jordan and Bostic had an analogous encounter.

Reconciles With James, Urges Group to Face Problems as Men, Members Confront His Assaults from Behind

In W 110 he reconciled with James. In W 133, after an absence from the record due to boycott of the group, in the context of a discussion of the need for faith, he returned with his dictum that the members face their problems like men, directly. In W 134, confronted by the doctor, he related his faith in the idea of manliness to the point of having his head shaved, then suffering catatonia. In a parallel transaction, he confronted Foster, conceding underlying good intentions and rectitude, followed by mutual reconciliation. Then he engaged in play with an attendant.

COMMENTARY

This rapid swing between character positions, authoritarian and obsequious, while derogating the alienation of the other from states of integrity, is illustrated here, but also marked by a new tendency to reconcile with members previously considered beneath contempt. I would infer that he is settling into acceptance of his homosexual identity.

Confronts Intellectually Acute Hollister re Homosexuality, As "Detective's Pimp"

In W 135, he identified Hollister's drive towards molestation of women as basically a pimping operation, based on that of an alienated, faultfinding man, a sexual detective.

COMMENTARY

This confrontation is from in front, rather than from behind, as he murdered his wife. One can infer that his bombast on facing stemmed from his problem in facing her directly. He wants Hollister to see through him,

Group Further Discusses Jefferson's Self Centeredness, He Gives Way to Sex Psychopath Morton

In W 138 members stayed with Jefferson re his self centeredness, and he gave way to Morton, as centerpiece.

COMMENTARY

Morton was a deeply regressed individual, whose alienation from self and sense of integrity was the object of concern.

Jefferson Asks re His Mental Telepathy, Feelings of Incipient Death, and Reconciliation with Family

In W 145, along with Hollister, Jefferson associated to his alienation from self and family, and reconciliation through parapsychological mechanisms, like telepathy. Members sensed his possession of an unconscious.

COMMENTARY

Through this transaction with Hollister, Jefferson is moving into position of awareness of his alienation from self and family, and of a consciousness beyond his awareness, or unconscious. Hollister cites his awareness of a malevolent transformation in the juvenile phase, prior to which he was a good boy.

Jefferson Leads Group, Sees Problems with Self Esteem as Core

In W 153 he and Hollister acted as leaders, with Jefferson challenging members to live down their pasts.

COMMENTARY

He has swung solidly in the direction of therapy, and assumes his dominance.

Jefferson Surfaces, Subject of Scrutiny as Subversive

In W 172, in context of group-wide character analysis, Jefferson was singled out for his tendency to escape to his room, and accuse others of malfeasance.

COMMENTARY

He has been absent for some time, attending the Integrated Group and devoting himself to radio mechanics.

Jefferson Leads Again, Regrets Killing, Had "Lost My Head"

In W 178 he assumed leadership again, suddenly announcing he regretted killing his wife, had lost his head, and punishment was not a real deterrent.

COMMENTARY

He is edging forward again in his self inquiry.

Tearful About Going Home to Family

In W 179, became tearful, along with the group, when Foster brought up going home to family.

COMMENTARY

Foster has long been an opponent, and it is significant that Jefferson is empathetic with him, and about the prospect of reconciliation with family.

Jefferson Further Remorseful; Reveals Opposition to Mother

In W 183 he further revealed his remorse, going on to cite that he condemned his mother right back.

COMMENTARY

I relate this datum on his earlier fight with his mother to Hollister's turn against being a good boy. Sullivan introduced the concept of malevolent transformation. Jefferson turned from that malevolent transformation to that of "good boy" when he reported his time with a colored mammy. I am hypothesizing that it somehow is related to a breakdown of relations with his biological mother.

Forthright: Jefferson Fears Leaving the Hall

In W 185, I noted Jefferson's kingship problem, then Murphy commented on Jefferson's mode of breaking up his marriage, and later the topic turned out to be his fear of leaving the Hall.

COMMENTARY

The fear in both would involve outgrowing the autistic character trait what had brought him here, and what was keeping him.

Jefferson: "She Bewitched Me; Now God Keeps Me from Killing Right and Left"

In W 189 he interjected the thesis that his wife had bewitched him, and he woke up to the realization that God kept him from mass murder.

COMMENTARY

This revelation comports with my thesis of an underlying messianic character disorder.

Jefferson and Foster: Agitating Each Other, Regressing

In W 192 Jefferson, Foster, and the members agreed on their readiness to agitation of self and other.

COMMENTARY

In the offing is regressive plumbing that which is ego alien, resulting in exteriorization.

Jefferson Walks Through, Fly Open

In W 196, after leading a protest about the food, he came back from his room, smirking and fly open. He boycotted W 199.

COMMENTARY

Jefferson's regression is towards revelation of a homosexual identity.

Jefferson Asks Re Prejudiced Mind, Disappointed In Ideals

In W 203 he joined in discussion of prejudice, asked what was wrong with the prejudiced mind, knew the answer.

COMMENTARY

Important here was the recognition of the phenomenon of mind, leading to the inference that he was studying his own.

Jefferson Submits to Thomas's Perverse Leadership of the White Therapy Group

In W 206 Thomas, from The Black Therapy Group, stating that he was "worse than anyone here, perverse with those who wished it," led the White Therapy Group into exhibiting itself. It was in turn led by Jefferson, who marched in, in shorts, penis exposed. Others discussed the issue of knowing wrong from right. The issue of emotional upheaval as causative arose.

COMMENTARY

Jefferson, edging toward exhibitionism, turned out to be the most perversely susceptible. This susceptibility would be the other side of his obdurate, bullying character.

Jefferson Would Rather Be Dead Than Impotent; Weakness for Intercourse Led To Murder

In W 211, in the context of Morton's compulsive predatory sexuality, Jefferson declared he would rather be dead than lack his sex drive, later joking about the expansion of the anus in sodomy.

COMMENTARY

In this free association, he is settling into awareness of the polymorphous perversity that exists alongside his righteousness.

Jefferson Attuned to Foster, As He Becomes Aware of His Course in Sickness and Alienation from Family

In W 212, Jefferson was attuned and supportive, as Foster grew aware of his course in sickness, especially regarding reconciliation with his family.

COMMENTARY

Jefferson is vastly different from the formerly domineering role he has played in the group, and tolerant of a state of sickness.

Reveals That Was Sympathetic to Colored People, Raised by Colored Mammy

In W 216, after the group rebuffed Street and Thomas's attempt to join the session, Jefferson cited that he was sympathetic to colored people, having been raised by a colored mammy. He wanted to bring them into a state of respect. He also held that close to death, as on death row, they "wanted others to run for them, and vice versa."

COMMENTARY

The inference I draw from the statement about the behavior of blacks facing death would have to do with a messianic or psychopathic outcome.

Individual Interview: "The Majority of Us Are Holding Ourselves Here"

Everything I said was for the good. I was not excited, it was only making progress. I didn't want anything to happen, but what was good. I think you made progress, could have made more. I think eventually the groups and things will turn out all right, providing Dr. Cruvant doesn't get under the influence of certain individual old attendants and routine. The patients find it hard to understand, but they will get better and better.

You can live in this place, there's no getting around it. Nobody knew what group was all about. I never resented the group. You only got out of it what you put into it. Nobody was putting into it, just lost interest at times. I never resented it. It would have got further, if there was more order. I was the first chairman, politician, by holding on to it. I didn't want the chair, but if I could do anything helpful to get the patients understand the doctor and the doctors understand the patients. There is a barrier between the patient and the doctor. The patient wants the doctor to understand him his way. That gap had got to be let down by the doctor, to show he's for him. Not against and not for, that patient is holding himself.

The majority of us are holding ourselves here. You want to get out of your way. An example is Passell, who raise hell about medications. He knows he can get them, but not his way. He needs understanding with the doctor, and faith.

Being misunderstood upset me the most. They didn't want to understand me, my way. My intentions were good. You need to show me it in my way, that is my intention. Things were going better, and I did not want anything to happen. Got my screwing in the Court. I hit the calendar at the wrong time. About me being wrong mentally, they did not hesitate a bit. It just happened I got in a bad current. I've made a lot of changes lately; I have more will power, and can put myself in a good current, avoid evil currents. I can handle every situation if I were free. Under some circumstances, like drinking, there is a question. There is a question of marriage, what would be his reaction to another current?

It is a question of acting in an unconscious way, and I would know how to meet it without getting into trouble. My letters home, my people can see a big difference in me, in the last 3-4 years. They make it appear it is my age, that I am more stable now.

The whole human race is one of a kind; colored people don't upset me. Certain individuals are not ready for society, are disagreeable, without a common denominator, and don't give. Before I was locked up, a man lived, died, did the best he could, in justifying his own self. You made $50 dollars a week, and drank it up. I didn't neglect my family, as far as drinking is concerned. I am like better that average by patients and attendants, regardless of the ups and downs. I get around to some understanding, sooner or later. I don't take time to figure it out, to get along as well as I do, a man would have to be oversane.

On the outside, one would get away, not continue. When people don't understand me, it makes me upset. That runs in the family. I don't show meaning on the surface. The doctor mistrusted me. I have a certain trust in myself, faith, and do so in other people. That may have to do with my case. You can dwell on something consciously, and impress on your subconscious mind, and they can come out in your life. I had a dream of going to the chair, three weeks before doing it. I woke up when they were cuffing me in. I had never seen the fucking thing. I had no intention of hurting her. It might have been just a coincidence. My brain was tied up with the killing.

It came to me like that, taking a bath one night, when she said this, that and the other, why was that. I had tried to think of what happened. I felt like a damned fool. I told them about seeing animals. Must have been crazy. I felt bad, of course, felt pretty damn rotten about it. She had done a lot of things that pleased me. The good, kind things she had said, the little things she had done extra, stand out in my mind, like the attendant Henson. She had the opportunity to misuse me. I appreciate it. It is the same with Dr. Cruvant. He could give me a hard way to go, as far as the law is concerned, and justified. He tries to show me. I never justified myself in anything I have done wrong. In a few minutes, I know I did wrong. I don't condemn myself. I still feel a lot of good in and for myself. I've blown up here, but not the go ahead will to the extent that I can detour if shown the other way.

COMMENTARY

Jefferson here is in a philosophical, somewhat messianic mood. It could easily turn into a violent, paranoid one. But he is reporting of real ego gains. Here he is learning to take time to "figure it out," my theme in therapy. He is reviewing his crime, his experience of misuse, intentions, and experience of breakdown. He is experiencing material from his "subconscious." He reports his psychotic state as one of seeing animals, likely of regression to a feral identity. And he denies self justification, also realizing he did wrong "in a few minutes."

One can infer that his Don Juan hyper sexuality and death are related; perhaps one enables him to transcend the other. One can also infer that his sexual life is deeply and directly hedonic, hetero and homosexual. Jefferson does a quick switch of sentiment and position here, on sexual identity. The issue of "rather be dead" was present in Rampa of the Fort Knox group. I later formulated the theory that both hetero and homosexual hyper sexuality were manifestation of a psychic resurrection from a psychic death.

Jefferson here through projection identifies his problem in alienation from himself. Close to death when one would become honest with self and authentic he has the colored man manipulating others, exteriorizing. He is still "all over the place" visiting again his affiliation with blacks, starting with a colored mammy, then derogating them for their self alienation and lack of integrity, something he is having basic difficulty attaining.

SUMMARY

Jefferson has come a long way in self realization. Together with William Cohen, this man had an altruistic conception of starting group therapy on "his" ward, after a year of rivalry with the black therapy ward. It seems to me that Cohen, the more liberal, initiated that partnership. Together they formed a therapeutic alliance with me. As on the black ward, the leader becomes the subject of discussion of the followers, and he is gradually helped off his arrogance and superiorism. He let go of a Southern prejudicial stance, noted along the way to identification with a stereotypic authoritarian father, and in time admitted to having a black surrogate mother.

He yielded to the influence of the sexual psychopaths newly on the ward, revealing a homosexual identity, alongside a Don Juan heterosexual one. He began approaching understanding of his developmental arrests and the dynamics of his family of origin. He hinted at a delusory life, as well as prescient parapsychological traits.

Through lecturing others on facing problems like a man, he appeared to be progressing to action on leaving the security of Howard Hall, mourning his losses, and facing return to his family and useful life as a citizen.

WILLIAM COHEN

William Cohen, 25, was in Howard Hall for a year prior to this work, transferred from Mason General Hospital after he became a chronic management problem due to assaultiveness and histrionic emotional storms, lasting days, marked by loud verbalization of mortal threat to the Director of Mason General (something he characterized as blowing his top). He suffered from the delusion that the superintendent, Dr. Simon, had killed his mother, and that he had conspired to have a fake mother visit him. Prior to inception of the therapy on his ward, he had visited the Black Therapy Group during one of its sessions, voicing his wish for joint therapy. Immediately prior to its inception he was confined to his room in a multi-day hypomanic episode, having to do with feelings that his fellows were plotting to kill him. In between such episodes, he was lucid and cooperative, becoming a leading figure on his ward, alongside Jefferson.

Cohen Engages Members about Their Alienation from Blacks

In session W 1 he stated that group therapy on the ward is a good idea, but believed that the white and black patients should meet together, each helping the other out. Then Cohen argued with a rival patient, who Cohen felt was picking on him, and asked the group for their opinion. They stated that the patient in question has been bitten by a snake and does not want to be bitten again! Cohen did not take exception to this interpretation, becoming affable after he reported his position. Jefferson noted that both had too little to do, and that they were playing up to keep occupied.

COMMENTARY

Cohen took a position early as leader in reconciliation with the black population, and getting together to solve problems. As with Holden, that called for listening to one's fellows, and surrendering one's autistic separateness.

Cohen Asks For Help with Hatred of the Head Doctor at Mason General Hospital

In W 3 Cohen presented as a problem his conviction that he was condemned to death, and that Dr. Simon of Mason General Hospital had killed his mother, and that the lady who visited him was a plant. This was done in heated fashion, and he listened as the members argued about the validity of his assertion. Then, after another member cited that Cohen needed to be "approved of right away." Cohen responded that he never asked for sympathy. No one cared for him, hated him, even though he was condemned to death. He went on to cite that Bishop hated his guts, Jefferson opined that he was just irritated by him, asserting that Cohen was after him to say how much he liked him. He cited an episode of upbraiding him for pestering him about the time. Members cited their dislike for Cohen's fetching ways, Cohen avoided replying. A member warmly observed that Cohen "was trying the other out, by pushing that the other hated him." Cohen admitted hat he had a few friends, that everybody was not against him. The group thanked me for the session.

COMMENTARY

When the group argued the case he was able to separate himself from advocacy, and attain a certain degree of perspective. He was then able to study that aspect of himself that "lost his cool" and plunged him into psychosis. The underlying delusion of being condemned to death was not dealt with here, but the issue of the alienation of the members was, with the assumption by Cohen as a valid member of the treatment process, where there was hope for him.

Individual Interview: Trying to Knock the Chip off His Shoulder

October 7, 1947

Emphatic that he was about to blow his top, and convinced he was to return to Mason General and be executed. He then stated his mother was an impostor, was actually dead. Reported that hallucinatory voices were counseling him against blowing his top. I asked that we go back to the inception of his trouble and he reported that it started with his intransigence in the mess hall at Greenhaven, where he was beaten while in solitary, and on the rock pile. I noted that they may have been trying to knock the chip off his shoulder. He agreed and cited his inability to remember how he got to Greenhaven and then asked for another appointment.

COMMENTARY

This patient was able to confide data which he resisted in the group, such as his hallucination. He also readily went along with me on the "chip on his shoulder."

Further Individual Counseling: Desertion, Court-Martial, and Positive Conception of Self

Cohen remembered that he had deserted and was court-martialed.

COMMENTARY

In these sessions this patient demonstrated an ability to work into a therapeutic alliance, constructively conceiving of self in his life course, accepting character analytic interpretations. His delusion of imminent execution is of great moment, related to some inner crime, undoubtedly related to his delusion of his mother's death.

"Magic Trust" in the Doctor; Assumes Leadership in the Group While Presenting His Delusion

In W 11 he was voted in as proxy chairman, stating that he had "magic trust" in me. Members began asking for help, and joined in helping one another by bringing in their own problems and observations. In 154 he complained of an imminent assassination, when Spires described his liking for guns.

COMMENTARY

I take the magic trust to be Cohen's literate way of describing his messianic transference, which also involved a state of mutuality with me. Through his leadership qualities he induced similar states in the group. Alongside is his delusional state, and the messianism provides a platform, intrapsychically and interpersonally, for its analysis.

Cohen Turns from Poison Pen to Constructive Journalism

In W 14 he was roundly condemned for his vicious letters, attacking members for their problems, as in the case of James for his incestuous offense. Jefferson came to his defense, for meaning well, in general. This was the impetus for Cohen to approach the occupational therapist for help in establishing a newspaper he called The Howard Hall Journal, the name exemplifying his initials, HJH.

COMMENTARY

The switch from alienated, vicious identity, to altruistic, rational, was dramatic.

Individual Interview: Expectation of Imminent Execution Presented As Delusion

Cohen asked for an individual interview, but refused discussion of his problems, convinced was to be killed. However, he appeared calmer, more in possession of self.

COMMENTARY

It appeared to me here that he was touching base with me, just to see if I was with him, individually.

Further Discussion of His Delusion and Alienating Ways

In W 17 he brought up his delusions of persecution and his breakdown at Greenhaven and Mason General Hospital. He became exasperated in the group process, about to break away, settled down, and the session ended amicably.

COMMENTARY

Cohen accepted sharing of discussion time with James, and checking of his malignant and rivalrous pen, also in a boyish fashion accepting Jefferson's supportive role.

In Early Integrated Group, Cohen's Violent Complaint: "Can't Stand People Looking for Sympathy"; Jefferson: "He Hates Me, to See How Much I Like Him"

In I 7, when Cohen blew up at a patient, members discussed his situation. Cohen explained that though he was condemned to death, he did not ever seek sympathy, could not stand that in others. He asserted that Jefferson hated his guts, and Jefferson replied that though he was irritated by him, he generally liked him. He had blown his top at Cohen when he unnecessarily asked him what time it was. Cohen then calmly accepted a member's emotional protest that he did not like him and did not care who knew it. Another, with warmth stated that Cohen was always trying people out whether they like him, by telling them they hate him, a persecution complex. At this point Cohen yielded, that he did have a few friends.

COMMENTARY

In this seminal session, members reached across the racial divide, accepting Cohen for his simple humanness, differentiating it from his paranoid delusion of persecution.

Group Discuss His Bossiness and Sensitivity to Criticism; Dementia Praecox Discussed

In I 12, at Cohen's initiative, the members discussed his authoritarian manner and sensitivity to criticism. Then, in obvious reference to Cohen's and Jefferson's tempestuous natures, the members brought up the unsettling effect of the moon on one's moods, then Jefferson's conflict with his wife, resulting in murder. This was followed by discussion of a member who brought up his own diagnosis of dementia praecox, then asking if that was what was ailing Cohen. The members considered that Cohen did resemble him, but appeared to be working his way out of it.

COMMENTARY

It is of interest that this seminal discussion occurred in the Integrated Group, most likely continued from the White Therapy Group because Cohen was chair of the large group. Linkage was made between their authoritarianism and crime. His history of loss in early adulthood of early great promise is suggestive of dementia praecox. This is a feature of the histories of Street and Lauton.

Cohen Yields Delusion of Imminent Doom

In I 13, in the context of a self guided discussion, Cohen brought up his delusion of imminent doom, with response by a members of it as the product of an overgrown boy, another as a subjective sense of injustice, and a third as a product of provocative behavior. Cohen participated relatively calmly, as the members related it to insanity and how they "ask for it."

Cohen, Chair of Integrated Group Is Humiliated, Recoups

In I 14, members derogated him as a Jew. He became combative temporarily, then recouped and continued leading the group.

COMMENTARY

He is growing in self possession, receptive to guidance from without.

Cohen Reads Letter Re Commitment to Help Self

In I 17 Cohen read a letter in which he committed himself to helping himself, describing his changes towards a prosocial attitude.

COMMENTARY

Following this he applied his talent at writing to starting the Howard Hall Journal.

Cohen Ascribes Homosexuality to a Younger Patient

In W 28 Cohen commented on Reardon's problem as possibly homosexual.

COMMENTARY

I would infer that he was edging towards acceptance of that problem in himself.

Mutual with Jefferson, Who Praises His "Wonderful Work with Patients"

In I 22, Jefferson warmly acknowledged Cohen's work with the regressed patients in the Integrated Group.

COMMENTARY

This is an important development, what I call a "union in the ego ideal" of men formerly bitter rivals, especially significant in stabilization of Cohen's self image.

Citing His Problems as a Contribution, Easy Going Chair Cohen Sits Down

In I 23 he started leading the group in a more easy-going, relaxed manner. He cited his problems as a contribution, then sat down.

COMMENTARY

This is further evidence of stabilization of this man's ego.

Individual Interview: Cohen Evinces Faith, Reaches Out to Doctor

He did not want to talk over problems, stated he was ready to blow his top, also that he was to be killed. Nevertheless, he appears to be less disturbed than before, exhibiting the aspect of his personality that had faith, reaching out to me. His interview lasted two minutes.

COMMENTARY

This patient is turning around, converted to therapy and starting to deal with his delusional state.

Cohen Touts Virtues of Participation of White and Black

In W 26 he cited the virtues of the Integrated Group, for its capacity to work on problems, and the participation of white and black.

COMMENTARY

Cohen is emerging as an overall leader, in conformity with his editorship of the Howard Hall Journal. This has implications for the strengthening of his ego, versus the previous paranoid tendencies.

Becomes Chair of White Therapy Group; Discusses Jefferson's Jealousy of His Wife

In W 28 Cohen became chair, wheedled members to the point of begging and browbeating, on what they wanted to say. Members brought up both his and Reardon's homosexual trends as problematic. Cohen brought up Jefferson's murder, this time asking if he was jealous of his wife. Members joined him in that question.

COMMENTARY

Cohen is moving into experiencing the low self esteem underlying his jealousy, and ascribed to Jefferson.

Jefferson Reciprocates, With Analysis of Cohen's Jealousy

In W 29 Cohen resumed his arbitrary manner, and was told off by members. Jefferson held that Cohen was here because of his character problems, among which was jealousy. Discussion moved to the merits of American justice, and whether Jefferson should be condemned to death for his crime.

COMMENTARY

Both Jefferson and Cohen here point to each other's jealousy and a hypothesized death resulting. On the agenda for future inquiry is Cohen's conviction of imminent death. We have encountered such a configuration in Bostic's case, where he experienced an internal death, on rejection by his love object.

Cohen Loses Chair over Domineering

In W 35 he lost the chair, second to his domineering, along with discussion of his paranoid fears.

COMMENTARY

He is regressing, unable to sustain the pace of progress he has been making in both groups and his newspaper. However, in time he will incorporate the sense of integrity manifested by the members who disassociate themselves from his tyranny, similar to that of Jefferson. Jefferson has given us a glimpse of a tyrannical father, with whom he identified. We do not have data on Cohen's father.

Cohen Seeks Chair Again, Asks Rival to "Spill the Beans"

In W 40, Cohen again vied for the chair, blurted out for his rival to spill the beans.

COMMENTARY

I would infer that he sensed data, the beans, emerging within himself. In Jefferson's instance, he did spill the beans on himself, when he praised his father for whipping him, when he, in his jealousy, intransigently challenged him.

Cohen Tells the Presidential Assassin to Speak for Himself

In W 64 Cohen challenged the presidential assassin to "speak for yourself" when he declared his independence of authority.

COMMENTARY

Ostensibly Smith was speaking for himself. My inference is that Cohen, who had plotted to assassinate Dr. Simon, the head of a Mason General Hospital, identified with Smith, and discerned that he was not speaking for himself in his defiance.

Seduction by a Middle Aged Woman: Screen for Cohen's Own Material

In W 85, in the context of the presidential assassin's call for data on what the members saw that could be called sick, Cohen related a story of seduction by a middle aged woman, with her husband nearby with a shotgun.

COMMENTARY

I infer that the story was a screen for his own material.

Asked for Individual Session re Identity of His Mother, Tearful in the Group re Reproaches for Denying His Mother

In W 86 he asked for an individual session, to work on his delusion re the identity of his mother, in which asserted that she had been murdered. He also noted his murderous hatred of the Commandant of an Army hospital. In W 87 he asked for help with his problems and a member asked him to ask for forgiveness of his mother for denying her. Another member, on being asked, stated Cohen should "commit suicide as the only way out, and to quit asking like a child." Jefferson shamed Cohen for denying his mother. The member who spoke of suicide described Cohen's denial, where Cohen, "though smart with us, is unable to help himself." Cohen, sobbing, asked for more time to straighten himself out.

COMMENTARY

This material centers about Cohen's deathly alienation from his (possibly seductive) mother, his childlike regression, and their relationship to his murderous rage towards a father figure. We are left with questions on a centrality in his family of origin, configuration we have encountered in Jordan, Jones, and Bostic.

Cohen Leaves Howard Hall

In W 88, on the occasion of another member's graduation, members spurred Cohen to talk about his fear of leaving the Hall. The presidential assassin stated it revolved about the fear of a tie in reality, reacted to in fear. Dr. Cruvant reported that Cohen exhibited severe, almost paralyzing fright during a recent visit to Cedar Ward.

COMMENTARY

It is of great interest that it was the presidential assassin who intuited Cohen's fear of reality. Cohen had most to fear from himself, a monumental temper and peremptoriness with men and vulnerability to women. Both Smith and Cohen had murderous designs on a head man. Had I been consulted, I would have recommended further analysis, as I did with Bostic.

SUMMARY

While we do not have the details of Cohen's inner life we were able to access in Bostic's or even Jefferson's cases, it is apparent that he underwent basic changes in the group. Much occurred in the Integrated Group. First, he plumped for the group process as liberating. Then he yielded his arrogant, superior position, becoming a "regular" member of the group. He became aware that his conviction of imminent execution was a delusion, as was that his mother was dead. He worked through a state of compulsive jealousy. He was on the verge of exploration of his central inner conflicts, when he was discharged. The newspaper he founded flourished, and helped ground him in reality and the esteem of his fellows and authority.

JAMES

This 46 year old white patient was resident in Howard Hall for five years, for paranoid schizophrenia. His family had called his incest with his 15 year old daughter to the attention of authorities, and remained completely alienated, as was his daughter. He openly held that, by introducing her to sexual life, he was protecting her from the depredations of other men. Found to be schizophrenic, paranoid, he was given a wide berth by both patients and personnel.

After Accusing Doctor of Intrusiveness, James Reverses Self, Asks for Help

In W 13 James led a generalized verbal attack on me as being intrusive. By the end of the session, he reversed self to ask for help, stating strongly that the group was the agency of understanding.

COMMENTARY

This ambivalence was characteristic of this man, expressed in logical, oddly unemotional terms. But when he expressed messianic hope, his manner became emotional and his eyes took on life.

Attacked By Cohen for His Incest with His Daughter

In W 14, Cohen read a letter, attacking James for his incest with his daughter.

COMMENTARY

James is moving from his schizoid apartness, and this attack by Cohen is bringing him into the mainstream of discussion.

James's Position: "It Is My Right to Treat My Family Any Way I Want"

In W 18, when another member brought up James's incest, he replied that it was his right to treat his family any way he wanted.

COMMENTARY

This brings the discussion closer to the hegemonic delusory position expressed by Jones, and enacted by Jefferson and Bostic.

Criticizes Sex Psychopath for "Lackeying" Lack of Integrity

In W 19 he was critical of Reardon for going into his case and his Don Juan behavior, which James.

COMMENTARY

An inference is that James possesses a sense of integrity, in contrast to the others. This fits in with his position, re his daughter, on the perfidy of men.

James's Sick and Well Selves, and His Passively Motivated Loom

In W 67 the members, discussing his unique loom, that had a shuttle cock propelled by gravity. It was constructed in occupational therapy, and demonstrated in the group. Smith, the presidential assassin and Jefferson were drawn into the discussion, which James seemed to enjoy.

COMMENTARY

In the relatively benign messianic context, James is accepting discussion of both positive and negative aspects of his character.

Reveals He Has Been Hallucinating

In W 70, in the context of acceptance by the members of self as faulted, he brought up that he had been hallucinating for years, stating he had discerned they knew no more than he did.

COMMENTARY

He is edging up on his motivations towards incest.

James: "Relationship with My Family Is Unchangeable"

In W 72, in the context of group discussion of life patterns, he cited that his relationship with his family was unchangeable.

COMMENTARY

I would infer that he is contemplating change of relations with his family.

James: The Doctors Are Trying to Drive Me Crazy

In W 73, in the context of discussion of family life, James inserted that the doctors were trying to drive him crazy.

COMMENTARY

I would infer that his changing sense of self, from altruistic possession of his family, a paranoid position, would lead him to decompensate, and feel he was going crazy.

James Cites Allegory of Jealousy of Unfaithful Wife, Failure as a Man, and Family Destitution

In W 79, after group wide denial, James asked why a man would emasculated himself, then went on to tell an allegory of a man who, a failure, was jealous of an unfaithful wife, lost his job with destitution of his family.

COMMENTARY

The story he is telling resembles his own.

Speculates On Suicide as a Voluntary Act

In W 82, in the context of discussion of irresistible action, James speculated on whether suicide was a voluntary act.

COMMENTARY

The inference would be that he contemplated suicide.

Smith and James Voice Despair and Hopelessness

In W 83 Smith and James voiced their despair and hopelessness.

COMMENTARY

It is of interest that he arrived at this position with the presidential assassin.

Dispassionately Discusses Parricide

In W 84 he presented a newspaper piece on parricide, in an understanding manner.

COMMENTARY

While still harboring his positions of paranoid and incestuous nature, here, mimicking me, he introduces a topic of seminal significance.

James: Evil Intent in Mental Illness; Member: James Helpless In Sick Course

In W 86 James answered Smith's query on mental illness, imputing an evil intent. Later in the session, Smith noted James's helplessness in his sick course, prior to hospitalization.

COMMENTARY

James is sharing data on his case with Smith and Jefferson, to tolerance.

James to Foster: "Your Sex Urges Are Not Under Control"

In W 89 James answered Foster on his query as to what were his, Foster's, faults, that his sex urges were not under control.

COMMENTARY

I would infer that James was in part imputing his own issues to Foster.

In Integrated Group, James Reveals His Wife "Won the Battle for Control"

In I 49 in the context of a report by the patients that the attendants were saying that the colored patients were taking over the Hall, James volunteered that his wife had won the battle for dominance in his family.

COMMENTARY

In this allegation of subversive dominance, he is revealing another item in his account of deviance.

White Therapy Group in Resistance, James Vigorously Defends Therapy

In W 92, members were openly anti-therapy, playing checkers instead of discussing problems. James asserted the value of therapy, and Jefferson allowed as how he was pro-occupational therapy. Smith asked for transfer to another unit, because he was made uncomfortable by the sessions.

COMMENTARY

Something is stirring, and the members are displaying more affect, James one of them.

James Remorseful About His Crime

In W 94, in the context of discussion of remorse, James stated he was remorseful, and wanted to be accepted by the members.

COMMENTARY

This is the first essay by James into analysis of his crime.

In Integrated Group James and Lopez Report on Alienation from Their Families

In I 51 James cited how hopeless he felt about getting on good terms with his family, planned to live by self, away from his family. He stated sadly that they did not want him anymore. This frank statement was in contrast with that of Lopez, who inserted a written statement, "no home, no family, no children," in one of his political treatises.

COMMENTARY

James's display of sad affect, hopelessness about loss of his family is in marked contrast with a previous position of hegemony, will run it any way he pleased.

James: For Encouraging Relationships, One Insane Man Renders All Helpless

In W 96, in the context of members' testimonies protherapy, James spoke positively re the need to encouraging relationships, and re Tex, how pressure on him hindered his self expression.

COMMENTARY

I would infer that he is here identifying with this severely regressed member.

James Reveals Wet Bed as a Child, Then That Was Incestuous With His Daughter

In I 52, a member exposed his rear to Miss Shannon, a visitor, followed by revelation by James that he had wet his bed as a child, and later that he had been incestuous with his daughter.

COMMENTARY

It appears that he is reaching into his developmental course, in grasping the significance of his incestuous deviance. Both of these revelations were relatively affectless.

Cites Obstinacy towards His Punitive Father, Then Displays that Anger towards Provocative Patient

In I 53, he responded to a film strip on father-son relationship with revelation that he had obstinately evoked punishment by his father, then turned around to chastise a provocative patient in the group.

COMMENTARY

His transcendent affectlessness is giving way to both revelation of his rebelliousness and punitive side.

Advocates Calm Nerved Approach to Discussion of Sex Problems "Coming To Us All"

In W 102, he advocated calm nerves in non-castigative discussion of sex problems coming to us all.

COMMENTARY

He is edging onto analysis of his offense, and the suggestive items are "calm nerves" and the universality of the problem. Through transcendent calm he avoids the turbulence within, and hides the intrapsychic dynamics apparent with Jordan, Cohen, Bostic, and others.

Sees Foster as Still a Wolf

In W 103, saw the wolf in Foster.

COMMENTARY

Again, I would infer he is imputing to Foster his own alienated feral identity.

James: My Father Ignored Me, Interested Only In Intercourse and Work

In W 105, after complaining about his father in the Integrated Group, James further complained that his father had ignored him, interested only in intercourse and work.

COMMENTARY

He is voluntarily reaching into what he considers as the life circumstance genetic to his crime.

Led By James, Members Engage in Kaleidoscopic Reflection on Their Careers in Sexual Deviance

In W 108, James displayed a graphic drawing of female genitalia, on the thesis that one needed to look sexual problems squarely.

COMMENTARY

This pornographic display resulted in a profound perverse pressing by members on each other, the opposite of analytic inquiry.

After Short Absence from Group, James Reconciles with Jefferson

In W 110, Jefferson and James reconciled, to catcalls by psychopathic members.

COMMENTARY

Jefferson and James had been thoroughly alienated from each other. My inference is that both had alienating fathers who specialized in the bad in their sons.

James Assumes Leadership in Debate on Hope; Jefferson Begins Regression

In W 112 Jefferson and James debated on hope, with James in the affirmative.

COMMENTARY

James is assuming a leadership role here, as Jefferson becomes a member of the group, ready to regress.

James, As Leader, Advocates "Natural Way of Speech" and "Common Sense"

In a controversy in W 114, on formalization of the group, with chairman, secretary, and rules of order, James effectively stood for continuation of the past way, in favor of a "natural way of speech."

In W 116, he emerged as a master of common sense, also holding that the members needed to, by their normal behavior, set an example, to "infect the attendants."

COMMENTARY

He is here displaying a capacity for wisdom, most likely stemming from messianism, that will stand him in good stead, as he faces the magnitude of his offense. He sees the patients as furthering an already inherent regressive orientation of the attendants.

Espouses Religion as a Unitary Experience

In W 119, he joined with a sex psychopath in espousing religion as helpful, citing it as a unitary experience.

COMMENTARY

I would infer here that the union of sex psychopaths and psychotics is of seminal significance, related to his internal dynamics, the coexistence of scrupulous conscience and sexual deviance.

Cites His Vulnerability to Homosexual Experience Early In Howard Hall

In I 57, in the context of a convivial discussion of black and white patients re spontaneity, James cited his seduction by a black patient, then related how had fought off a homosexual assault in the Army. When a member alleged he wanted a homosexual experience, James bristled and challenged the member.

COMMENTARY

His underlying deviance and alienation are coming into view.

Edging into Affect, James Becomes Bordering Assaultive as Members Address Plagiarism of Songs

In W 125 James asked for help, and the members went into his plagiarism, resulting in his feeling that the members went into it at his expense. He became borderline assaultive.

COMMENTARY

I would infer that the plagiarism, re authorship of songs, was in good part based on his hegemonic tendencies, similar to those of Loren Jones and Vince Jordan, earlier. In the borderline assaultiveness he is edging into affect, a break from his affectless reasonableness.

Hollister, Sex Offender, Reaches into James's Hegemonic Problem

In W 151 Hollister, the sex offender who had joined James in agreeing on the helpfulness of religion in their problems asked James what he was doing, that the police took him out of his house. James snapped that it was his personal business, and that Hollister should attend to his own improvement. Members cited that both were improving.

COMMENTARY

They are edging further into yielding the hegemonic arrogance we have encountered with the others, in which the individual has a transcendent mission that entitles them to purview over the other, and susceptibility to others. James would be susceptible to his daughter, as well as experience sexual purview over her.

Brings Up Difficulty in Changing, Abstinence from Pathological Specialness

In W 153, led by Jefferson, the members discussed their difficulty in changing. James asserted that he could not change peoples' minds about him. Jefferson with feeling asserted that James was better.

COMMENTARY

We do not know what Jefferson had in mind here, but the issue under discussion was whether Jefferson would be a murderer the rest of his life. At issue essentially was their insight into the autistic, transcendent position that led to the incest and murder. The feeling Jefferson displayed would be the human link whereby they could help each other, through despair, abstain from their pathological specialness, to rejoin a simply human status.

Holds That Society's Shortcomings Impede Facing Delusions

In W 178, Jefferson cited his regret over killing his wife, lost his head, and that one needed to face oneself without delusions, but that society's shortcomings was an impediment. James supported him concerning society's role.

COMMENTARY

The affective link with Jefferson is perhaps playing a part in moving closer to facing his delusions, and part in the incest. Intensive individual psychoanalytic treatment is a necessity here.

Identifies With Patient Struggling To Leave Past, Remorse over Murder, Acceptance in the Present

In I 77 a chronic patient dramatically exemplified the dilemma of the group in admission of guilt, fear of rejection, James sympathetically citing the world's lack of sympathy.

COMMENTARY

James is edging towards grasping the nettle, the deeply vulnerable state of a prideful, alienated individual, reconciling with past, present, and future.

Introduces Reconciliative Relationship with his Daughter by Letters

In W 187 James presented a letter from his daughter, in which she cited her love and acceptance. He eventually came to exposition of his possessiveness towards her, versus how the church had preempted his family from him. The members emphasized that his daughter's feelings came first. After protesting his "lawful right of possession" of his family, James agreed to the need to respect her feelings first, and stated hat he had answered "in a nice way."

COMMENTARY

Basic here was the preemptive nature of his concept of the role of a father and head of the family. At the inception of the group, he had declared that he could do anything he wanted with his family. This was a regressive, patriarchal at best, delusional in reality, position similar to that of Jefferson, Jordan, Jones and the others. The earnestness of the discussion here matches that with Vince Jordan in the other group. The members are painfully shedding their autistic beliefs in reconciling with their families. A family therapy group would be of seminal value here.

James: Trust In the Group and Take Your Medicine

In I 81 James joined with others advocating, in the face of disillusionment, trust in the group, and taking one's medicine.

COMMENTARY

James has been quiet of late, as the members struggle back and forth with regression.

Reports That Members Victimizing Others Homosexually; Street Agrees to Invitation by Victim

In I 83 as the members associated to the issue of victimization brought up by the film slide series, James noted that Certa did that with others, agreeing with me that there might be invitation by the victim. Street surprisingly also agreed.

COMMENTARY

My inference is that James is here edging into an underlying ego vulnerability. In a previous session, a member had pointed out James's passivity tendency as exemplified in his construction of a loom whose shuttlecock passively moved back and fro, responding to gravity as he lowered and raised its sides.

Members Confront James on His Plagiarism as Harmful to Self and Others

In I 85 members brought up James's claim of authorship of popular songs, asserting how he was harming himself and others in doing so. After resisting, he voiced doubt regarding himself and others.

COMMENTARY

Remarkable here was how the members devotedly "stayed" with him in this encounter, reaching him, with the appearance of doubt in a formerly perfectly sure individual.

James: The Hall Is Under "The Hypnosis of Hate"

In I 86, in the context of ongoing revelation of members of their problems with reality, James noted that people in the Hall were under a hypnosis of hate, and it came from ignorance, not accepting him as he was.

COMMENTARY

Like Vince Jordan, he is swinging between a dawning awareness of his intrapsychic and interpersonal reality, reached through doubt of his delusional state, and what he called he experienced as hypnosis. Bostic has given us data on the foggy in-between state.

SUMMARY

James has come a distance from initial empty passivity, through assertion of his right to hegemony over his family and incest, to inquiry into his vulnerability to his wife. At end of the work, he is moving into position to deal with what he called a hypnotic state and its accompanying delusions. He also is moving towards reconciliation with his family and his incestuous object, his daughter.

In this course, he moved from the position of an alienated and superioristic isolate, acceptance of an initial nadir, or bottom position as in the group, allying with others, eventually becoming chair, based on constructive aspects of his premorbid personality.

REARDON

This 24 year old somewhat immature appearing white male was admitted to Howard Hall under the Miller Act for homosexual solicitation. He also had a history of extensive experience with prostitutes. We have little data on his background, except that he grew up on a farm, and had fought with his father on the proceeds on its sale. He quickly became acclimated to the Hall, good naturedly joining in the program, discussion and occupational therapy. His even temperament, engaging manner, yet verbal pertinence played a part in the successful integration of the program for psychotic and psychopathic members.

Admitted to the Hall, Reardon Engages in Therapy in Integrated Group

In I 10 Reardon, a new patient, lost no time in asking for help in the Integrated Group, Cohen coming to his aid, helpfully.

COMMENTARY

This was a brief appearance in this group of 70, in which he came to the microphone, to state that he needed help, giving no further details.

Asks For Help from the White Therapy Group

In W 19 Reardon started the session, asking for help of the members. He characterized himself as compulsively aiming for sex with both men and women. James criticized him for "lackeying."

COMMENTARY

James appears to be focusing on Reardon's sense of sexual integrity. At the same time, Reardon will turn out to focus on the lack of a sense of integrity in the members.

Again Asks for Help from Integrated Group

In I 11 he again made a brief appearance, stating he appreciated the acceptance on the part of the members.

COMMENTARY

He is adapting to the messianic mutual helpfulness atmosphere of this large group.

Group Works on Reardon's Wandering

In W 20 Reardon revealed history of wandering, use of prostitutes in each town. A member attacked Reardon and myself, as though we were allied. I was focused on Reardon's bisexual Don Juan status.

COMMENTARY

It appears to me that the member who attacked Reardon did so to accuse him of betrayal of the prisoner's code of psychopathic integrity.

Reardon's Struggle with Father, Characterologic Problems Discussed

In W 24 the members noted his peculiar way of collaborating, arriving at his fight with his father, over the proceeds to the family farm. Cohen sensed that he was homosexual, and then Jefferson noted his difficulty in taking initiative on his own.

COMMENTARY

I would infer that Jefferson is beginning to be aware of the impotence underlying his potency in the group. Reardon's struggle with his father was emblematic for Jefferson and Cohen.

Reardon to Cohen and Jefferson: "Why Don't You Boys Quit Fighting and Help Me Out?"

In W 25, the most boyish of the patients, Reardon called on Jefferson and Cohen, the ostensible leaders, to quit fighting and help him out.

COMMENTARY

I would infer that he attained the superior position from which he criticized Jefferson and Cohen through messianism.

Reardon Is Chair of the Integrated Group

In I 13, sporting a black eye, which he would not discuss, he was elected Chair.

COMMENTARY

I would infer that he is becoming "one of the boys," standing up when verbally assaulted. He had just advised Jefferson and Cohen to quit fighting. He helped himself, in the manner of the Hall.

Members Work On Reardon's "Ill Chosen Dependency on Men"

In W 37 members battled, psychotic versus sex psychopath, over chairmanship, and settled on work on Reardon's homosexuality and dependence on men.

COMMENTARY

Reardon is working into accepting membership in the group, not setting himself critically against it. He now is a homosexual among homosexuals.

In Context of Film Series on Life Course, Reardon Relates His

In I 20, Reardon began relating his life story, in context of a film series on the subject, and in response to my challenge after he badgered me. I guided him to continue in the White Therapy Group.

COMMENTARY

Reardon is getting the idea, of figuring himself out.

Reardon Badgers Group to Help Him

In W 41 he badgered the group to help him, discussing his tendency to badger. It turned out that he had badgered his father. Jefferson resisted helping him, stating that all that mattered in life was money.

COMMENTARY

The badgering way of initiating inquiry into his problems is an initial representation.

Reardon Challenges Members Who Decry Facing Court

In W 42 Reardon again takes on the group, stating he was going to face the Court and fight for himself.

COMMENTARY

This stand for his sense of integrity is moving him closer to collaboration in therapy.

Reardon Criticizes Forthright for Discrepancy, Chastised By Group

In W 45, Reardon interrupted Forthright while he was relating his life story, criticizing him re an alleged discrepancy. The members chastised him, which he accepted.

COMMENTARY

This is an example of the badgering he had previously identified, and of his working out transference issues in the group.

A Psychotic Member Reacts to Reardon's Homosexual Advance

In W 47 Certa jocularly described Reardon's homosexual advance. Reardon admits to it, wishes to explore it further.

COMMENTARY

This would have formerly been a fighting matter. It is of some moment that Certa is doing the confronting, since he is similarly constituted to Reardon, polymorphous perverse and at the same time wishing to live in reality, respected by others.

Reardon Speaks Of the Alienation That Leads To Homosexuality

In W 49, in the context of Smith, the presidential assassin's report on his hopelessness, "nothing there," Reardon with feeling spoke of the alienation, "not caring about oneself anymore," that leads to homosexuality.

COMMENTARY

This example of Reardon's dependency on Smith tellingly focuses in on the issue of alienation from self and others.

Reardon has played a pivotal role in the collaboration of psychotic and sex psychopathic patients, at working on their problems. He vigorously from the first plunged into the program, though small of stature and boyish, standing up to the members verbally and eventually physically, in the manner he described in his history of a fight with his father.

He opened himself self to the members, taking the lead on analysis of his passive-aggressive personality. Starting with opening up by badgering me in a telling manner, Reardon acceded to analysis of his personality problems. The members followed with identifying his rivalry, of his need for ascendancy over the other. He impetuously demonstrated that trait with members. Certa, himself impetuous, pointed it out.

He was the first to make it back to Court, under the Miller Sex Psychopath Act, successfully.

FORSYTH

This 47 year old white male, edentulous, 6 feet 4 and muscular, played an important part in both the Integrated Group and in the White Ward Group. Whatever he did was at the same time dramatic and introspective, with a deep absence of identity between. He had been in Howard Hall for many years, and his diagnosis was hebephrenia. I have no forensic data on him. In his production, he spoke of a wife, but I have no data on a continuing tie. Jefferson in his mayoral capacity did speak of Forsyth's wife later in this account. It was clear that he was retained in Howard Hall because of dangerousness.

Forsyth: Doctors Are "Chronic Calendars"

The data start with session W 60 when he appears on the scene as a member selected by the personnel from a back ward who seemed to talk nonsense sense that the group might understand. He was clothed in overalls whose buttons had been systematically torn off to the point where personnel allowed him that habitus, and also allowed him to be barefoot. He wore an amused, wry smile that reached hilarity when he was making a point. Those points were almost poetic in cast, but very cogent, as in the first session, where he, on being asked by group members what he thought of the doctors, called them "chronic calendars." Patients were "flowers of despair." The group was "actualizing'" and when he shook hands with me, it was "raking it." He went on to cite that he did not give a damn for himself, and had no thoughts of his own, others were liars, and he had to be shrewd, stay ahead of them.

COMMENTARY

As this man spoke in a mock oratorical manner, his smiling face became depressed, and his tone depressed and angry. He did not reach the state of subjectivity and tears of another hebephrenic individual with whom he partnered, Lopez, or come out with biographical data like him, but appeared to edge towards that. His representations moved from amusing and entertaining for the members, to representing core intellectual and emotional data. He would lead the group in song and dance, and was quick to embrace me, in a manner befitting reconciliation of alienated family members. It was evident that he possessed considerable intellectual capacity concerning life course issues, could lead the group in discussion of them, but at the same time was deeply regressed towards habit dilapidation, with the stereotypical appearance one found on back wards, down to nudity and fixation on oral and excretory function.

In the course of his participation he found a place in the group, especially the large one, which had entertainment as a built in function, There he was clown and wise man, entertainer and audience.

Composes and Sings a Song of "We Are Trying Together"

In I 29, in the Integrated Group, encouraged by Cohen, he sang a song on "we are trying together" then asked that I speak on confidence and fear.

COMMENTARY

The members moved from regarding him as a fool, and he appeared to be gaining in confidence, speaking of his own despair, not giving a damn for himself, and not having thoughts of his own. He thought of others as liars, and his need to be shrewd, to stay ahead. Like Perez, he is sneaking in allusions to his life course and inner state and concerns.

Forsyth Begins to Speak of His Problems with Women

In I 45, during projection of the Flux series, in which life courses were correlated with the seasons, Forsyth associated to the hands of a woman there as that of the Madonna Savior, and the others as malevolent. He persevered in that behavior, interfering with the singing which followed. He appeared to be mocking reality, and protesting the hopelessness of taking up the material. He had to be removed by an attendant, and was borderline assaultive. In the course of this scene, a previously mute catatonic joined him in a duo of dancers.

COMMENTARY

Forsyth reacted to the images on the screen in a very vivid manner, as if he was back in school class, and teacher's favorite, plus the class bad boy. This is the beginning of his exposition of his ambivalent relationship with women. Also, he evidenced his leadership role in the group, in bringing out collaboration by a previously mute catatonic patient.

Forsyth Identifies a Woman as Causative of his Breakdown

In I 50 I asked him what had brought him to the hospital, and he replied with a question, "A woman?" In I 61, his back to the group, he sang with the chorus.

COMMENTARY

He is edging towards discussion of his inner life.

Forsyth Cites Perverse Relationship with his Mother, Sister, and Father; Lopez: We Are "Simply Human"

In I 62, during a pregnant pause, Forsyth raised his hand, stating he wanted to take up a problem. In a hypomanic, word salad fashion, he launched into what had bested him, giving details about his mother. He called her vile names and talked about his offers to her of sexual intercourse, and her refusal. He then called himself a series of equally noxious names, including "sister raping." This was interspersed with songs which he had composed, and were rife with neologisms.

The members responded with calls for him to sing, statements that he was crazy, and serious contemplative listening by members such as Donald Street. I got up and stated that he wanted the members to tell him how the group felt since he had mentioned the group many times in his talk. Mr. Forsyth agreed, and I outlined what the reactions had been, namely asking for songs and that he was crazy. A member walked up to make a remark, and Forsyth continued his self derogation. I interrupted him, and pointed this out, and he agreed. I asked for somebody to say how Forsyth felt. Lopez raised his hand, came up, began gesticulating and shouting, in his usual harangue. I noted that there were two members who had difficulty expressing themselves and perhaps they could help one another.

Certa asked Forsyth to read Lopez's prepared statement. Lopez agreed to my query on that. Forsyth read it, slightly mocking Lopez, with about one third of the group in hilarious laughter by the end of the reading, including Lopez. Forsyth went on to other material of Lopez'. Lopez began his harangue again, saying that all of the people in the group, including he and Forsyth, were ordinary working people in trouble and noted the importance of 1922 and 1942. He then stated he was through, and sat down.

Forsyth continued with gibberish talk, aping Lopez, and then went into material about his father and about homosexual experiences with him. The members became restless, and one of the band members asked if he could continue playing. He tried to get the microphone from Forsyth, who stated he wanted to keep it. I came up to ask for a vote on who was to continue: ten for music and two for Forsyth. Forsyth would not accept the vote. An attendant came up and was beginning to lead him away, when members asked that he stay.

Forsyth sat down, and became attentive to the music. Later he got up and danced and clapped and sang with the music, in imitation of the behavior of the black patients, along the way doing a strip tease, while balancing a chair on his nose.

COMMENTARY

I have included the details of this session for their pertinence in depicting how this man began to leave the thrall of his hebephrenia for the group's reality. He begins by volunteering presentation of his problems for discussion, depicting his mother as incestuous and perverse, with a corollary state in himself, which extended to sexual molestation of a woman he identified as a sister. At that point he broke completely from his manic, perverse attempt at the reality of problem solving, into word salad and song. I noticed the rapt attention paid to him by Street, a similarly constituted individual.

To maintain the structure of this friable transaction, I referred it to the group, and eventually Lopez the politician responded, abetted by Certa, who was ready to engage in whatever action and emotion was present, outside himself. Forsyth then read a tract by Lopez that simultaneously referred to political and personal issues, transcending them by hilarity. Lopez eventually cited that they both were simply human individuals, noting two dates of importance in his case. Forsyth went on to cite his father as regressed to homosexuality. The members became restless at this point, and the inquiry into the dynamics of Forsyth's family of origin was over for the moment. He then played the role of Bottom from the Midsummer's Night's Dream, centering his identity on his nose, as supportive to a chair, reversing reality.

Members Induce Revelation of Despondency and Regression

In I 74, in the Integrated Group, he enacted leadership of the singing was induced by the members to open up about his despondency, homosexuality, murderousness, and cited himself as a "cruel Caucasian." He then stated he could not be helped in a hundred million years. He noted that he was helping Miss Williams.

COMMENTARY

Again, members, as I did initially, take the initiative of drawing Forsyth out on what is transpiring in the midst of his manic state. When he spoke of his low and murderous state he edged towards their expression.

Forsyth Sings Out That Did Not Give a Damn, Obstreperous, Leads Group to Reality

In I 76 sang obstreperously that he did not give a damn, to the point that Jordan asked that he be removed from the group. The group held an animated discussion on that issue, and Forsyth became quite vituperative towards Mr. Jordan. Then, quizzical, he offered the microphone to all who wished to speak.

COMMENTARY

In identifying with me, handing the microphone to members, he appeared to move towards reality.

Forsyth Attentive On Mention of a Supreme Being

In W 137 Forsyth dropped his hebephrenic grin and became soberly attentive when I mentioned a Supreme Being.

COMMENTARY

This is a straw in the wind.

Appropriately Dressed, Forsyth Visits the White Therapy Group

In W 173, appropriately dressed, he returned to the group, citing "invincible, invisible, this is a group meeting," to applause. As the meeting progressed, he appeared increasingly serious and sober.

COMMENTARY

Apparently, he had asked collaboration of attendants for this event. The applause is indicative of the underlying mutuality, I hold, of messianic nature.

Climbs on Table in the White Therapy Group, Wants "Understanding"

In W 176 he impulsively climbed on the ward table, standing there, stating he wanted understanding.

COMMENTARY

He is edging closer to revelation of what he has in mind.

Indirectly Indicated Wish for Response by Others

In I 78, he commented favorably on Murphy's wish for direct reflection by others, itself in the context of his agitating others.

COMMENTARY

Still mute, he is indicating a wish for expression of his underlying feelings, and response by others

Forsyth Passionately Attempts To Bring Order to the Window Shades

In I 84, during discussion prompted by visual aid on the raising of children, Forsyth became deeply agitated, straightening out the window shades that were blowing in the wind, and reordering the positioning of chairs. He had to be removed from the group.

COMMENTARY

My inference is that his deep and morbid inner concerns were mobilized by the content of the discussion, family life and the raising of children. He was acting the part of a fanatically proper parent, disciplining errant children, the flapping shades and askew chairs.

Forsyth States His Fear of Speaking, Edges Towards Direct Expression of his Inner State

In I 94, in the Integrated Group, after leading in singing, Forsyth was again central, after revealing to Miss Williams his fear of speaking. He then demanded I tell him what was on his mind. He went on to cite that he had been born a woman, but had a machine gun. Chisholm then spoke of Christ's sacrifices.

COMMENTARY

I took the statement of being born a woman, yet possessing a machine gun as commentary on alienation from himself, in favor of the dramatic spontaneity of hebephrenia. I also took it to be reference to a rebirth, after an original death of self. It was not the direct expression I took he was in fear of enacting. That would have brought him into the sort of fear Vince Jordan experienced in defying his voices, themselves expression of his Godhead. That factor appeared next in the transaction in mention by a member of Christ's sacrifices. Forsyth's dilemma smacked of sacrifice.

Forsyth Again Notes his State of Fear

In W 179, after Dr. Powell asked what held the group together, fear or reason, Forsyth, flush faced, stating he was leaving out of fear, not reason, quit the group. In the session, Jefferson went on to state his regret for killing his wife, a possible indication of where Forsyth had gone in his revelation, had he been able to stay.

COMMENTARY

My inference is that he had to leave because of massive anxiety, but here he was able to defy that element of his personality generative of the fear, by noting the presence of fear.

Jefferson Induces Forsyth to Speak of his Wife

In W 180, Foster, who came closest to him in agitated behavior, turned on his antics. Jefferson and Murphy defended him, asking him to explain what he meant by his repeated word, "actualization." Jefferson then induced him to speak of his wife and his concern re her, since her husband had recently died. Forsyth became both more agitated and edged towards pertinence through massive denial. He stated it was "up to others to do anything about it."

COMMENTARY

Jefferson, whose wife was dead, is motivated to evoke from Forsyth where he stands on reconciliation with a now available former mate. Again, Forsyth is able to act counter to his fear by citing that somebody else would have to solve that problem. It is of note that Jefferson knew of the ongoing history of the members of the group, as the Mayor of Howard Hall, and here as a therapeutically concerned, intimately related member.

Forsyth Points out That Foster Manipulates Situations

In W 181 he joined Jefferson in his reservations about election of Foster to the Board of the Howard Hall Journal, citing Foster's manipulativeness.

COMMENTARY

Here Forsyth soberly is acting as a member of the group, and pointing towards a personality characteristic that is prominent in his own makeup.

Forsyth: "Complainers Lack Appreciation for What Is Done for Them, Unable to Understand Their Bad Impulses"

In W 201, during discussion of complaint by an adolescent patient of mal-treatment, Forsyth shouted that the complainers lacked appreciation for what was done for them, that they were unable to understand their bad impulses.

COMMENTARY

Again, Forsyth is moving towards participant membership in the group, without dramatic display of rebellious alienation and savioristic role assumption.

In his actions this regressed hebephrenic man exemplified the dilemmas of the other patients. Massively alienated from himself, Forsyth nevertheless responded to the challenge of the therapy by becoming devoted leader and resistant follower. He revealed what was going on inside him in a fragmented fashion, "word salad," chopped up, as well as with the great pith of poetry. He was able to make paradoxical emotional contact with the group through an intellectual humor laden channel, as a clown. But he did reveal his grief at loss of his life with his family, in the context of a diad with a similarly griev-ing patient, Lopez. Through telling exaggerated lying stories about his family members, full of sexual perversion, he gave some indication, in his relation to me, of deeply idealistic ties to them. A member intuited that Forsyth was emotionally locked in a room, impelled to destroy it to escape.

Forsyth had presaged the regression to silence of the last period by stating his fear of speaking. But he is signaling his preoccupation with matters feminine, awaiting further initiative on the part of the members to reach through to him.

Of all the patients in Howard Hall, this man comes closest to dramatically exemplifying the inner situation and motivation of Rampa, what was locked inside.

FOSTER

This 40 year old white patient was transferred to Howard Hall from the D.C. Jail under the Miller Sex Psychopath act. He displayed superioristic behavior from the first, annoying the patients not so much by his words, as his manner. His history was one of molestation of children.

Asks For Help with His "Faults"

In W 89, he asked James, Smith, Jefferson, and myself for help with his faults. James replied that his sex urges were not under control, and the group moved the discussion into issues in sexual traumatization on arrival at the Hall.

COMMENTARY

Foster did not reveal his "faults," but succeeded in evoking discussion by the members of theirs. James did come out with his experience of sodomization early in his residence in the Hall.

Along With James, Asks for Discussion of Homosexuality

In W 90, along with James, he asked for continued discussion of homosexuality. This was followed by a deep silence and change of subject.

COMMENTARY

I would infer that both the requesters and the members are resisting.

States Knows What Needed To Do: "Stand Trial, Go to Jail"

In W 96, in the context of an anti-therapy swing on the part of the members, Foster stated he knew what he needed to do, get a lawyer, go to court, then jail.

COMMENTARY

He is becoming a member of the group, yielding to its dominant member, Jefferson.

Negative with Group: "Sorry To See You Here, Glad To See You Go"; Group Noted His Stubbornness

In W 97, after display of antagonism to therapy, members became critical of one another, then re Foster for his stubbornness that put him beyond help.

COMMENTARY

The members are turning towards therapy again, and noting Foster's character problem of stubbornness, noting also that it keeps him from being helped and helping himself.

Foster Asks the Group in What Way He Was Sick

In W 102 he asked "in what way I am sick." Members replied that he lied to the doctors. Jefferson stated that he had caught him in a lie, then on his changeability, switching from one position to the other. Then they brought up a peculiar story he had told them of having paid a little boy in a cowboy suit a nickel to let him shoot his bow and arrow. In W 103 the members commented further on his stubbornness, lying to himself and general malevolence. Jefferson sensed that Foster suffered from guilt re the sexual problems he was concealing. James characterized Foster as a wolf, hurt by a shepherd, still after the sheep. Foster answered that he would "crack without my defenses." He had been once been hospitalized at Perry Point, and "that was on my mind all the time."

COMMENTARY

The members here benevolently sparred with him, until he yielded, admitting to his sickness, without providing specifics. But he is beginning reference to his mind, and referred to his former breakdown as seminal.

Foster Espouses Discussion of Feelings, Members Accuse Him of Soliciting Fellatio

In W 108, spurred by James's poster of a woman's genitalia, Foster noted James's feelings of loss "hurt" when removed from the position of chair. In a ribald discussion of sexual issues, members accused him of solicitation of fellatio.

COMMENTARY

In the turbulent discussion, the members are bringing up, in fragmentary fashion, the pieces of the puzzle of sexual psychopathy and its genesis. Foster here brings up loss and psychic trauma. The members focus on perversity and character disorder.

Defending Group and Against Accusation as Child Molester, Foster Assaults Jefferson

In W 109 Foster defended the group's validity and his reputation against Jefferson's attack on both, by assaulting him.

COMMENTARY

Here he is challenging the father figure of the group, becoming a valid member, and entering discussion of his problem as a child molester.

Tells Member Was Fortunate for Not Lying to Come to the Hall

In W 111, in context of a passionate session in which members avowed concern for one another, Foster with feeling stated to a new member that he was fortunate not to have lied to come to the Hall.

COMMENTARY

I would infer here that he is making up his mind to come straight.

"I Know My Problems and It Is Pretty Easy To Know Myself"

In W 114 he sauntered from the periphery to sit next to me, stating, "I know my problems and it is pretty easy to know myself." Jefferson stated that it was a "bunch of shit and he knows it." Foster displayed childish hurt, and could not understand why Jefferson would make a remark like that.

COMMENTARY

I would infer that Foster was in a regressed, childish "good boy" ego position here, something Jefferson is to attain later.

In Discussion of Dementia Praecox Experience, Foster: "Exactly What Happened to Me When My Mother Died"

In W 118 during discussion of dementia praecox experience, its occurrence in adolescence, with loss of feeling for self and purposiveness, substituting ideals and their converse, Foster declared that was exactly what happened to him when his mother died. The furor he raised in school at the time resulted in continuation in an industrial school.

COMMENTARY

This was a pivotal session, in which Foster was reached in his ego ideal. It was apparent that he had an idealistic tie to his mother, dealing with the question of mourning by reversion to a psychopathic identity.

Related Story of Impatiently Quitting Job As Trolley Man When Repeatedly Questioned by Passenger

In W 121 he impulsively left the group, returning to tell a story of quitting his job as trolley driver, because a passenger repeatedly asked to be let off at a certain stop.

COMMENTARY

The impatience in the group and the story seemed to have to do with the issue of a driven state that brooked no interruption. This was exemplified best by Jefferson and his bullying.

"Tired of Sex Crammed Down My Throat"

In W 124, during presentation by Hollister of his sexual misadventures, Foster blurted that he was tired of having sex crammed down his throat. Members replied that he had that problem, was ignorant of it. The discussion turned to asking for the other to aggress one.

COMMENTARY

The metaphor Foster used is quite descriptive of his behavior towards others, and becoming apparent to the members.

Member Pursues Foster for Not Facing Self, Irritating Others

In W 126, a member pursued Foster verbally for not facing self, turning to something else, and irritating others. That session, a member obdurately attempted to humiliate me.

COMMENTARY

The cheese is becoming more binding, the focus on the verge of reaching him.

Foster Again Asks For Help, Defensive Re Agitating Others: Defended by Other Patient

In W 128 he grew defensive about agitating others, in a pointed manner. A new member acknowledged that he himself was an agitator, recognized Foster to be such, but that he was improving.

COMMENTARY

The combination of asking for help, and pointedly bringing up his effect on others, is significant. If indeed he is improving, it might be an indication that he is usefully aware of that character problem.

I would infer that his alienation is giving way and that he is allowing members to identify with him.

Opens Up In Integrated Group

In I 59 stated he was "better, do not need any more treatment." In I 60 he asserted that he needed to go into his problem "in its totality."

COMMENTARY

He is embarking on a systematic inquiry into his difficulties. It is remarkable that he is initiating it in the Integrated Group, and my inference is that the frank messianism there and the black members are further along.

Asks "How Analysis Goes," Gives History, Early Ambitions and Initial Courtship

In W 131, together with Hollister, gave history of early ambitions and plans, frustration when his girlfriend became pregnant by another man.

COMMENTARY

He has developed the idea of grasping the idea in therapy of contemplation and inquiry into his life course in positive terms, and is relating historical details, re his ideals and outcomes.

In Integrated Group, When Jordan States Despair, Asserts He Is Allright

In I 63, when Vince Jordan stated he was in despair about getting anywhere, was still the same person, Foster asserted that Jordan was all right.

COMMENTARY

I take this to be an empathic supportive statement, not a contradiction.

I Cite Foster's Improvement; He Denies, Citing His Depressive State

In W 141, I noted Foster's improvement, which he denied, citing his depressive state, and that he was still agitating others.

COMMENTARY

Nevertheless, in denying my assertion, in his depression and honesty he is showing improvement.

Cites Loss in His Family, Alienation of Siblings

In W 144 he sadly related the alienation of his siblings, despite what he claimed was his loving care. Members speculated that they had turned against him because of his agitative ways, and he replied that he had turned "flippant" only after incarceration. Hollister noted that Foster takes people's seats when they go for a drink of water. Members counseled him to lay low, work his way from his scapegoat image.

COMMENTARY

He is identifying the circumstances of the onset of his psychopathy. He is also letting the members counsel him.

Upset by Unscrupulous Presenter

In W 146 Foster became agitated by a member who had taken advantage of a woman thirteen years his senior.

COMMENTARY

I would infer that Foster is now no longer in his psychopathic identity, and is messianically idealistic.

Insists That I Work with Member Who Broke Down in Prison, Heard Voices

In I 68 he insisted that I work with a member who had broken down in prison, in the course of a fight over cigarettes.

COMMENTARY

He is becoming deeply involved in the therapy of other members of the group, still in a domineering manner.

Foster's Righteous Intrusiveness Discussed

In W 150 members discussed Foster's fight with a member whom Foster had called a punk. Foster righteously claimed that the member had performed passive sex with a colored patient, and left. The member admitted wished homosexual sex, but felt shoved around by him.

COMMENTARY

The language is the same as that utilized towards Hollister earlier, protesting that he was shoving sex down his throat. At issue here is Foster's arrogance, towards a prosocial end. It may be why his siblings are alienated.

Members Discuss Foster's Dominating Ways

In W 150 members objected to his domineering ways, one citing him as a square shooter, but objected to his obnoxious ways. Foster admitted to this, and members reassured him that he "should feel as good as the next man."

COMMENTARY

He is coming off his arrogance, through benign transaction with the members, like many before, starting with Holden.

Speaks of His Dual Personalities and "Orneriness"

In I 72 he brought up the issue of his dual personalities. The members focused on his orneriness, and he ascribed it to maltreatment and isolation from others. He left, when the members cited his personality as inadequate.

COMMENTARY

He exemplified the issues at hand, starting cooperative, then turning psychopathic when the members cited him as inadequate. This carried the connotation of homosexuality and femininity.

Boasts That Hired "Over" an Experienced Venetian Blind Worker; Members Inquire Into Previous Hospitalization

In W 160, in attempting to reassure Bolster re his doubts re obtaining a job after discharge, Foster boasted how he had been hired over an experienced worker. Members then elicited data from him about a previous hospitalization, which turned out to involve molestation. Members then inquired into his still present agitating behavior, in which he had called one of them a punk.

COMMENTARY

Members are engaging him in some depth on his psychopathy and superiorism. He remains engaged, yielding to the group, in the process.

Jocular Game with Hollister, Giving and Taking of Cigarettes

In W 166 Foster and Hollister played a jocular game with Hollister, having to take what the other offered, both compulsive and on principle.

COMMENTARY

He is moving from an alienated, agitating stance, to one of conviviality.

Voted In As Chairman

In W 170 members elected him chair.

COMMENTARY

This was partly in response to Murphy's high handedness, but nevertheless a mark of confidence on the part of the members. He has come a long way.

Re Jefferson: "You Have To Give In To Him"

In W 179 he criticized Jefferson, after one of Jefferson's regressions to antisocial sentiments, that he was eccentric, squawking, had to have his way. Jefferson responded that Foster mumbled and got in people's hair.

COMMENTARY

They are monitoring each other's regressions.

Nomination to the Board of the Howard Hall Journal

In W 181 he was nominated to the Board of the Howard Hall Journal.

COMMENTARY

This is testament to the favorable character changes he is undergoing.

Threatened Assault by Impulsive Patient

In W 184 a hypersensitive member, who had been lobotomized for violence, threatened assault, for agitating him. Foster denied it.

COMMENTARY

My take on this is that the member in question sensed Foster's still present agitative ways.

Looking Out for One's Proper Feelings

In W 187, in discussion of James's reconciliation with his daughter, with whom in childhood he had committed incest, Foster noted the paradox of looking out for the feelings of the victim, also one's own, ultimately "all that was important."

COMMENTARY

He is here, from a position of nascent wisdom, attempting to grasp the issue of guarding one's own integrity and that of the victim.

Members Work on Foster's Hypomanic "Thinking, Agitation, and Noisiness"

In W 189, after members confronted him on his inner and manifest agitation, Foster, feeling condemned and forlorn, was close to tears and somewhat paranoid. Jefferson came out with that he had been bewitched by his wife, prior to the murder.

COMMENTARY

The members are emotionally holding him, and he is yielding and revealing an underlying depressive state. I sensed that the bewitched material that Jefferson revealed was pertinent to Foster's hypomanic state, as a state that possessed him.

Foster and Jefferson Face Their Mutual Problem

In W 190 Foster pointed out Jefferson's agitative and dominating ways with Certa. In W 191 members helped Foster and Jefferson compare their agitative ways and awareness of an underlying "hot potato," manifested in Jefferson in readiness for violence.

COMMENTARY

Remarkable here was the grasp the members had of the need of each for dominance.

After Criticism, States the Group Had Done Him a Great Deal of Good

In I 81, members were at first critical of his domineering, and he later asserted that the group had done him a great deal of good about himself and the mistakes he makes. Earlier he walked out, citing that the group was against him.

COMMENTARY

His capacity to take criticism is increasing.

Foster Is Recognized Leader, "Walking Properly down Life's Path"

In W 209 Foster led the group in the topic of dealing with life course issues, "walking properly down life's path." In W 209 he urged Morton to unburden himself.

COMMENTARY

He is gaining in wisdom, versus his former "wise guy" ways.

Foster Tells Story, Tearfully Reconciles with Self and the Members

In W 212 he tearfully unburdened himself of his story of becoming sick after his wife died, confused in longing for her, drinking made it worse. Regressed, he urinated in an alley, encountered by a boy who went to the police. Deeply tearful when related admission to St. Elizabeths. Realized that he was trying to be boss when agitating others, and that his family was not against him, but for him. Certa noted that Foster's weakness and inability to carry through as a man.

COMMENTARY

Foster has been moving in the direction of unburdening self. He is providing leads to further inquiry, namely his depression following his wife's death, and his problem in mourning her.

Individual Interview, Requested by the Patient

"I get pointers from group therapy. I have problems in getting along. I am a quiet sort of fellow, can't get out a good conversation. I am ignorant about consequences, like syphilis. I am not guilty of my charge; I am here to be cured of syphilis, then go back to jail. I have no mental condition."

"I had no difficulties on the street. From the group therapy, I learned about sex, and about v.d. I have a tendency, I know about approaching women, by talking with men. First I thought I was a big shot, big bluff like Jefferson. I called his hand, that making a big showing did not work. Jefferson tells the small guy to shut up when he opens his mouth. One has to be quiet, prove that difficult. People down on a patient because he kids the wrong way. I learned from what the other person sees in you, that you make a fool of yourself, by being a big shot. I did not realize it at the time."

"They did not give a hell. I had a tough break in life, lost my mother. I was at the St. Mary's Indiana School, didn't give a hell. When I was out on the street, there was nothing to look forward to. This group meeting helped, I had people to talk to. My brother and sister did not give a hell about me. I don't want to look for them for help then. After I last my mother and dad, I let myself go down in a rut. I see things now. I have a girl friend now, and a good life ahead. On Ward 8, I had a fight with Certa, had asked him 4 times, he got mad and slung a chair at me. I walked away from him. I transferred to 8. I want a doctor, they all go away."

"Jefferson is not responsible for whatever he does. He has funny ways."

"I dream of my mother and dad, and about something that happened during the day. I dream of going to the beach. We did go the beach. It was pleasant."

"I get distressed by colored people patting my ass, dirty talk, sticking somebody in the ass. It is terrible for some of these patients, what they are doing to him, the new patient."

COMMENTARY

This material spilled forth from this patient, without asking for response. It was as if he lay down on my couch and, troubadour-like, related his tale. The new patient he mentioned is Bostic, and I am not aware that he was molested. Foster was anything but quiet in the groups, and is doing a thoroughgoing job of denial. He provides leads for individual exploration, like loss of his mother, and his subsequent course, letting himself "go in a rut."

At this point in the project, Foster is increasingly sober and appropriate, leading the group constructively. He has largely shed his polymorphous perverse ways, and gives evidence of mourning loss of his wife and family, and inquiry into subsequent regression into perversity and paranoia.

Of the members most helpful to Foster, Jefferson stands out, through his paternal Deep South ways. He guided him towards shedding his agitative ways, which had resulted in isolation and alienation. He then traversed through to awareness of his childhood tendency to narcissistic hegemony, and vulnerability to loss, and began mourning. At the end there was still analytic work ahead, having to do, as in Bostic's case, with the idealization that preceded perversity.

DORMER

This 34 year old black male was admitted from the DC Jail for study of his capacity to stand trial, pending trial for an assault on his wife. He stated that he had lied to get to Howard Hall, because he knew he needed treatment. He gave a story of a psychiatric discharge from the Navy, after he developed severe headaches while going to fire fighting school. He made a quick adjustment to the program at Howard Hall.

Jordan Expresses Fear of Dormer' Directness

In B 238 Jordan expressed fear of Dormer' directness, antagonism, and superior feeling.

COMMENTARY

This is the first appearance of Dormer in the record, and here he stands out as stating it as he saw it. I would infer that Jordan is really afraid of reversion to his assaultive self.

Dormer Calls Crawford a Perpetual Liar, Getting Away from Self

In B 240 he stated that Mr. Crawford was a liar in claiming he had killed three people.

COMMENTARY

Dormer is moving from resistance to accepting members on their psychotic and psychopathic terms, to searching for the person behind the screen identity.

Mentioned Assault on His Wife and Prior Psychosis in the Navy

In B 242 he brought up his assault on his wife and his prior psychosis in the Navy. The discussion then moved to inability to meet one's obligations with the family.

COMMENTARY

He is moving towards what turned out to be a fragmented, yet continued exposition of his difficulties.

Moves into Helping Members, Further Revelation of His Violent Tendency

In B 245, after protesting his own innocence, he stated that Vince Jordan's problem was his sentence. He needed to help himself by getting it dropped. In W 254 he counseled Jordan to engage Dr. Karpman in analysis of his dreams. In W 255 he stated that disappointment by a woman lead him to wish to hurt her. In B 257, he sympathized with Vince Jordan; "all he needed was a break," in the context of discussion of helping oneself. In 258 he lauded the freedom from conformity to one's family experienced in jail. He noted that one of the members is a thief, going on to state that no one is free.

COMMENTARY

After perfunctorily noting his assault on his wife, he remains superficial, until he opens up with the philosophical statement about freedom: no one is free.

"Lost Soul, Too Much of a Rat to Get Along with Anyone"

In B 260 he stated that he is "a lost soul, too much of a rat to get along with anyone," has been writing that to his wife. Had lied to the doctors to get to prison, to get the self punitive heat he put on himself off him.

COMMENTARY

At first brutally honest, Dormer softens, to tell his story of being a lost soul. He is revealing his self punitive side, an important development.

Individual Interview

"When I first came, I heard a lot of talk about the group wasn't nothing, mostly for attendants. I have learned a lot about myself and other people. A lot about myself and other people and how to govern my temper. I didn't like when people ride a fellow. Hood is the main man riding the doctors. I've got sense enough to know the doctor is trying to help the fellows. Most of them is talking—I leave pretty satisfied when I talk to them, except for Dr. Bever. I like a regular fellow, baseball, football players."

"I was 32 years old before the trouble. First time I knew about those people was in '46. I don't think much of it. Not guilty. The shadow, I feel something is behind me, and when I look, seems like a shadow passes over me. It is there practically day and night. I am not afraid. Women don't come to my mind, unless I see one and the boys started talking about it. Most of the feeling I've got now is I'm worrying abut my kid. Not guilty toward him. He is getting some money. His teeth are bad. My sister is not loving what she should. I've asked her to put braces on them. I did get pretty angry out there. They don't understand what to talk about when a man is here. The kid spit up blood. Joe did this and that, so bad. If he's bad, they made him bad. He's a good kid, if he is bad, they made him bad. I've been pretty peed off with them. It made me—they could have come here to speak with me. Like a mad dog, leaving me stuff, and not speaking to me."

"I wrote one, tore it up. Then I wrote one better. I don't want to hurt their feelings. I wrote they shouldn't leave things here for me, like a mad dog.

COMMENTARY

The shadow Dormer notes as a constant presence may be what I came to call an advent phenomenon, announcing mourning, for what Freud called a revenant, returned from the dead. Dormer is focused on his son, and denies the guilt he is edging towards, "for failing him."

Further Inquiry into His Breakdown: Close Attachment to His Family, Break from It

In B 263 I guided Dormer to memory of the onset of his headaches, with sharp pain he thought was a stroke. This was during firefighting school in the Navy, and stress re his family occasioned by attendance at a dance. Attachment to his wife, their intense letter writing emerged. His memory returned, painfully. In W 267 he related that his mother in law thought him crazy, and that he had not given her any money. In W 298 he revealed another fragment of memory, that his wife's pregnancy was pertinent to the onset of his headaches.

COMMENTARY

I played a vigorous role in guiding and evoking his reenactment in memory of this crucial material. What became apparent was a deep tie to his wife and family, combined with an alienating drive towards freedom from that tie. A key element, that of a Romeo-Juliet mutuality with the victim, here resembles that in Bostic's case. His alienation from his mother in law is significant. The context of this inquiry was resentment in the group of non-giving authority.

Asserts That Would Be Homosexual in Prison; Denied God's Rule

In B 270 he asserted that he would "go with men, while in prison, regardless of what anyone thought." He went on to state that there was no such thing as righteousness, that it was between people, helpful to one another, denying God's will.

COMMENTARY

It is becoming apparent that his break from his family to becoming a somewhat psychopathic playboy again at the dance in the Navy would stem from deeply held beliefs that would alienate him from his religiously based marital vows. Bostic had a similar conflict.

Tearful about A Potential Killer's Caring

In B 280, after the members became tearful re my caring for them, Dormer stated that a member, who threatened to kill another member of the group, really cared for him.

COMMENTARY

I would infer that Dormer is reflecting on latent caring on the part of a potential killer, which could be applied perhaps to his caring for his wife, in the context of his assault on her.

Castigates Jordan for "Foolish Talk"

In B 286 he repeatedly castigated Jordan for hegemonic claiming of women and obscene talk. In W 289 he reminded Jordan that he already had a Cadillac. In W 308 and 309 he derided Jordan's claim to a Cadillac.

COMMENTARY

He has assumed the role of corrector of deviance in the group. In this, he is moving intrapsychically to the other polarity of his personality, good, conforming, and responsible for the other.

Deeply Involved with Jordan Re His Delusion of Possession, Trades Nightmare Experience

In B 309, after deepening derision of Jordan re his possession of a Cadillac, Jordan tearfully came out with his homesickness, then report of a dream of undergoing a rat bite, in turn followed by report of Dormer on awakening in a cold sweat. On Thomas's, in a little boy's way query on "What is insanity?" Dormer angrily shouted, "He's explained it many times, you fool."

COMMENTARY

He is verging on regression to the psychotic level of fixation of Jordan, having ostensibly to do with entitlement and an early symbiosis with mother. The multiple letters exchanged with his wife point in this direction.

Asks Re Motivation of Man Who Rapes 5 Year Old Girl

In B 318, critical of religious motivation and arrogant men, he initiated discussion of a man who raped a 5 year old girl, followed by speculations by the members of "sex on the mind," "lost soul," and sexual subservience. In B 320 he asserted that holding his own with men meant homosexuality.

COMMENTARY

I would infer that he is dipping, through curiosity and trial assertion, into his psychotic, perverse depths.

Asks For Help, Remembers Post War Alienation from Family, Current Killing Impulse towards Doctor

In B 326 he asked for help again, but was unable to remember anything beyond his post war alienation from his family. Jordan felt violent towards the non-giving doctor in Dormer's story. Dormer then remembered being up all night, killing Dr. Bever.

COMMENTARY

Under his defensive façade of rationality, he is recalling his alienation from his wife and family, also, with the associational aid of the group, his murderous hatred of an authority figure experienced as non-giving.

SUMMARY

In this man's hospitalization, he found a place in the program, mostly helping others, but also had made considerable inroads into his problems. He appeared to suffer from a post traumatic amnesia and confusion like Bostic. He did realize his vulnerability to loss of his ideal, messianically tinged, in men and women, subsequent rage, and assaultive danger. He was beginning to work on a possible homosexual component at the end of the work. It is apparent that he is reconciling with his family.

HOLLISTER

This 42 year old single white male entered the program under the Miller sex psychopath act for repeated molestation of women. His occupation was that of taxi driver, and he had used that platform for his depredations. He had left a university just short of a Bachelor of Arts degree, and had a work history of low paying jobs. He was alienated from his upper middle class family of origin.

In Discussion of Dementia Praecox and High Ideals, Jefferson Contested Those of Hollister

In W 117, I had stated that boys prone to dementia praecox appeared to have high ideals and aspirations in adolescence, and Hollister responded that as his situation in life. Jefferson derogated it, citing that Hollister wanted women as much as anyone. In W 118 he brought up religion as helpful.

COMMENTARY

I would infer that Jefferson is fighting off awareness of his praecox tendency in adolescence, through assertion of masculinity, but that Hollister is initiating awareness of his disorder.

Participant in Integrated Group: Supports Jones in Movement from Alienation

In I 56 he supported Jones, who had complained of rays from the Federal Buildings, in his movement in the group.

COMMENTARY

This intellectually elite member is teaming up with a regressed black member.

Sensitive to Women with Suppressed Desires, Accused Wrongly of Molestation

In W 121, in a bizarre revealing/concealing manner, "to fill in the blanks," he cited his getting like a violent patient, and related an episode of wrongful accusation by a woman who jumped out of his cab, called the police. He later cited "sensitivity to women with suppressed desires," secondary to experience with five maiden aunts, whom he had to take care of. The members of the group were quizzical and negative about his account. Hollister's demeanor vacuous, as discussion proceeded.

COMMENTARY

The way he presented his problem, asking for help, yet not asking would be as important as the material that emerged. It is apparent that he is deeply alienated from himself and others, somewhat bizarre, dependent on women, and vaguely messianic towards them. The members are suspicious of him.

Cites Disgust over Members' Debate on Homosexual Vulnerability

In I 57 he stated that the discussion, debate on vulnerability to homosexual advances, was nauseating.

COMMENTARY

The members are in intimate wrangling, in which Hollister participated in a vague way.

Sexy When Woman "Coarse"; Hollister Self Immolative in Group

In W 121 he related episode of sexual excitement with mentally defective woman who stated, "horsenuts." Members became verbally aggressive towards him, and I asked whether he induced such action.

COMMENTARY

It is increasingly apparent that Hollister is masochistic in the group, inviting attack and derogation.

Hollister Out to "Get" Abnormal, Panicky Women; Members Note His Low Self Esteem As Cabbie

In W 130 he vowed to "get" abnormal, panicky women who rode his cab, even if it cost him $1,000 apiece, also related further his staging sexual encounters with disordered women. The members focused on his low self esteem, with his educational attainment, in driving a cab.

COMMENTARY

He is inducing the group to look at him, as he did towards self, as disordered as the women he molested, in the context of identification with violent, alienated men.

Reports Subjected to Homosexual Advances; Accused of Such by Jefferson

In W 135 Hollister cited homosexual advances he had repelled in Howard Hall, while Jefferson stated he had been propositioned by Hollister, stating that he had it in mind, in the first place. He further alleged that Hollister could not make up his mind, and "acted like a detective's pimp." Hollister corroborated the detective allegation, stating that many women thought he was a detective on sexual matters.

COMMENTARY

Hollister's complexly perverse personality is becoming apparent. The detective aspect is being enlisted in the treatment.

Hollister Is Elected Chairman; Cites Bad Boy Background, Recently Evil

In W 145he told of how he had put girls' pigtails in the inkwell, looking forward to being told was bad. Recently sensed the world thought he was evil, no good. Closely watched men to keep them from being his enemy.

COMMENTARY

I take his election to chair as indicative of his shedding the bizarre shield of weirdness he had manifested on admission. This is related to the datum he came out with in this session about watching to see that men did not become his enemy. It points to a state of alienation, in which he would be man's enemy. That alienation would have begun in his juvenile period, one that Sullivan noted as one of malevolent transformation. Hollister is forming a collaborative relationship with Jefferson.

Members Discuss Hollister's Previous Act of Wiping Ashes on Just Cleaned Floor

In W 146, in the context of discussion of members' fall from their social position through perversity, members discussed Hollister's past act, soon after admission, of wiping ashes on a just cleaned floor.

COMMENTARY

This is evidence of his previous bad boy ways.

Settling For a Low, Hum Drum Job

In W 148, in the context of discussion of the meaning of the loss of position of a former relatively high government official, Hollister cited his fall to a low, hum-drum job.

COMMENTARY

Hollister is entering discussion of his underachiever status. Significantly, he is doing it secondary to discussion of another's problems.

Re-experiences Loss of Family through James's Fall from Grace, Eviction from Home

In W 151 Hollister brought up James's forcible eviction from his home.

COMMENTARY

Hollister utilizes others' problems to reflect on his own, and the account of James's removal from his home by the police was emotionally jarring.

Further Work On Sexual Career: Man's Work on Farm Versus Perversity with Women; Passionate Vow to Not Leave until Solved Problem

In W 152, after I brought up the argument that terminated his work on irrigation ditches on his uncle's farm, he stated that his preoccupation with sex followed. Then he passionately avowed that he would not leave the Hall until he solved the problem. This led others to make declarations, positive and negative about their core problems in alienation.

COMMENTARY

He is now a leader in the group, and passionate about recovery. I am inferring that when he abandoned work on the irrigation ditches he regressed to perverse dependence on/domination of women.

Collaborates With Captain Bolster on Their Job Careers

In W 158 he collaborated with Captain Bolster on their difficulties in their jobs careers. In W 158 he threw his election prospects.

COMMENTARY

Both were underachievers. In collaborating they are pro-tem abandoning their autistic ways. He has been attentive to members' job problems all along. He perversely illustrated his problem by throwing the job of chair.

Hollister and Bolster Separately Expound On Their Rage

In W 161, separately Bolster and Hollister detailed their rage, assaultive in Bolster's case. Hollister asserted that he avoided getting people to blow their tops by use of Anglo Saxon terms re sexual matters. He especially raged against communists, mocking their use of language. He sensed I had trouble blowing my top.

COMMENTARY

He is edging closer to the underlying alienation and rage he harbored, attributing his defensiveness to me, in an *ad hominem* fashion.

Agitates Friend, Re Fellatio, Is Struck, Responds

In W 162 he agitated a friend from whom he had become alienated, to the point of being struck, fought back.

COMMENTARY

His previous *ad hominem* transaction with me is of a piece with this one, with the agitation of the other as an attempt at reconciliation. This pattern has been displayed by Cohen and Jefferson, Bostic and Jordan, and others. I sensed it was present in my relationship with Rampa, of Fort Knox. He is moving closer to the alienation underlying, leading to his alienation from self, resulting in abandonment of his life purposes and underachiever status.

Reconciles With *Ad Hominem* Opponent; Discussed as an Outsider with Suppressed Perversity

In W 163 he reconciled with the former friend he had agitated into striking him. Member discussed his alienative ways, secondary to feeling like an outsider, with suppressed perverse feelings.

COMMENTARY

In having his perverse feelings out in the open, he is becoming more of a member of the group.

Hollister More Responsible, As Howard Hall Journal Board Member Candidate

In W 164 he allowed himself to be put forward as a candidate for the Board of the Howard Hall Journal.

COMMENTARY

This is significant re his motivation as an underachiever, and the analysis of the motivations underlying.

Compulsive Offering and Taking Cigarettes with Foster

In W 166, in the context of discussion of Bolster's isolation from others, to "solve" his problems, Hollister and Foster brought out their jocular confusion re who offered and who took cigarettes, citing their adherence to high principles.

COMMENTARY

Bolster's schizoid way of hiding from his inner concerns is here contrasted, in the group's dialectic, with the almost symbiotic confluence of Hollister and Foster, in which, on principle, they acted on.

Brings up Story of His English Professor, Who Dwelt in Poe's Dark House

In W 167, in a private conversation with me, during the session, Hollister brought up the situation of his English professor who lived in Edgar Allen Poe's house, a hypersensitive man, and shutting one's eyes to people one could not stand.

COMMENTARY

I would infer that here he is moving to autobiography, of hypersensitivity, enclosed in a dark house, extreme intolerance of others. Again, this points to a developmental crisis, resulting in alienation from self and others. We have come across this earlier.

Espouses Indian Cause against White Man's Inhumanity

In W 168 he railed against the white man for exploitation of the Indians, advocating restitution.

COMMENTARY

He turned against family relevant striving when he was repairing drainage ditches on his uncle's farm. Since, he has been an underachiever, alienated. Here he is alienated against the white men, his people. He could not stand them in the previous session.

Identifies with Man Who Had Killed His Mother

In W 170, after ambivalence towards me, he identified with a man who had killed his mother.

COMMENTARY

This isolated bit, in the midst of a confused session, is ostensibly of interest in regard to this man's self alienation.

Joins With Members on Their Fall from Grace

In W 196 members, including Hollister, went into the sad, skid row feelings they experienced in their fall from middle class grace.

COMMENTARY

Again, Hollister is utilizing the other members to track through his life career. In this instance, he entered into his depressive feelings. On the other hand, he is allowing himself to be one of the boys.

This underachieving early middle aged man, obsessed by impulses to expose himself and molest what he called needy women, through confrontation with his sex psychopath and psychotic peers is identifying a polymorphous perverse identity, in alienation from a messianic "good" self. The therapeutic alliance is growing in strength and capacity, as he moves from an outsider to an accepted position in the group, both as leader and follower.

MURPHY

This 36 year old white male was admitted to Howard Hall under the Miller Sex Psychopath Act, for molestation of adolescent girls. He had a college education, was married, earned his living as a middle tier office executive. He appeared of considerable intelligence, and early appeared to identify with me, taking notes during the sessions. He was extremely tight lipped about his offense, however.

Opens Self to Discussion by Hollister: Relationship of Delusions Re Mars to Exposing Self to Women

In W 137, he opened himself to discussion, chiefly by Hollister, a fellow sex offender, after he detailed his theory about Mars (closer to the sun, larger than the earth, and that matter was softer the further from the nucleus). He accepted Hollister's interpretation that the theory and his self exposure to women were related.

COMMENTARY

Hollister's inference was that Murphy suffered from some defect in his manhood. Both are launched on their voyages of self inquiry.

Passionate Vow to Stay, Change, To Make It with Wife

In W 152, after Hollister testified with passion that would not leave the Hall until solved his problems, Murphy a new patient, with equal passion vowed to stay in Howard Hall, until changed as a person, not do indecent acts. He would become a drunkard, gambler, criminal, not make it with his wife.

COMMENTARY

This man's conversion to therapy extended to adoption of the doctors mannerisms and his note taking. This resulted in conflict with his peers.

Called "Dr. Murphy," Is Nearly Assaulted

In W 154, he was called Dr. Murphy, countering that the other was a homosexual, and narrowly missed being assaulted.

COMMENTARY

The member was evidently attempting to smoke him out, resulting in association to a homosexual identity.

Acts As Mentor of Meaning to the Group, Re Despair of Getting Spoken Answer, So Wrote

In W 167, after involved and elaborate charades, Murphy referred to a patient's despair of getting an answer through speech, so kept on through writing.

COMMENTARY

Murphy here is referring, through great indirection, to his alienation from the self that could tell his story straight.

Sets Self against Jefferson in Election to Chair

In W 169 he moved to oppose Jefferson, the self styled leader, in obtaining the election to the chair position, doing so in an irregular manner. He continues taking notes on the sessions.

COMMENTARY

Murphy is beginning to act out his story, exhibiting some psychopathy.

Murphy: Defending the Group by Fighting Jefferson Who Beat Him Down

In W 170, when attacked for his note taking, defended by Hollister, testified to his dominant honesty, then passionate against Jefferson for beating him down.

COMMENTARY

He is picturing himself as a David against Goliath.

Murphy Is Attacked Further About Note Taking

In W 175 he was attacked by Forthright and others for his taking of notes. The discussion moved to what was incriminating there, with Forthright's murder of his wife referred to in a note by an attendant.

COMMENTARY

The members are becoming aware of the crimes and personalities that might be in the notes.

Members Cite Murphy's Identification with the Doctor

In W 177 the members pressed Murphy further on his identification with the doctor and acting like one.

COMMENTARY

The encounter on this score is becoming increasingly ad hominem.

In Ad Hominem with Foster, Confronts Him on His Self Defeating Way

In W 189, after Foster was in tears on confrontation about his agitative ways, he counseled Foster that in attacking Jefferson he was continuing them, in a self defeating way.

COMMENTARY

This is his first action, pro therapy, as alternate to the doctor, in which he helped another patient. In this instance, Foster is close to his basic feelings of forlorn alienation.

Murphy Opines That Speech Regression is Akin to Masturbation; Getting Down to Brass Tacks

In W 197 he confronted a member who spoke in the high flown manner Murphy had exhibited in the past, stating it was akin to masturbation, and that one had to get down to brass tacks.

COMMENTARY

Again, through the other, he shows intention to come out with his problems.

In Integrated Group, Murphy Brings Up His "Problem"

In I 81, in the context of discussion of "big shot" superiority, he stated he wished to bring up his problem, following which he stated that the members were missing the point, the need to believe in the treatment, that one could not hear until that happened. He captured the rapt attention of autistic members like Forsyth, at this point.

COMMENTARY

Murphy has been attending the Integrated Group for some months, but this is the first time he has taken a hand in its dynamic. I would infer that he is consciously attempting to grasp and deal with the superiorism underlying his alienation, by acting as a leader in the Integrated Group where that is in full flower. This is an instance of the usefulness of treating psychotic and psychopathic populations together. The psychotic enable the psychopathic to reach their alienation from self more surely. Later, Murphy cites how he learned about his superiorism from watching Thomas. Here he is referring to the psychotic "big shots," and their incapacity for belief in the doctor.

Murphy Brings Up His Pedophilia; His Superiorism Discussed

In W 199 he volunteered discussion of his pedophilia, in those terms, and members set to in critique of his manner of bringing it up. He revealed he was asserting himself at Dr. Karpman, the dream analyst's direction. He also admitted that he was threatening to the others through his note taking.

COMMENTARY

The members are attempting to close the gap between this deeply superioristic man and themselves. But he is responsive and has taken the first professed step in dealing with his psychopathy.

Murphy: We Must Change Ourselves to Protect Young Patient

In W 201 re the danger of sodomy with a new young patient, Murphy led the members by citing the need for self change, then attacked Jefferson for challenging members to "pull your pants down."

COMMENTARY

Murphy is becoming a leader of the white therapy group, dealing with Jefferson with impunity, and engaging in unselfconscious discussion of perversity.

Murphy Tells Group What Has Learned Re Keeping Self in Trouble and Harming Self

In W 202 he volunteered that he wanted to tell the members what he has learned about keeping himself in trouble and harming himself. He had got himself in jail and felt that people were down on him. He had learned actually that he was doing something to get people to act that way towards him. Dr. Karpman had asked him to tell why he had gotten arrested. He had gone through successive stages in writing it up, and revelation of himself as a no-good person, who had done things to harm others.

He had realized that in playing sexually with a girl, though she wanted him to, he was doing "a wrong thing to her future thoughts about herself." He had realized that Jesus was his guide.

COMMENTARY

This revelation was at Dr. Karpman's instance, and he is seeing himself through his eyes. Since he so closely identifies himself with the doctors, this apparent advance is suspect. However, he has opened himself to the group, and to his membership in the sex psychopathic contingent. Of central moment is his new found messianism.

Jefferson Attacks Him as Omniscient, "Acting like A Doctor," and Denying The Feelings of Others

In W 203 Jefferson attacked Murphy for omniscience, acting like a doctor, and denying the feelings of others.

COMMENTARY

In acting like a doctor, Murphy has ostensibly empathized with members. Jefferson here is ascribing his own superiorism to Murphy, but still engaging in a step towards penetration of Murphy's defense.

Individual Interview

"I am getting disgusted with the people who are keeping me here. I have been disgusted with myself, but now I'm well. You're not as quick to use things against me. They know how to find out what is wrong with a man, not what is right. The group meetings have taught me the necessity of getting along with people. On the outside I had trouble. When locked up on jail I knew I had to hunt up something to divert me from concentrating on sex. I lived on sex all of the time."

"I hunted up some philosophy books to divert my mind. Am able to think of sex when want to, knock it off when want to. I can control any emotion now. I can get mad, fuss. It don't mean nothing. I can stop it, in an instant. I am sorry that the group meeting is losing you for the man they are getting. He does not have any more control over his emotion than I or the patients. Even though he isn't saying anything, his face changes. That is not good for a group therapy. It is a bad influence on the patients. The patients will follow him; subconsciously have a tendency to follow his good behavior."

"When they strike a note of sanity, it helps them. I thought this AM before I make a decision, think a time or two. I've had control of my emotions for 5-6 months. These homosexuals have a lot of talk, don't affect me much. They have personalities I don't like, take advantage of someone else, not considerate of other people. But they do not interest me no more than anyone else. They don't engage, and I am not fanatically against it. I would not care to associate with people in that practice in any way. There's an abnormal emotion in themselves. Sex soothes and stimulates nervousness. Homosexuals are unbalanced."

"I am upset the most by Jefferson. He is domineering. He wants, tries to be a homosexual tendency all the way through. He wants it run his way. Dr. Cruvant permits him to get away with lots of things other patients couldn't. That's what I used to do. He runs around with his dick hanging out, runs in front of people. I used not to dislike it. I want to dislike it. The people want to change, but want to experience the pleasures of the past, and not get into trouble. I want to change, want to give it up. I don't want so much to do it. I could have thoughts no matter where—sex, exposing self, fooling with girls, pleasurable. I want to be like you, not like that. I think I have. Nothing interests me along that line, even my wife doesn't interest me, with sex, like a sister and a mother. My desires were in the past, emotional and sexual. Now I have no thought of sex. I don't know if you have changed me. If you don't want a thing, you don't miss it."

COMMENTARY

Murphy is displaying empathic and intuitive capacities, and in direct identification with me, distancing himself from his sexual obsession.

Murphy Contributes That Relieved Tension by Surmounting Danger

In W 203 Murphy contributed to the discussion of Certa's near drowning by stating that he relieved tension by surmounting danger.

COMMENTARY

He is letting himself act in a self revelatory way, regressing inwardly, in an analytic manner.

Murphy: Had Raped Women, Sexually Perverse with Wife, Played Sexually with Girls

In W 205 he volunteered that he had been sexually perverse with his wife, had raped women. A member asked him why he was sexual with girls, when had intercourse with his wife, and Murphy stated that was one of his problems. He also stated wanted to stay in Howard Hall until he had changed so that he would not do the same things over again.

COMMENTARY

He is now in transaction with the members on their level, a significant change.

Murphy: Learned Had Been Fool As "Know-It-All"

In W 205, in the context of perverse enactment on the part of the group, at the instance of Thomas, a black patient from the Black Therapy Group, Murphy hinted at knowing the wrongness and loss of control of his perverse actions. Then stated had learned how had been a fool, watching Thomas act as a know-it-all.

COMMENTARY

Murphy is reaching into his motivational dynamics in increasingly pertinent fashion, as a member of the group, versus its doctor. In fact, Murphy acted as the group's leader, defending its sense of integrity.

Murphy Stands Ground with Jefferson on Domineering Versus Submission

In W 207 Murphy stood his ground with Jefferson in a review of the events of last session, with particular reference to submission to Thomas's perversity.

COMMENTARY

My inference is that Murphy is reaching through to his sense of integrity, in the heat of this exchange.

Murphy Closer to Discerning Problems with Self and Others

In W 208 he counseled a member on his vague and high flown language, as similar to that he had employed in the past. He then criticized those who criticize authority.

COMMENTARY

He is acquiring perspective on his earlier behavior.

Members Inquire into Murphy's Subjective States of Powerlessness

In W 214 members inquired into the defenses of members, including Murphy, against attacks, non-caring, and powerlessness.

COMMENTARY

Murphy is letting the members identify with him in his disadvantaged inner states.

Murphy Idealizes the Doctor

In W 215 Murphy idealized me, followed by Reston's statement of his past idealization of alienation as a way of life.

COMMENTARY

Murphy is here entering into analysis of this important superiorism, crucial to his treatment. Reston dialectically is providing a lead to its dynamic and possible genesis.

Murphy has moved from an extremely tight lipped, superioristic person, who though idealistic in his marriage, "had to" transgress in a perverse manner. He managed to induce the group to react to him as his father did, emotionally beating him, while exploring the underlying dynamics. He sought out the collaboration of Dr. Benjamin Karpman, for individual analysis, and gives evidence of attainment of insight into life course issues, such as how he deviated from his own proper family building to a career in molestation of young girls. The data on his family of origin are fragmentary, none on his relations to his mother, a bit on his father, who beat him, and allegedly set him on a course of alienation.

His relations with his fellow patients gave evidence of a bad case of exceptionalism, in which he acted like the doctor. We have no data on the anlage of that almost delusion, just as we have none on how delusional he became in his alienation from self. But it has become evident that he has learned to be a patient among patients, becoming sober and in current reality, realizing the severity and basic nature of his illness, and motivation to both reveal it to himself and Dr. Karpman, and in time to his fellows, and to sequester it, so he can work out productive ways in reality, as in work on the Howard Hall Journal.

In my work at the Atascadero State Hospital, a half century later, I applied lesions learned in private practice with the severely disordered. I offered patients like Murphy a specially designed group, called Living In Reality, where they could systematically comprehend their life course and pathology, also an ongoing experience in individual psychoanalytic work, to their tolerance. More on that in the Summary.

BOLSTER

This 48 year old white patient had been hospitalized while on duty for the Civilian Conservation Corps, prior to WWII. He was then transferred from a Veterans Administration hospital, to Howard Hall, after he had murdered an attendant. An officer, he had in his illness become violent towards authority for its failings. Resident on a ward for chronic patients, he was proselytized by members of the White Therapy Group, chiefly Cohen. He had been known on his chronic ward "Captain Bolster." His diagnosis was paranoid schizophrenia. Medium in height and build, he appeared ten years older than his stated age, gray and edentulous. He was largely seclusive, emerging to inveigh loudly and at length against authority. In the midst of his harangues he would pause to assume the military stance that led his fellows to call him "Captain Bolster."

Bolster States That Needed to Go about Self Analysis

In W 63, together with Forthright, he stated that they needed to go about self analysis.

COMMENTARY

This attestation is part of the new practice on the part of the members, led by Jefferson and Cohen, of adherence to the therapeutic mores. It is significant that Bolster, a deeply schizoid member, chose Forthright, an even more chronic and loner, to come out with this pronouncement. Their affectlessness made the act even more poignant.

Afraid He "Might Hurt Somebody" in OT; Asks To Partner with Doctor in Nature Community

In W 87 he asked for a discharge, so he could make his own way. He then revealed a fear of OT, where he might hurt someone, then cited his past murder while in a "disturbed state." He then launched into a dream of, with the doctor, building a community in the woods, where in a new life, each would learn to respect one another, work out their problems and the doctor do his therapy. I challenged him to start now, and he demurred in favor of waiting until we left. Mr. Jefferson attacked the idea and hope of therapy, and when I cited his bullying as a problem for Captain Bolster in his design for recovery, he came out with positive counsel to Jefferson.

COMMENTARY

It is of moment that Bolster partners with me here, as he did with others, in his initiatives towards therapy in the group. He is also in an ego position to conceive of the nature of problems, and to ways through them. He is emerging as a leader in the group, and a challenge to Jefferson. In such emergence, he is positioning himself into his premorbid personality, with its considerable assets.

Presents His Case, Building On It with Each Session

In W 122, after a pregnant silence in the group, he volunteered re his case, murder of an attendant. He touched on his hopelessness, his self condemnation, and then became tearful. He went into his terror and fear of other people's opinion of him as a murderer. In W 132, he joined with others in insisting on talking about faith, versus the sexual concern of Hollister. In W 135 he reported his rage over an instance of an injustice of seeing a home torn down in the vicinity of the CCC to which he had been assigned. He asked me if he was right to have become so angry. In W 138, in the midst of general resistance, took the initiative to describe "landing in the Canandaigua Veterans Facility," after discharge from the Army, secondary to resistance to authority. In W 141. together with Murphy, he was quite anti-therapy, after Mrs. Sheridan's denial of mimeograph stencils to a member. In W 142 he expounded on his theory that there were "nerves in every cell," and that fresh air was the answer to his "nervousness."

COMMENTARY

This man starts out as "flat" emotionally, in accordance with his diagnosis of paranoid schizophrenia, but, enabled by both his and the group's messianism, he shows increasing emotion, starting with sadness, building to monumental rage, ostensibly at injustice. He is beginning to grasp his emotional situation, now as nervousness.

Individual Interview

"For the future, I don't see any future. When I was trying to get out and do something, to put myself on my feet, they wouldn't listen to me. Not from my standpoint, from their standpoint. I was trying to get out. Somebody would walk out with what I had. I wanted to be put on the payroll. They wouldn't let me get there."

"My experience has done me absolutely- if they had put me on an outside ward, the moment they slammed me in here. I would to God have fought it out on the outside. First thing, they put me on detail in the dining hall. Go away, we don't want you. The little stuff I had was picked up. They haven't roughed me because I haven't roughed it. Every paper I had was lost."

"The treatment here has meant to me riding along as best I could. I appreciate these group meetings. They are good from this standpoint. I don't know what is being accomplished. At first I tried to take part in the discussions. They said, 'You're talking too loud,' so I sat down to self. From the educational viewpoint, it seems a hold off. All the talk in the group meeting won't do anything for the numbness of my hands."

"The purpose is to get a man on his feet, keep a job. But the attitude since I came here was, don't you pick up a spoon, etc. If the attitude had been a man could go about a business, instead of being penned in every minute. I want a garden, 2 acres of land, and it would be different. Of course I'm critical. These associations would break me, and I'd land up dead."

"To determine what's going to put me out of here, it's impossible. You're an incompetent menace. You can't write, contact relatives, people. If you express yourself, you're blowing your top. I don't see what has been accomplished to get these men outside. They need the camp life, what they were used to."

COMMENTARY

As noted earlier, Captain Bolster was called that by patients and personnel, continuing recognition of his prior officer status in the Army and still present intimations of authority. In his breakdown he had lost his identity as such, and like Cohen became homicidal. Unlike Cohen who was virulent bluster, Bolster had choked an attendant to death. Perhaps the numbness of his hands is related to the murder, and an avenue to inquiry into it.

Bolster Brings Up Case of Prominent Person

In W 149 Bolster urged the group to discuss the case of a prominent person who had fallen from grace.

COMMENTARY

I would infer that he did so to bring out the instance of a prominent person, and his fall from grace, a situation analogous to his own, as an Army officer.

Moving Towards Exemplification of His Crime, In His Current Behavior

In the course of his exposition, Murphy interrupted him, and he blew up at Murphy for interrupting. Jefferson supported him, stating he had thrashed a boy, in front of his father, for spitting on him.

COMMENTARY

This sort of blowup had resulted in murder of the attendant at Canandaigua. Bolster and Jefferson join in righteous rage here, as Bolster becomes a member of the group, about to let go of his autistic superiority, a position that Jefferson had exemplified.

Enters Depression, Ostensibly Occasioned by Loss of Teeth

In W 151, Bolster went further into his experience at Canandaigua and the murder of the attendant. He became sad, and broke into tears. After some sobbing, he stated it was about his loss of teeth on coming to St. Elizabeths. Members laughed at him at times during this account, and he stated that was his life, and he could do nothing about it.

COMMENTARY

This man's pitiful status is in contrast to the image held by the patients, who called him Captain in respectful terms. They have intuited the man in his premorbid status. I sensed it when he related his story at Canandaigua, and the humiliation he suffered there. I was not surprised when he ventured that we form a partnership in a therapeutic community on a farm.

Bolster Declares Self as Criminal

In W 155, he dramatically declared himself a criminal, skipping over to his need for freedom, using Foreman as a foil, concerning a hypothesized placement in South America after discharge.

COMMENTARY

He is simultaneously confessing his guilt, while in fantasy living a life in an alien land, after discharge.

He Pursues the Inequity in Foreman's Case, A Job beneath One's Dignity

In W 156 he pursued the alleged inequity in Foreman's case, then espousing a farm position for himself as his salvation, and mentioning his difficulties with members of this family. He later joined in discussion of having a job beneath one's dignity.

COMMENTARY

He is edging up on his alienation from his competent self, hinting at difficulty with his family members.

Joins with Hollister, In Discussion of Job Problems

In W 158, he used Hollister's discussion of his jobs beneath his level of competency to hint at his own.

COMMENTARY

Both Hollister and Bolster edged into facing issues through edging into them. Here the issue is competency and loss.

Hollister and Bolster Discuss Their Rage

In W 161 Bolster brought up his assaultively rageful response to provocation by a patient at Canandaigua, in contrast to the simple rage he exhibited when provoked by Murphy. Perrow admitted he got people to rage at him, by use of provocative language, then exhibited rage at the communists in this country.

COMMENTARY

Again, Bolster utilizes a fellow patient's situation to bring out his problem, but here he couples it with further account of his course at Canandaigua, leading to his murder.

Bolster Cites Jews as Grasping

In W 164 he ended the session by citing the Jews as grasping.

COMMENTARY

I take it that Bolster was ascribing to the Jews a characteristic of his own, perhaps a sign of his coming back to himself, as ambitious.

Bolster Expounds Further On the Jews and His Economic Difficulties

In W 165 he expounded on the role of Jews in his economic difficulties.

COMMENTARY

He is edging further into data on his breakdown.

Group Discusses Bolster's Isolation

In W 166, the members touched on Bolster's isolation, wanting to solve his problems by himself.

COMMENTARY

He moves back towards his sensitivity to intervention by the group.

Absent from the Group for a Period, Bolster Resumes Account

In W 192 he brought up his impasse with the doctor at Canandaigua, over a mathematical query he had put to the doctor to test his competence. Members joined in sympathetically, but Bolster, disgusted with himself, walked off.

COMMENTARY

At issue was Bolster's perfectionism and ad hominem superiorstic confrontation with the doctor, something he has already displayed with me. I would expect a similar confrontation with me, in the next cycle with this man.

Doctor and Bolster Exchange on His Mummified Status

In W 201 he grandiloquently called me Abraham Lincoln, who exhumed mummies, from some ancient time. In like jocular manner, I challenged him to take off the wrappings of hate and alienation, and he flushed.

COMMENTARY

This therapeutic transaction may be accounted as a success, inasmuch as he experienced massive anxiety tinged with rage, but did not quit the group, or assault me. In characterizing me as Abraham, he is playing on my last name, in a positive manner. He mentioned ancient time, and I infer that he is investing me with messianic import.

Agrees That Has Erected Wall of Hostility

In W 204, after inveighing against authority, he came around to, on his own, the wall of hostility which he has encased himself.

COMMENTARY

Here Bolster is taking initiative at analysis of a characteristic I noted to him in W 200, versus rote hostile detailing of authority's failings.

By the end of his course in treatment, this middle aged ex-officer had altered his isolative and paranoid behavior to the point of leadership in the group at self analysis, and helping others in theirs. This was in response to my challenge, after he appeared in the group, proselyzed from a chronic ward. He began his course, coupling with another like-minded murderer, urging him to analyze himself. He then asked for discharge, to make his own way. I challenged him to do something about his still present temper; he proposed partnership with me in establishing a therapeutic community out in the wild, where we would help the members solve their problems. This resulted in a negative reaction from the group leader, Jefferson, whom Bolster then counseled.

Bolster then presented his case, with hiatuses, the circumstances leading to the murder, and the role of his perfectionism, demand for equity, and irritability, which he labeled as nerves, in which they literally called for fresh air. Along the way he called himself a criminal, and went into his terror of other's opinion of him as a murderer. At the end to the work, he was working on his seclusiveness, and his wall of hostility. In the process he is leading and being led by the members.

CERTA

This 22 year old Alaskan Indian was transferred to Howard Hall because of impulsive and violent rages that his local hospital could not manage. He joined the group late in its life, displaying none of the rages, but mood instability, and a need for constant action. His diagnosis was psychopathic disorder with psychosis.

Certa Edges towards Therapy

In W 153, Jefferson asked who was ready to leave, and when Certa raised his hand, provocatively stated that he would be back, for the rest of his life, that he was changeable and lacked self respect. Certa agreed, wanted to hear more. In W 169 he asked me to take his chair.

COMMENTARY

He is turning towards affiliation with the pro-therapeutic faction, and committing himself to the self inquiry and self affirmation in reality I have been urging on the members.

Nominated For Position on the Howard Hall Journal

In W 173, members jokingly nominated Certa's for position on the Board of Directors of the Howard Hall Journal.

COMMENTARY

This reflects Certa's self mocking ways, but also that the members sense his growing seriousness in the group process.

Foster Points out Jefferson's Agitative Ways with Certa

In W 190, Foster pointed out how Jefferson derogated Certa.

COMMENTARY

I would infer that Foster is affiliating with Certa, in their struggles with his bullying, steps toward their autonomy in the group. Jefferson's bullying also had an affectionate quality, homosexual in nature, where Certa would be "his boy."

Certa Cites Low, Alienated Life of Reston; Asks for Help, Lonely for Home

In W 195 he described his experience in Baltimore, lodging at Reston's home, his drinking and low life. This led him to ask for help and report his loneliness for home.

COMMENTARY

From a stance of mocking emotion, after engagement in helping the other, he feelingly asks for help, then reports his loneliness for home.

Should I Have a Lobotomy, What Is Psychopathic Personality with Psychosis?

In W 204, he asked re his diagnosis, whether the treatment should be lobotomy, his fear of telling others his troubles, and inability to think about himself seriously. He went on to tell of his crime, grabbing a woman's pocketbook, his waiting for her to catch him, his jailor informing him he was psychotic. A wonderful student, it all changed when his mother threw him in the gutter, he became unconscious, broken nose. She was an alcoholic, had beaten him black and blue and had died when he was young. Earlier he had stated he did not care for his father, and that he would fight anything.

COMMENTARY

This story of a malevolent transformation following assault by his mother was blurted out by Certa with a great deal of affect, involving the members towards sympathy, and statements of wishing to help.

Certa: "My Brains Are Hot"

In W 205, in the context of discussion of alienation and perversity, Certa pointed to his head and stated that his brains were hot.

COMMENTARY

He is here linking his emotional alienation and perception of his brain and mind. He is moving towards report of the experience of malevolent transformation that Harry Stack Sullivan described in juveniles, and that I relate to the dementia praecox outcome.

Challenges Jefferson on Malevolent Nature of Society, "Blaming Others for What He Did"

In W 211, he challenged Jefferson's inveighing against society, focusing on that he blames others for what he did, himself. He went on to cite weakness as underlying not being able to carry on as a man.

COMMENTARY

Certa is surfacing as a leader in the group, in self scrutiny.

Individual Interview

"The group is not important to me. I go there to pass time, as far as helping individuals with problems. As far as mine, I feel ashamed to discuss them in public. It has learned me to control myself, not fly off the handle, into 10, 000 places. Ever since the group was stopped, I am going back to my old stages. It makes me feel desperate, if I can't talk my problems over. I want to get out so I blow my top. Ever since the group meeting, I got mean, desperate. I always think of getting out before the group meeting starts. When it starts, I think of hitting somebody. When somebody says something I don't like, they have to say the right things to get along with me."

Talking about my mother, or calling me names, from certain people, like Foster, I want to kill him. Cohen agitates you in a constructive way. He calls you mother fucker names. I agitate people like, constructive, who can take a joke. When people gang up on you, sometimes I take your side, sometimes the other."

COMMENTARY

An American Indian from Alaska, Certa exhibited wide mood swings, and psychopathy. He would attack patients on impulse, and here we have a clue to his motivation, supervising what his fellows say. That sounds like his mother's behavior towards him. He is struggling for insight. He carried himself at first like a hyperactive psychopath, acting the fool/wise man, as is done by hebephrenics. The members patronized him at first, then accepted him, as he coherently came out with his account of his course from premorbid to pathological.

SUMMARY

From being locked in an alienated position in the group, as the group's fool and depraved homosexual object, this Alaskan Indian is moving towards valid membership in the protherapy faction, acknowledging his alienation from self and his life course. He is relating his story, finding support from the members. Apparently, he came from a family of alcoholics mother and father, both brutal. The story is fragmentary, but it is likely that his father abandoned the family, and his mother in her rage assaulted her son for affiliation with his father. Certa dates his loss of feeling for himself as a good boy from that time, his alienation from self becoming fixed when she died, under unknown circumstances.

He was able to do a certain amount of grieving in the group process, on his own and in the course of participating in the accounts of others, particularly Reston and Foster. Like many others he fought an oedipal-like battle for autonomy with Jefferson.

And like so many others, he could have profited from systematic individual analytic attention.

FORTHRIGHT

This 42 year old white male was in the Hall for a schizophrenic state noticed while he was in jail for murder of his wife. Like Captain Bolster, he had resided on a chronic ward for years, and had been sought out by his fellow patients and also the personnel for participation in the White Therapy Group. Slight in build, he nevertheless carried himself in a menacing manner, not afraid of anything or anybody. He was extremely seclusive and taciturn.

Individual Interview

October 14, 1947

The interview began with the accusation of "You have been calling me a liar for a number of years." He went on to state that I had been laughing at him. He then showed me a rough sketch of a landing barge, stating that those punks in the Navy Department, plus others, had grabbed the credit for this invention. He then showed me copies of artificial harbors. He went on to state that the statements he had made about "those perverts were to knock those doctors. When a man is a nut and calls another man a nut, you have to knock them back. It takes recrimination; they smeared me up right. One of them suggested I murdered my own wife." Then Mr. Forthright showed me a gun barge; "why load a ship with something which won't stop anything. Mobility, fire and accuracy. It is too dangerous for me to fight with my fists. I'll kill somebody."

About the group, "you people have locked me up and created an animosity toward you. You couldn't do anything to help. I took it that you people did not have anything to do with it—none of your damn business. You did not want to listen, wanted me to back out. You particularly wanted me to talk about sex perversion, not about anything else, from the first. I don't like that kind of talk, and don't like any kind of smut.

You don't want to talk about my ideas, only about sex. Why should I bother to understand them; they got in trouble. Most of the people who came to these prisons are guilty. A majority are insane because they think they are going to obtain benefit by pretending they are insane sick bay rats."

"The group worried me, because it demanded that I be there, take part in the discussion, which was distasteful to me. I am supersane, to take this. I'm going to full value, vengeance. I'm going to take vengeance if I can. For the future, we've got to live, that is all. The thieves, they grabbed it. It's a prison for me, no asylum. No change, I'm not superman. I'm not going to back down on those charges. Not upset by any particular person in the group. They are trying to get out, lying to you as much as they could. They talk to me about it afterwards. I got several out, and the worst one did not say thank you. What I would like to do is to get my people to come up here and help me—my sister is in terror of me, and I did not do anything. They won't even answer my letters."

COMMENTARY

I sensed some human affect when Forthright spoke of his sister, and frustrated idealism, similar to that of Captain Bolster, who had killed an attendant at a VA hospital. Forthright had asked for this interview.

Joins with Bolster, Both Chronic Patients, In Prospective Self Analysis

In W 63 Forthright joined with Captain Bolster in discussion of how they needed to go about self analysis in the group.

COMMENTARY

Both had been proselytized for therapy by Cohen.

Forthright: "You Have to Pull the Skunk by the Tail, So That Everyone Can See"

In W 77 he made the statement at a critical point, re intention in therapy, "you have to pull the skunk by the tail, so that everyone can see."

COMMENTARY

This statement of forthright confrontation with the problem of alienation, citing a feral identity and low estate, with public airing, is characteristic of this man.

Joins Discussion of Actual and Psychic Enslavement, Noting Revolt and Return to Former Ways

In W 122, he spontaneously was drawn into discussion of the multiple ways of slavery, revealing the thought that ran through his mind, about the idol under the altar when he was wed in Nicaragua. His wife had the same concern. He later stated that the Indians wanted to revolt, kill their masters, to return to their former ways.

COMMENTARY

This man had killed the wife he mentioned in his account, and here mentions a previous mythic loyalty for which one would kill.

Forthright Attempts to Engage With Dr. Meza about Roads In South America, Thwarted, Leaves Angrily

In W 153, Forthright left in anger, when Hollister as chair asked for an end to "private excursion" on Forthright's part in attempting to engage with Dr. Meza re roads in South America. The topic at the time was the difficulty one experienced in self change.

COMMENTARY

This may very well be an example of Forthright's all or none way, in temper breaking off when he was attempting to be convivial, cut off for the moment from the rest of the group.

Comments on Silence in the Group as Quaker

In W 174, he broke the silence by commenting on it as Quaker-like, later advising a member who was revealing personal data, "not to bother Hollywood people."

COMMENTARY

He is edging back to participation, and I would infer that not bothering Hollywood people has to do with kow-towing to people who sell out to the system.

Forthright: The Doctors Have Taken Everything from Me; Now Ask Me to Admit to Delusions

In W 178 he blurted out that the doctors have taken everything from him, now ask him to admit that he is suffering from delusions. He later agreed with Jefferson on the need to give up delusions, then alleged that a member had gone home to kill his father in law for having intercourse with his sister.

COMMENTARY

In the swim in the group's associations, he is both unburdening himself of his delusions and fighting off enunciating them. He is following Jefferson's lead here. Jefferson is at the point of confession of his murder and his regret.

Forthright: Others Had Murdered His Wife

In W 180 he confided to an occupational therapist attending the group, that others had murdered his wife, and that he was writing a novel about it. He advised Jefferson not to reveal its contents.

COMMENTARY

I would infer that he is advising Jefferson to abstain from further revelations re his murder.

Forthright: The Shame Handed Down In the Family

In W 182, Forthright spontaneously engaged with Miss Williams, the occupational therapist, stating "the shame handed down in the family," with a contingent veiled threat to the lives of others. I was then able to elicit from him that his wife and one of his sons were dead. The other son wrote to him, respecting him to that extent.

The members of the group accepted this line of inquiry, but Forthright fought it. Certa the formerly brilliant student showed interest, and confronted Forthright re his "point in the problem."

COMMENTARY

I sensed the spiritual component of his marital relationship, stemming from his previous statement about the idol under the altar at their wedding, and asked whether she was dead in spirit. What I had in mind was the issue of alienation on the part of the son supposedly dead, on the way to differentiating it from actual death. We have encountered this conundrum in the cases of Bostic and Cohen, where both suffered from the delusion that their mothers were dead.

Defends Jefferson's Right To Murder

In W 183 Forthright defended Jefferson's right to do as he did, ostensibly murder. In consonance, Jefferson went on to cite that when his mother condemned him, he "condemned her right back."

COMMENTARY

Certa and Jefferson are consonant with Forthright in his categorical unto death defiance of authority. We have encountered this stance in Rampa, of the work at Fort Knox.

Forthright Holds Jefferson Afraid to Leave the Hall; Death as the Way

In W 185 Forthright contradicted Jefferson in his derogation of the union of the Prince of Wales and Mrs. Simpson, then asserted that Jefferson was afraid to leave the Hall, then going on to a member's escape attempt, terminated by a broken rope and "the rope is dead." He then commented that "everybody might try to leave by that rope."

COMMENTARY

Along with the thesis of shame on the family, this assertion of idealism of a higher order led to positing that Jefferson was afraid of facing reality and reunion with his family. This has implications re his own internal dynamics.

I Report That Forthright Fantasized Killing All the Negroes; Jefferson: That Is Going Too Far

In I 79, in the context of discussion of dog eat dog ways, I commented on Forthright's previous statement on killing all the negroes. Jefferson responded that was going too far.

COMMENTARY

Forthright has been silent for some time, and I here attempted to reach him, somewhat provocatively, "grabbing he skunk by the tail," as he had earlier asserted. He did not respond, but Jefferson did, with care.

SUMMARY

Forthright became passive in therapy eight months before the end of the work, and absent from my dictated accounts. I had made a point to include every scrap of information about him, because I considered him representative of the alienated leadership, the members who sat in the rear, silent and schizoid. I would infer that he was on the verge of mourning his wife and the alienation of one of his sons, and too autistic and proud to reach out to his family, for reconciliation.

In his individual interview he mentioned his alienated sister, showing considerable affect. Analytic family therapy would have been a major avenue of work with this man, also pastoral therapy. He has displayed considerable sensitivity to spiritual issues. The group work was distasteful to him, and individual analytic treatment might have been easier. Again, he was on the verge of some real work in grieving his wife, and systematic analytic therapy aimed in that direction was indicated.

HOLSTER

This 52 year old black minister was admitted to Howard Hall under the Miller Sex Psychopath Act. He had molested women parishioners and engaged in sex with several. He soon joined the discussions, in a self revelatory manner.

In B 261 he stated that the "group is lost to itself," going on to state that thievery was justified by those cut off from care for others.

COMMENTARY

He is here back to his role as preacher, but is reflecting back to it on the issue of self alienation.

Touts God's Will as Determinative of Righteousness

In B 270 he passionately asserted that it is up to God whether one is righteous, quoting Romans to the effect that he punishes whether one is righteous or not. Members were in discussion on their right to what they considered as ideal objects, as exemplified by Jordan's right to his Cadillac.

COMMENTARY

Holster is moving towards exposition of his departure from felicity.

Tearfully Reports Reconciliation with His Wife

In B 271 after I noted the morality and hopefulness of the last meeting, Holster tearfully reported reconciliation with his wife, later defended me, as making sense.

COMMENTARY

He is moving further towards analysis of his alienation.

Disgorges Self of His Sexual Preoccupation and Enactment

In B 275, in a pressured confessional, he disgorged himself of his recent massive sexual preoccupation and enactment with female parishioners. He ascribed it to evil spirits. Members joined him, inserting their material. In B 276 Holster confronted a member of the group on his resident evil spirit.

COMMENTARY

Holster is engaging in a revival mode of communicating his experience, joined by members of the group. Thomas later engaged in an analogous experience with the White Therapy Group, but enacting perversity itself. In pressing his pastoral function on that member, he risks analysis of his own evil spirit.

Members Encounter Holster on His Murderous Intent towards Wife

In B 278, in the context of discussion of the human anger versus holy rage of a patient who bit others, Holster revealed his anger at his wife, and intention to murder her by a gun.

At his own and other's instance, Holster is opening up and becoming subjective, as opposed to preaching, using himself as an example. This is an important development, evidence that he is yielding his superiorism, as have so many others in the group, starting with Holden.

Claims Was Wrong in Murderous Reaction to His Wife Unfaithfulness

In B 283 he stated he was as wrong as anyone would be wrong in the situation. Indignant and murderous, on his wife's unfaithfulness. Together with Vince Jordan he later urged that the members not agitate a member of the group.

COMMENTARY

Here he is both preacher, helping a disadvantaged member, and regular citizen, admitting error in his private life. In the offing is further analytic inquiry into his character and the dynamics of his marriage.

Holster Attacks Doctors for Turning Wife against Him and His Fits

In B 305, in the context of discussion of reconciliation with one's family, and one's alienation from it, Holster burst in with an attack on the doctors for turning his wife against him, that he was not to be trusted, was not there all the time, and had fits.

COMMENTARY

His mode of inquiry, of grasping his nettle, is tinged by paranoia, but he is reporting data on his own untrustworthiness, alienation, and whatever is meant by fits, ostensibly rages over items of controversial nature in the marriage. The impact of his professional transgressions is undoubtedly of moment here, but is left ambiguous.

SUMMARY

This middle aged black preacher, here under the Miller Act for molestation and other sexual transgression in his church, rapidly became an active participant in the Black Therapy Group. Caught by its messianism, he acted like he was in church, asserting that he was reconciling with his estranged wife. then passionately confessing to his transgressions. The members began inquiry into his personal life, centering on his relations with his wife, and he revealed his intent to murder her for her infidelity. Then he turned to deeper inquiry, involving his emotional absence and fits, ostensibly of anger.

The record stops there. His characteristic way in the group was to emit fragments of his story when the group dynamic evoked it, or when he could bring up his problem, as a contribution to the others. It is evident that systematic family therapy was called for, as well as pastoral therapy and individual psychoanalytic counseling.

LOPEZ

This 50 year old Filipino male had been transferred from a ward in St. Elizabeths some years ago for his combativeness. He remained seclusive, muttering incoherently to himself. On institution of the Integrated Group, under the encouragement of Cohen as leader, he emerged from his chronic, passive status, as a leader, joining in a series of sessions with Forsyth in making personal representation and giving expression to the concerns of the long term patients.

Lopez Makes Political Speech, Warm to the Doctor

In I 38 Lopez came to the fore with a letter which he read, with my assistance, detailing defects in democracy in the Philippines. He stood up to Cohen's criticism of the appropriateness of the letter. Lopez then shook my hand, and stated his wife would come to Washington to see me. He then touted the Jehovah Witnesses, and their approach to life.

COMMENTARY

The letter was largely in schizophrenese, and I picked my way through it to communicate the essence. He appeared deeply grateful, shaking my hand warmly, and then appeared to anticipate family sessions of reconciliative sort. It is apparent that in the surge of mutuality, with messianic features, he obviated the alienation from his family that is to reappear in subsequent sessions.

Again, Political Speech on the Philippines

In I 41, in the context of a deeply paranoid phase of group representation, Lopez gave another speech on the Philippines.

COMMENTARY

He regressed from his representation of his personal situation to a stereotypic paranoid stance.

Makes Speech on the Great Depression, Complete with Economics

In I 48, in the context of paranoid representations by the members, he got up and made a relatively coherent speech about the Great Depression, complete with economic data. He then sat down. There was no reaction from the members. A black patient then organized an impromptu seminar on the deleterious effect of racial prejudice.

COMMENTARY

My inference is that Lopez did affect the members, by its seriousness and the fact that he was broaching the topic of depression. He is through a semiprofessional approach, Harper and all, edging towards his personal problems.

Lopez Reports on Alienation from His Family

In I 51, in a warm, *ad hominem* fashion, Lopez early approached me to ask how I was, handing me a sheet of paper. On it, in the midst of schizophrenese, were the statements, "No got home. No family. No children." followed by reference to a job, the depression, and loss of his family. After the entertainment phase, he got up and started his harangue on the Philippines. I brought his back to the text of his message on his family.

A member stated that Lopez' family had not visited though they lived in Brooklyn. Lopez corroborated this. Jones alleged that the problem was from without, not within. Lopez then revealed his own problem with ambivalence towards his family, that his wife had killed his son in 1926 in the Philippines; the son was reborn in America in 1929. He then agreed to my inference that he was stating his feelings in political terms. I remarked on the artistic talent he showed in his posters. This was accompanied by interjections by members concerning their problems.

COMMENTARY

He is acting as a leader now in presentation of his problems. His greeting to me, man to man, in the Philippine open hearted fashion, is of great significance, to act as his entrée to reality.

Lopez: The Members Are Ordinary Working People

In I 62, Lopez laughed with the group during Forsyth's hilarious reading of Lopez' political statement. He then stated that he and Forsyth were ordinary working people, in trouble, and the dates were 1922 and 1942. He then sat down.

COMMENTARY

Remarkable here is the coupling of Forsyth and Lopez, who in a schizophrenic way are enjoying each other, and edging towards reality.

Comes to the White Therapy Group, Presents His Problems

In W 137, Lopez made his way to the White Therapy Group, and started the session with presentation of his problems, with me as interpretive assistant. He stated that July 4th was his day of deliverance, then turned to the Watchtower, asking me to read about The Supreme Being. Forsyth paid particular attention.

COMMENTARY

Lopez and Forsyth are beginning to form an existential partnership of value to both, in representing the regressed, chronic members of the group, as they gain the courage to hope for restoration to reality.

SUMMARY

It is becoming increasingly suggestive that this man is suffering from a fall from grace and social position, similar to Foreman, Hollister, and Holster. His greeting to me early in his work had the feel of a highly placed Phillipino. He was transferred to a hospital in New York City.

It is also apparent that he had begun emerging from regressive chronicity to assumption of leadership of the chronic patients, along with Forsyth. Family therapy would be an important avenue to reality, along with pastoral counseling.

MORTON

This 46 year old white male was admitted under the Miller Sex Psychopath Act, for molestation of young girls. He was edentulous, small in size, ostensibly affable, carrying himself in a boyish manner that seemed at odds with signs of middle age, stooped posture, graying hair, jowls.

Morton Is Drawn into Discussion of Self and His Alienation

In W 138, after an intense discussion of Jefferson's egocentrism, Morton was drawn into exposition of his life as a hobo, now wanted only the most mundane of considerations—food, bed, and roof.

COMMENTARY

His description of his life as a hobo drew the interest of the members, due to its color, indicating a considerable thoughtful person.

Tearful About Loss of His Home, Had Not Molested

In W 140, he denied he had molested "the old girl," then cried about loss of his home.

COMMENTARY

The molestation had been with young women. In his psychopathy, he cites an older woman, and links it to loss of home. An inference might be that his molestation might have to be with female counterparts of a feminine self, itself related to a mother figure.

Morton Presents Self as Truthsayer, "Gave Up On Life"

In W 157, members confronted Morton, who admitted he had gone to bed with nude young girls. He defended himself as impotent, had given up on life. He then retreated to the toilet, supported by Jefferson and others, who empathized with his difficulty in bringing out his feelings. In W 159 he revealed that he had a urethral obstruction since age 21, which ostensibly interfered with intercourse. The members were quite sympathetic, Morton sober.

COMMENTARY

Remarkable here was the leadership he was able to assume in engaging the members re submitting his feelings on alienation, to the group. He follows that with physical data specific to his capacity for intimacy with women.

"Preyed On by Girl," While Asleep

In W 210, urged by Foster, he related that he had been preyed on by a girl, who was being followed by the police. The members countered that he was covering his guilt.

COMMENTARY

He is closer to elucidation of his offense, and his motivations. The members are extending themselves to take him in hand, versus a long period of passivity. Foster is close to reconciliation with himself, and perhaps senses a similar tendency in this man.

"Would Not Change in a Million Years"

In W 153 he volunteered that he would not change in a million years, and that what happened 100 years ago was to blame. The members went on, about the intractable nature of their problems. Forthright had preceded Morton's exposition, angrily leaving the room, on exercise of authority by Hollister.

COMMENTARY

Again, this unlikely individual is a leader in enunciation of the problem of categorical alienation, and its attendant feelings. That capacity for leadership led me to think that he had the capacity to reorder a life and self he had given up on much earlier. I sensed that, under his alienation, lay a deeply sentient individual, one who could trace his alienation through the generations.

It is becoming apparent that this patient is on the verge of analysis of his character, in what way is he impotent psychically, and its relation to his presumed urethral obstruction. Also, exploration of his impotence with women. He offers a lead in citing an event a hundred years ago. The increasing sobriety carries with it the beginnings of sadness and genuiness.

THOMAS

This 38 year old black patient was admitted under the Miller Act Sex Psychopath Act, for molestation of adult women. He apparently had more education than the others, and at one time mentioned being in the pulpit. As is borne out in the record he arrogantly considered himself "somewhat of a psychiatrist."

Thomas and Rival Search the Flaws in Each Other's Character

In B 259, Thomas and another member, in rivalry, discerned the deviance in the other. Thomas cited him as an Uncle Tom, for his exploitation of young girls with a big shot attitude. The rival saw him as a thief. In B 260 he supported Dormer, who had discerned members as lost souls, as helpful to others.

COMMENTARY

Thomas's superiorism is combined with a messianic orientation.

One Needed Self Esteem, Belief in God, "The Blacks Are Jews"

In B 299 in the context of discussion of fighting for oneself, Thomas stated that one needed self esteem, belief in God, adding that the blacks were really Jews.

COMMENTARY

Thomas is starting to preach in the group, citing his race as messianic.

Under Guise of Helping Other, Introduces Own Perversity

In B 304 he related story of drunken farm inmate, like himself, who was initiated into alcoholic and sexual perversity by a woman. He then touted his intellectual superiority. The members were active in bringing him to reality.

COMMENTARY

Thomas is dramatically exhibiting his perversity and intellectual delusion.

Thomas Enunciates Need for Members' Clarity of Speech

In B 306 he became champion of therapy, group opposing his superiorism, in making people over.

COMMENTARY

Members oppose his assumption of specialness, as they have done with Holden.

In Tune with Jordan's Autism Re Cadillac, Reaches Him; Asks "What Is Insanity?"

In B 308, verbalizing mocking autistic material like Jordan's Cadillac delusion, Jordan came out with the Henry Aldridge, "Coming, mother!" sexual allusion. This train of association, joined in by the doctor, led Thomas to opine that Jordan suffered from the need to transcend his low estate, to something higher. Jordan eventually came out with that the doctor was destroying his soul, illustrating with being treated like a child. In B 309, in a childlike manner, he asked me to explain what insanity was, "bit by bit."

COMMENTARY

I would infer that Thomas is messianically in tune with that aspect of self he wishes to transcend, through delusion and character defense of specialness and superiorism.

Teams with Dormer in Counseling s Member to "Get the Anger Out"

In B 310 he supported and counseled several members on bringing their feelings out, particularly anger.

COMMENTARY

He is acting as a leader, accepted by the members.

"Too Bossy," Denied Position on the Howard Hall Journal

In B 311, he accepted the criticism of the members and denial of the position on the Boards of the Howard Hall Journal.

COMMENTARY

This bit of character analysis is of seminal importance.

Begins Analysis of His Sexual Perversion

In B 313 he brought up his cunnilingus and asserted that all the members masturbated. Many agreed, citing that it stemmed from the absence of women.

COMMENTARY

In altruistically leading the discussion, he is engaging in revelation of his perverse tendencies.

Asks For an Invitation to Visit the White Therapy Group

In B 317 he labeled the doctor as racist when he avoided extending an invitation to visit the White Therapy Group.

COMMENTARY

Here he is messianically and audaciously moving towards racial integration, also acting in a perverse manner towards me.

Hears the Voice of God All the Time; Sensitive to Derogatory Babbling

In B 318 he reported that he heard the voice of God all the time, the doctor is an ignoramus in not acknowledging that superior being. Later, reported that struck Street for derogatory babbling.

COMMENTARY

I sensed that there was a relationship between Thomas's transcendent position and his sensitivity to Street's derogatory babbling. He had earlier demonstrated capacity to reach into Jordan's autism.

"Sex, Sex, Sex in One's Head Overpowers Everything"; Believing One is God

In B 319 Thomas stated that the man who raped a 9 year old girl did so out of sex, sex, sex, overpowering everything, evil. He went on later to report on the background stems from lack of a solid family, lessened manhood, "lost to himself." The woman senses it, looks down on him. Members cited him as hypocritical for his fanatical religiosity. He went on to state that Father Divine had elected himself as God and the people believed him.

COMMENTARY

Thomas is free associating into revelation of his grandiosity, as well as his perversity. Thomas is jointly reaching into his sexual psychopathic identity and a messianic imperative. He is edging into identification of his alienation from self, resulting in a messianic/satanic status. Again, individual therapy would have been indicated. This patient has great leadership quality; potentially of value in reaching to the compulsive "had to" I was investigating.

But first he needs to come off his superiorism, however helpful it might be to others, and track through the marital experience for the breakdown it apparently suffered. He already is edging into his helplessness there, and some regression.

"Being the Great I Am"

In B 321 Thomas denied having any problem, then a member affirmed that it was being "The Great I Am.

COMMENTARY

In the context of discussion of the need to solve specific problems, Thomas denied his, and a member enunciated that it centered about his grandiosity.

Thomas, Black Patient, Leads White Therapy Group Re Perverse Sexuality, "Worse Than Anyone Here"

In W 206, Thomas came up from downstairs, was greeted by a member who was berating the others about talking about sex, when the real problem was race relations. He went on to describe his problems with alcohol, and Thomas went into the subject, citing it was pleasure, in his case related to boredom, and "one could not let it go." He did so in a manner that resulted in eruption of the group into a range of deviant activities they considered pleasurable. In one, Jefferson walked through the ward with his penis exposed. Thomas eventually told that he was worse than anyone in the group, engaging perversely when people wanted it. He had masturbated when a white woman excited him, a Pullman porter. Murphy demurred mixing the groups, citing that Thomas was "some sort of psychiatrist." Thomas waxed sarcastic about the quality of the white group.

COMMENTARY

In this telling session, cited more fully in the account of the White Therapy Group, Thomas cited his addiction to perverse sex and through his charisma induced the group to regressively engage in such.

Thomas and Street Return to the White Group, Rebuffed

In W 216, Thomas, along with Street came into the White Therapy Group, seated themselves. Members objected immediately, and Thomas went to the bathroom. The attendant asked them to leave, and Street readily yielded, then Thomas.

COMMENTARY

I take this to be a manifestation of both Thomas's and Street's capacity for leadership, an underlying concern for the integration of the Hall. They were able to accept the reality of the moment. My inference is that Thomas was impelled by profound messianism, akin to Father Divine, or Martin Luther King, later. Of interest is Street's partnering with him in the venture. Of note is his capacity to reach across the racial divide, like Cohen earlier, to leadership of both groups. In further inquiry, the natural history of his self alienation, or "lost" status, resulting in disjunction in his marriage is a starting point.

SUMMARY

This man was soon converted to therapy, through his evident messianism, exercising it in analysis of his Satanism. His capacity for leadership shields him from subjectivity and analysis of his profoundly regressed, omnipotent character. Standing him in good stead is his capacity to identify with the regressed ego positions of the others, as early with Jordan, in his autism re a Cadillac. Individual and family therapy would be a great stabilizer here.

FRANK FORSTER

This 42-year-old black patient has been in Howard Hall for six years, transferred from the hospital for persistent assault. He carried the diagnosis of hebephrenia, and had exhibited periods of profound regression. He joined the group from a chronic ward in Howard Hall, at the proselytizing instance of Cohen and others.

Individual Interview

"I was here the day you came, and when you opened up, you were perfect. Your first address was perfect. An open door, to grasp the opportunity, or you're it. What can one do with crippled feet? I said to the boys to grasp it, and they said to have your other leg broken. I don't represent freedom, another planet, where there are no trees, or anything. I don't think I'm worth anything, a small moth in the worth of eternity, not worth discussing.

The more you turn your head, the more you see. Nothing in the group upsets me, it doesn't have any order, because there are 60 minutes to an hour. There is no individual who has got me upset; behind walls gets a man excited. When they tried to break my neck, electric neck, probably I'd do the same thing in their position. But in public meetings you've got to have order. I was going to ask the doctor where he was going to transfer me. He should transfer me into time—no death there. Just look at the sky. My brother is supposed to be a graduate from Howard University. I'm in here because he is ashamed of me. He's one of the greatest public speakers in the U.S. I beat him in special time. He's ashamed that I can take a little lot and raise more than him. I'm in here because he's ashamed. He figures there's something the matter in my mind—could catch up with me—a man can't fight another on his own territory. I have no stake in this time, without metal or oxygen.

I have done a lot of clowning, don't represent this world. The group has done me more good than harm. If they are satisfied to play ball, they are not prepared to go to my house where quality is important. The group gave me the difference between value and other things. What is baseball? An intelligent man like myself has no difference between colors—roses, cows, an ant. I am an ant by nature. I am not a colored man.

Expression repeatedly is people's living. A person who plays ball would rather play ball then eat. I want to play ball too, but you have got to have the equipment. Need food, baseball food. They serve hospital food here. I appreciate my way of living. I learn by what they enjoy. I talk about shoes they catch the ball in shirt. But I don't pay no attention to my feeling. I need space to construct.

I have no connection at all with the opposite sex, because they can't keep up with me. I live alone to deal with nature. Intense heat and intense cold. When they switch on you, you've got to be prepared."

COMMENTARY

Frank Forster is in part hebephrenic, and I was looking for any trace of emotion, as with Donald Street. In this interview, we came closest to it when he talked of shame and his brother, "I'm in here because he is ashamed."

Forster Breaks in With Tale of Beating by Mother and Brother; "Bad Will Show Up in Several Generations, I Don't Feel It"

In B 148, in the context of discussion of Bostic's murder, Forster broke in to tell of being beaten by his mother and brother, going on to cite that "bad will show up in several generations, but I don't feel it." He went on to state that "a murderer did so because he thought he could get away with it." After he told about being beaten by his mother, a member stated that he knew what was wrong with a man who killed his mother, and he stated he would commit suicide if he killed a woman. He went on to state that he liked life in the Hall, was never out of his mind, even when was wild. Later the members returned to his liking for the Hall, and with tears he retracted that sentiment.

COMMENTARY

My inference is that he appreciated the asylum Howard Hall afforded him from his violence, that was sensed by a member who stated he knew what was wrong with a man who killed his mother.

Forster Cites His Lack of Fulfillment and Smallness; Walks Out In Anger

In B 154 he cited his inner state of lack of fuifillment and smallness as causing his overeating. In B 155, with Jordan, he quit the group, on criticism by a psychopathic member.

COMMENTARY

He is beginning to experience subjective feelings.

Members Work On His Superiorism

In B 158, Forster opened up further about his compulsive eating, followed by query by the members on his above it all superiorism

COMMENTARY

He is actively engaging with the group, concerned about his overeating. The members focused on his stance of superiorism.

Tells His Life Story

In B 161, he engaged with the group almost the entire session, on his life story, centering on his mastery of English, which he taught.

COMMENTARY

As important, was his emotional capacity to evoke concern, and his coherence. His superiorism appears to center on his profession as a teacher.

Reveals Bizarre Fantasies and "Craziness""

In B 167, he related his periods of regression, with cophrophilia and catatonia. He stated that he "was acting crazy in a crazy house," experimenting with himself.

COMMENTARY

He is delving deeper into his life in the Hall. Again, he is edging up on the affect behind his alienated thoughts and actions.

Knows Ahead Of Time, the Other as Infantile

In B 178, he held forth on his capacity to know ahead of time, in a visionary capacity, then alleged that a rival in the group was infantile. In B 179, the members jocularly discussed his rival's interest in the feminine behavior of his cats.

COMMENTARY

I would infer that he is edging towards that which was genetic to his hebephrenic state, and the relevant infantile emotions. His rival exhibited homosexual behavior.

Forster Deeply Emotional Re His Low Self Esteem and Homosexuality

In B 181, he engaged the members emotionally concerning his low self esteem and homosexuality.

COMMENTARY

From his superioristic ego position, he is now deeply condemnatory re his life course and especially his homosexuality. The affect is one of sadness.

Condemns Homosexuals as Murderers, Since Did Not Procreate

In B 184, he condemned homosexuals as murderers, since they did not procreate.

COMMENTARY

He is moving closer to the family dynamic underlying his hebephrenia, and the role of alienation.

Bostic Cites Forster's Alienation from Human Self

In B 185, after Smith stated that he needed to solve the problems of fish and insects before his own, Bostic, who had received language instruction from Smith, stated that Smith had no voice of his own.

COMMENTARY

Bostic had gone through a state of alienation from self in his psychosis, marked by muteness, and I would infer that he intuits a similar state on Foster's part, relative to that aspect of language which revealed one's inner state.

Points out Member's Member Lives in Different World

In B 203, he pointed out Sullivan's unwillingness to face his malevolence and deviation from his own sexual mores, also that he lived in a different world. Sullivan confirmed and elaborated on this, stating his wish to be helped further.

COMMENTARY

Forster apparently intuited and comprehended Sullivan's situation, similar to his own, complete with life in an alien world.

Isolated to His Room for Perverse Combativeness, Talented Chef, He Chews on Mattress

In B 204, after Forster complained about the meals in his room, the members reflected on his many peculiarities, including chewing on his mattress.

Preaching good will and understanding, Foster was further criticized for jealousy and combativeness.

COMMENTARY

The members are comprehending his inner dynamics of perversity and how he turns on himself.

Absent Four Months, States Was "Like a Fish, Gills and All, In Need of Cleaning"

In B 314 he coupled with Thomas, in mock-serious hebephrenic way announced was a fish, gills and all, in need of cleaning. Thomas then asked if fish meant homosexual, which Smith denied, asserting that Thomas was a murderer, who, jealous of his prowess with women, had tried to kill him. He went on to cite that he, Forster, was a manufacturer of corn cob pipes. Hairy Thomas and niggers were inferior, Niggers were inferior. He then brandished a chair over Thomas's head to make him understand. Both claimed they were of sound mind.

COMMENTARY

Forster is at, or close to, nadir, and in claiming he was of sound mind, calling attention to Thomas's hard head, which needed to be softened by the chair, and to his own stubbornness. In calling attention to the doctor as lording it over others, he is possibly thinking of being a regular member of the group. In both aspects, he is in the position analogous to that of Holden, giving up his superiorism. He would then let go of his superior, God-like position, and as a human, mourn. Systematic individual therapy would have been central to his course.

DENNIS SMITH

Dennis Smith was a 43 year old white male, who appeared well educated, carried himself in a jointly menacing and dignified manner. He appeared aware of his significance on the national stage of attempting assassination of an American president. He was found mentally ill, remanded to Howard Hall, and was kept on Howard Hall 6, under close surveillance because of possible danger of assault by others. He was seclusive from the first, holding himself to be superior, in some undefined autistic manner.

Individual Interview, November 1947

"When we scrapped, it was as tough on you as on me. That place kept me in a white pitch. I was too sick to do anything but watch out for myself. There are a number of men representing family associations throughout the world. Their subconscious memories of themselves are in a state of conflict. When they are sick and you are sick, you get sick from it yourself. They are here for one thing. The person who strikes against himself keeps himself in constant turmoil. That understood, is being lived out.

It is a case of how to treat self and others, or reduced in mental self. It has reached a certain point, where all can be expected to take. Took a medical degree here. Subconscious understanding will have its way out, couldn't realize what over there for. Catch emanations from the rest. When they can't accept the group session, it still has a subconscious effect. It has a physical effect on me, when it reaches that effect, it bothers me.

This place has changed, it used to be strict. I have a memory for all things. Now it is social acceptability, to change self. To be accounted for. To be considered concerning his activities. Subconsciously stirred up, beyond this world, that makes him sick. He needs to be checked. I don't make a great effort to. I am too weak to resist, we lost consciousness of ourselves at times. Dangerously ill.

One man affects me completely, is too loose mouthed, Jefferson. I have to consider myself his doctor in that relationship. All the other doctors are my assistants. It is better to stay away from it. If he doesn't come back to a memory of self, all it will do is to aggravate himself. He represents something in this world he has lost. He uses his authority, with minor principles. Until he overcomes that minus effect on himself, he can't be overcome. He has been supported by other people. He needs to recognize, and then leave this institution. But there are other people outside. He forces other people to recognize him. It is not his ways, but his effect on the universe. He considers only himself. It is a father-son relationship, where the son comes here as support to the father. He doesn't go to church. I do. I recognize his effects."

COMMENTARY

Smith had attempted to assassinate Roosevelt from Lafayette Park. Here he has himself as doctor to the patient Mayor of Howard Hall, Jefferson. Here Smith is analyzing him, as alienated from his memory of self, representing something lost. He states that "recognition of self" is the key to leaving Howard Hall.

Smith: I Am Nothing to Start With, Can't Possibly Do Anything with Myself

In W 49 Smith surfaced, holding forth on that there was nothing to start with, could not possibly do anything with himself, and was a permanent threat to the President.

COMMENTARY

This statement was in the context of a discussion by the members of the role of prospective death in their lives. His statement of impossibility of self change speaks volumes for self and others.

Smith Opens Up On His "Burdens of the Past"

In W 75, in the context of complaint about authority, he began revelation of his problems, citing his "burdens of the past, and excitement."

COMMENTARY

Beyond "nothing to start with," he finds a *nidus* of hope for self in report of what he characterized as burdens and excitement. He is joining the others, in telling his story.

Illness Caused by Someone Else; Vitriolic About My Lack of Understanding

In W 82 Criticizing the nominal leader of the group, Jefferson, re his politics, Smith went on to cite that illness was caused by someone else, then turned vitiriolic against me, for lack of understanding.

COMMENTARY

He is leaving his transcendent stance, to enter the reality of the group, attacking its authority and myself, pro tem focusing on the other as the cause of his illness.

Downplays Jefferson's Hope and Pro-doctor Orientation, Voices Despair

In W 83 he downplayed Jefferson's hope and belief in the doctor. Then, with James, separately voiced despair and hopelessness.

Asks For Help Re Members Saw in Him Was Sickness

In W 85, Smith asked what the members saw that the doctors considered his sickness. The discussion edged towards low self esteem and fear of the other's low esteem. Had nothing to do with sex. James identified with Smith, in his alienation, stating that his troubles were forced on him by incarceration.

COMMENTARY

He is edging further towards admission of his illness.

Smith Asks Purpose of Mental Illness, Notes Incest Offender's Helplessness In Face of His "Sick Course"

In W 86 Smith relented further, in cooperative manner asking the purpose of mental illness, and noting the helplessness of James, the incest offender, in the face his sick course.

COMMENTARY

He is now next door to allowing himself to conceive and experience his illness.

Reveals Delusions about the President's Family

In W 189 in a joint session with Dr. Cruvant's administrative group, Smith related that he had a relationship with Mrs. Roosevelt, in which a little girl came out of a toilet in a Lafayette Park, after Mrs. Roosevelt entered it.

COMMENTARY

Smith has been boycotting the White Therapy Group, and happened to be attending Dr. Cruvant's Administrative Group. He here is continuing his course in self revelation, but through revealing his delusions. He undoubtedly had used the toilet in Lafayette Park, preparing for the assassination attempt. The emergence of Mrs. Roosevelt as a little girl would have required a transformation. If he as stated had a relationship with Mrs. Roosevelt, the suggestion is that he underwent some sort of transformation. I sensed that Smith, as with Bostic, Jefferson, and others, had a feminine cast, and the presence of a little girl is further suggestive.

It is little wonder that Smith, whose sense of honesty would require him to "say it like it was", became massively resistive to further revelation of his internal dynamics.

SUMMARY

Of all the individuals cited, Dennis Smith was the one most in need of individual psychoanalysis, were we able to establish a therapeutic alliance. He formed attachments to James and Foster, citing his despair and hopelessness with the former. Had I scheduled regular interviews with him, he stood a chance of forming a relationship with me.

I would infer from his first sentence in the individual interview, "it was as tough on you as on me," that he could and sought to intuit at least a portion of my feelings, in an ad hominem way. He goes on to cite his sick state. He conceives of a "subconscious" and inner conflict. He cites his memory "for all things." He realizes that his self is overwhelmed, "lost consciousness of ourselves at times." He goes on to cite how, super sensitive to those in authority; he is susceptible to Jefferson's failings. But he also is studying him, for representing something "in this world he has lost." Smith feels like son to the father, here, also refers to a Heavenly Father in whom he believes.

He goes on in the group to confess his nadir and helpless status, a matter of hopeful import for the therapy. He hints at burdens from the past, then indicates his violent feelings re not being understood, to his standard. Together with James, he voiced despair and hopelessness. Then he asked for help with the illness ascribed to him by the doctors. Then he refers to James's sick course, and his helplessness, a step away from reporting his own experience. Then, after an extended absence from the group, he reported his delusion re the President's family, and his relationship with Mrs. Roosevelt. My inference was that he was edging into the dynamics of his alienation from himself, something he reported sensing in Jefferson, in the first interview of this report.

HARVEY

This 20 year old white male was transferred to Howard Hall for long term care after undergoing a lobotomy while in St. Elizabeths for violent, impetuous behavior, marked by long, hypomanic episodes of three years duration in which he assaulted others and tore at his skin. He made an uneventful adjustment to the White Admitting Bolster, readily accepting the group therapy.

People Agitate One Another to Drive Them Crazy

In W 187, Harvey reported that Murphy had been hit on the head by a saltshaker thrown by Certa, whom Murphy had agitated. Harvey then stated that people agitate others to drive them crazy.

COMMENTARY

My inference is that Harvey, who had shown the effects of agitation in his behavior, might be suffering from some overpowering internal state that led him to exteriorize.

Individual Interview

I would like to get out of this place. You have operated on my head. It is no good. My right arm gets pains at night, and my head hurts. I got along in the group all right. I learned not to fly off the handle all the time, to listen. I was messed up with the fellow who talks all the time. Learned to walk away. Murphy would give me a lot of long words, and then turn around and tease me. I quit teasing others because they told me I would be hit in the head.

The group at first was too noisy, but it wasn't. They said go to the group meeting. I went to listen. I found they were talking about something, so I listened. They talked about sex, but that isn't going to get you out. But a man ain't no good, that don't work. Everything went blank, listened to you all talk. I'd get mad, not want to go upstairs, but I'd go, and listen. They'd talk about popping a window, get you into a room, but it takes something more that that. Also about cold packs, it doesn't do any good. I used to figure this is a bunch of shit, don't do no good. Finally go it so it's all right.

COMMENTARY

The key here is his experience of "everything going blank," in reference to his sense of reality and self esteem.

Asks Me about Helping Assaultive Members

In I 51 Harvey asked me how he could help members who had problems with assault. I counseled him to share with them on his restlessness.

COMMENTARY

He was markedly rational in this approach to me. I inferred that he was in a messianic mode, and encouraged him in that regard, on the way to further inquiry into his course in illness. I inferred also that the lobotomy had been addressed to a satanic state.

"I Have No Brain, The Doctors Took Mine Away"

In W 197: Harvey blurted out that he had no brain, the doctors had taken it away, and needed to return it.

COMMENTARY

I inferred that he identified his brain with an accustomed paranoid state.

Harvey Threatens Hospital Photographer

In I 54 Harvey threatened violence to the hospital photographer who took the photo illustrating this volume.

COMMENTARY

I would infer that Harvey was in a presumed position of authority, protecting the group, a paranoid position.

Asks to Play Piano, Dances and Sings with Black Patients

In I 56 he came up to me, asking about playing the piano, then joined with the black patients in singing and dancing.

COMMENTARY

Since an attendant joined the dancing later, I would infer that Harvey was able to exert leadership function here. His paranoid based taking responsibility for the group earlier is of a piece with this development.

After Forsyth Demanded I Tell What Was on His Mind, Harvey: People's Actions Keep Them in the Hall

In I 75 Harvey followed Forsyth's demand I read his mind with statement that people's actions keep them in the Hall. He later encouraged a regressed member to come out with his delusions about a female form and machine gun.

COMMENTARY

Again, he is in a messianic mode, acting as my therapeutic associate.

Speaks in Agitated Fashion, Ascribing Hostility to Others

In I 77 Harvey spoke in an agitated fashion, about the hostility of others.

COMMENTARY

It may very well be that Harvey has incurred hostility for his exceptionalism, perhaps like Murphy, who also elected to become my therapeutic associate.

Starts To Tell His Story: "Wild" After Argument with Father

In I 79 told story about argument with his father re stealing cars, getting drunk, hospitalized, refused to eat, wild, broke windows and had to be in restraint for 20 days. Members scoffed at Harvey.

COMMENTARY

Harvey has not reached the lobotomy phase of his account, but apparently he had been in a driven psychopathic state, terminated by the argument in which his father reached him, resulting in a fulminating psychosis, terminated by lobotomy. His earlier complaint about members' hostility is borne out by the negative reaction of apparently psychopathic members of the group

SUMMARY

This white man, in early adulthood, had apparently avoided psychosis by embracing a psychopathic course. The psychopathy was intentional, interrupted by an argument with a father with whom Harvey had a sufficiently close tie to allow him to reach him, deflecting him from a driven psychopathic course. The psychosis was interrupted by lobotomy, and he was transferred to Howard Hall for continued care. He found a place for himself in the group. He preferred the Integrated Group, with its warmth and entertainment, which he joined. He elected to act like me, helping members who had his past problem with assaultiveness. He ran into difficulty with the psychopathic contingent, perhaps in a manner similar to his father. Again individual psychoanalytic work was indicated.

REVIEW OF THE INDIVIDUALS IN THE GROUPS

Of the 125 people under treatment at Howard Hall these 23 stood out as representative of that small society. We were able to engage them as collaborators and in effect train them to be leaders in the establishment of what amounted to a school for living. Those that go un-named are identified through their characteristics—behavior patterns, traits, appearance. In establishment of the school for living, our 23 helped themselves, in the course of helping others. In this review I shall retrace their dramas of unlearning the ways of alienation as well as those of education in social ways. I have drawn inferences of intrapsychic, political and sociologic nature, as we proceeded.

The first of the 23 to appear in the record, Vince Jordan, identified himself as a King, demanding that I give an accounting of myself, or die. The second, Loren Jones, identified himself as God, and possessor of the Hospital, demanding that I free him from his manacles. Both appeared thoroughly alienated from themselves.

The reader is reminded that this account is one of a search for the motivation, the "Had To" underlying that alienation. As I have noted earlier, my motivation in the work first appeared in relation to an exemplar of that alienation in the prisoner Rampa in the book, *Turning Lives Around,* an account of work in rehabilitation of military prisoners done in the 2nd World War. Rampa "had to" do as he did. He was a man possessed, in a thrall in which he gloried in his role as rebel leader. He lived and died for his cause.

In the current account, the men detailed were in an analogous thrall. They were tortured souls who had transgressed, and in the process had just about destroyed their social lives. Society forced them into the special prison of Howard Hall, separating them from their families and the rest of the hospital, known the world over for its benevolent asylum to those afflicted with the then dreaded schizophrenia. There was no exit, except through reconciliation with a self from which they were long alienated. As criminal psychotics, they were doubly alienated from self and others.

Yet relatively early in this account, led by Holden, the third patient in the account, the black patients, lowest on the hierarchy, reached through that alienation, to their and society's reality. In time, the white patients of Howard Hall rose to their challenge, and formed their own treatment group. Later, we formed a large Integrated Group, encompassing all the wards of Howard Hall, both black and white.

CULTURAL "NORMALIZATION" AND PERSONALITY REORIENTATION

The psychoanalytic approach to the individuals went hand in hand engagement with them as members of their groups, in recognition of their living situation and mobilization of efforts at its alteration for the better. An early concern was improvement of their food. Chronic mental illness is attended by alienation from table manners, assumption of regressed modes of ingestion, and apathy amounting to anhedonia about food itself. The group therapy mobilized the patients' capacity for feeling, hedonia, resulting in hunger for the foods taken in prior to the breakdown. This would come in imperative fashion.

But not far behind was recreation, in which production of music was most prominent. They asked to do something productive with their time, calling for an occupational therapist. Then they volunteered to educate the less fortunate among them. All that activity led to normalization of the Hall, important in the development of the school for living we envisioned, replication of that achieved at the Fort Knox Rehabilitation Center during the war.

Led by an occupational therapist, an educator, and the patients themselves, that surprisingly sophisticated self help program resulted in publication of a nationally recognized newspaper, classes, book discussion groups, and an athletic program.

In constructing this new reality, the members both initiated and consolidated gains in therapy. These were made in the course of transaction with me, resulting in addressing and renegotiation of internalized autistic commitments that had resulted in psychotic and psychopathic personalities. They had arrived at these commitments in life and death crises experienced long ago, fixated and hardened in hospital and prison.

In the therapeutic re-negotiation, they had gone through crises again, through formation of a therapeutic alliance with me that in turn called for analysis of their psychotic and psychopathic personalities. The first patient presented here, Vince Jordan, King of an alien universe, whose mission in psychosis centered about revenge and collection of scalps.

Along the way, they combined to work on the delusions of their leaders, Jordan, Street, Jefferson, and Cohen. In time, they reconciled with their families, and prepared to resume their lives in society.

The District of Columbia was a pioneer in sex offender law, The Miller Act. It brought a trickle, then a steadily increasing number of sex psychopaths to a Hall populated chiefly by criminally psychotic individuals. Many psychotics were afflicted with prejudice against sex offenders. The ongoing therapeutic community served them well, and instead of the conflict found in prisons, here there was vigorous, family-like discussion. They learned to identify what they had in common, alienation from self, and to treat delusion and delusory behavior as problems that could be altered and solved.

Though we were handicapped in the endeavor by lack of systematic individual therapy, I was able to elicit specific data on self alienation in a number of representative individuals. Those data were revealed in a dialog analogous to that in psychoanalysis, in an interpersonal free association

That self alienation was manifest first in the way Jordan identified himself, as King. In an Army Prison, Fort Leavenworth, he had abandoned his current identity and regressed to the days of kings and court, obeisance and fealty. He was no longer the troubled Army private of the beginning of his breakdown, missing home and an entitled "consideration." He was no longer a bogus lieutenant, or hero in a wartime riot. He had gone through a nocturnal transmutation in prison solitary in which something in him gave way, and by dawn he emerged delusional and hallucinating, transcendent as King, Christ, President General, and Nat King Cole.

But in time, through forming a therapeutic alliance with me, he became a regular member of the nascent therapy group, although a special one, as the group recorder and keeper of the magazines and books donated by the Red Cross and personnel. He also played a hand in its formation and guidance, becoming a chairman. From that position he was supported by his fellows in the group, a succession of who coupled with him with a passion I describe as messianic.

He joined with them in soulful personal wrestling with other members of the group, to bring them into reality, versus their delusions, prominently Jones, Holden, and Bostic. He and they reentered into the regressed states, states of altered consciousness genetic to their disorder. An example was the one Jordan cited of nocturnal residence in solitary, naked, in which he first experienced hallucinations. He reported that they generally related to an identity of vastly superior or inferior sort. He did not say that the voices told him to kill, the issue central to Rampa's situation, in which he would kill or be killed by a guard. But my terror told me that he intended to kill me, in our first encounter. Then, early in his relationship with Bostic, he elicited the statement from Bostic, "You're going to have to kill me!" I would infer that Bostic, attuned on his own to such identities, discerned the killer in Jordan.

As he and his fellows gained a greater foothold in reality, his *mein* began to change. He looked less like Hamlet, less bemused, less self centered. He began to communicate with his family, and boyishly reported receiving goodies from his mother. After musings and ventures into homosexuality and split gender identities, he settled on thinking of himself as a man, possibly sufficient to self, less in the former Don Juan need to conquer and serve women.

He brought the issue of his messianism from an autistic nature into relative reality by becoming a minister by mail. His Christ autistic identity gave way to figures of popular culture, having to do with middle and upper class aspiration, like possession of an iconic car, or status as a performance star. Ever ready to pronounce one of their number as fit to leave, his compatriots held off, as he plaintively hung onto these remaining delusions by a thread. I feel confident that a mini dose of antipsychotic would have altered his already changing chemistry sufficiently to render him delusion free. As it was, the delay occasioned by the lack of such medications allowed this deeply wounded and autistically compensating man to heal more intentionally and therefore soundly.

Though impaired early in life in a narcissistic fashion, Jordan cited that he was a good student before his breakdown. The same could not be said for Jones, who stated that he was "this way," all his life, autistic in a hegemonic manner. Yet he was capable of emotional display unusual for a schizophrenic, relative to his losses in life. His underlying hegemonic delusion remained rock solid, despite effective relations with the group. He volunteered again and again for help by the group, despite administrative difficulties. Unlike Jordan, he did not grasp that he was delusional, though he did say he was not crazy, but tough. I would say that this man fell through the cracks of our experiment. Were I to do it over again, I would have paid systematic attention to him individually, attempted to seek out his family, and of course, attempted judicious pharmacotherapy.

Ron Holden was the first to graduate from Howard Hall. He quickly adopted me and my program, and his paranoid personality underwent a massive shift into a positive frame of messianic nature. His bent towards letter writing found use in initiating action towards becoming my brain trust, and his pre-psychotic experience in building roads, assuming administrative duties in program building. Then, his tendency to look at both forest and trees manifested in his paranoid character was useful in productively tracing the life course data that emerged in the group members.

The members turned the skills he had taught them onto him. They criticized the superiorism he took towards them, and Holden had to yield it to their analysis. He rebelled briefly, became depressed, showed insight, then assumed "regular" membership. He analyzed the temper that had got him into so much trouble, and was ready for discharge from Howard Hall to a ward in the hospital.

The members turned that analytic power onto Street, one of the leaders of the group, for his superioristic, alienating ways. He yielded sufficiently to allow access to data on an underlying low estate when Bostic appeared on the scene. Street played a chief role in Bostic's recovery of his memory and composure, devotedly staying with him and nursing him for four hours. He then pursued his role as chief critic, becoming agitated when subjective emotion that would in effect betray his cause of alienation, also criticizing Bostic in his affiliation with his fiancée. The members sensed that his meaningless gesticulation and mumbling was obstructionist and critical, and periodically would ban him from the groups.

His complaints of headache and sensitivity to noise subsided in time. He cited electroshock as the treatment he needed, pointing the way to awareness of an underlying depression. He did report "weakness," and hinted at feeling "bad," and preoccupation with his past. He admitted to humiliation of self, helplessness in facing his problems. He grew aware of his alienation from others and exceptionalism, reporting at one point that he was "just another member." In that exceptionalism, I sensed he was too proud to an autistic extent to accept membership in the group. In his hebephrenia, he plunged into its opposite, self humiliation. The members worked in a speculative manner on the relation of his domineering to his murder attempt.

Bostic and Jordan noted that Street lived in a world of make believe, which Bostic cited as manifesting idealistic obsession, involving proud, massive denial, leading to the crime. Street did admit to being "pent up inside," with murderous anger towards authority figures. After vying with Bostic for leadership of the group, he settled for the role of gadfly for the rest of the experiment, except when he joined Thomas in his effort at further integrating the races in Howard Hall. It is perhaps evidence of yielding of his alienating superiorism that he joined with Lauton in homosexual affiliation in the Integrated Group.

This hebephrenic individual both allied himself with me as a co-therapist, and most extreme opponent. At the same time, at the end of the work, his ready shift from hebephrenia to talking with me in an intelligent, person-to-person manner, led me to estimate that in time he would relinquish his psychotic world and stance, and return to reality. He was well aware of his lacks and still had plans of altruistic nature, to be a medical missionary. My thesis is that finishing the mourning behind his depression would release him from his dementia praecox like state.

In his recovery, Bostic led the group in encounter of self in one's life course and an inherent driven state and its relation to violence. Something deep and affiliative had been murdered by his fiancée, and he, enacting the opposite to his messianism, an evil state, had killed her.

He displayed the most coherent prepsychotic personality, capable of the quickest and most comprehensive recovery. In that, he resembled John Jefferson, who had recovered from a catatonic state, to emerge as a paranoid personality, liable to catatonic episodes. He enlisted the members, in what I call a messianic mutuality, in a passionate recovery of his memory and then traversal of his crime.

Once recovered, he assumed leadership of the group, at one time fighting Jordan for primacy and his honor. Importantly, he induced tears in Jordan, on the issue of leaving the world of make believe. He came closest to demonstrating the messianic aspects of his dilemmas in his coming preacher role, and conviction that he was a devil. Death and resurrection played a prominent role in his experience.

Family therapy played a part in working through his resistance to further analysis of his dependent vulnerability on his victim. He ended the treatment on a positive note, discharged to court, for trial.

The next significant patient was Lauton, a young sex offender, who resembled Street in intellectual capacity, but was not as alienated and effectively handicapped. Whereas Street was able to display only intellectual contrariness, down to muteness, Lauton could always talk, but in a vague manner. Also like Street, he acted as a weathervane relative to underlying emotions in others, as when he reacted strongly when Bostic began discussing his vulnerability to his fiancée, holding that she had provoked him. Earlier Lauton had revealed that he was trying to get in touch with his dead sister, through prayer. He identified with Bostic to the extent that he believed Bostic's mother was dead, and sensed how that death had affected Bostic.

He was guilty about masturbation, later felt sinful, and still later hinted at a "devastating interior fantasy life." Following this he regressed into initiation of open homosexual love with Street. This is similar to Jefferson's manifestation of his homosexuality, and this regression may be considered as a forward step in the integration of the personalities of both. Its frequent occurrence in the stories of these individuals led me to hold that as an important question to be investigated in my private practice to come.

Jefferson was a central figure in the work. Much of his changes were through character analysis, presided over by an eminently sensible and masterful superego that led to his designation as the Mayor of Howard Hall, in which capacity he mediated disputes of his fellows. He became the subject of a group in which he was the leader. He provided the most data about the relationship with a father figure. He cited him as brutal, and behaved like him in conflictual situations. Jefferson did not bring up his natural mother, and the relationship of his father to her, but he held a domineering orientation to women, but for the colored mammy who had a hand in raising him. She is most likely reflected in his very human side.

Thus what he considered "weakness" allowed him to progress to awareness of a homosexual aspect of his character, and affiliative relationships with the black patients. He endured the reproach of traitor to his heritage. He ended the work mourning his dead wife and tearfully facing the prospect of return to his family, while aware of his antisocial tendency. At the end, it was apparent he was about ready for discharge.

The next patient to appear in the record, William Cohen, worked closely with Jefferson. Through a positive therapeutic alliance, and with Jefferson's help, he accomplished a dramatic change from being a hypersensitive wild man with wide, threatening mood swings to sober collaborative citizen of the Hall who contributed most to its racial integration. He recovered from a bipolar state with paranoid and psychopathic character features. He reconciled with a mother from whom he was alienated, and about whom he had developed a delusion that she was dead.

The next patient, James, was a severely paranoid individual who joined the group in its 157th session. He was resident on a chronic ward, and on hearing of the existence of the group, asked for membership. Severely paranoid, he had committed incest with a daughter, to save her from evil others. His fellows gave him a wide berth. He joined the group interaction with some gusto, soon subjecting his incest and Cohen's paranoia to the group's scrutiny. He then compared his marriage to that of the others, and his autistic features became subject of the group's inquiry. After criticism of Jefferson's authoritarianism, he attained the position of chair, helping others, revealing aspects of his marriage, eventually remorse over his crime, yielding a feudal concept of marriage and fatherhood. He moved into reconciliation with his family and daughter, and like Jordan, was struggling with his delusions towards the end.

The next member to appear on the record was Reardon, a young homosexual. He is included in this exposition because of the pivotal role he played in the integration of the homosexual and psychotic populations. He had a pleasant, rational way and was manly enough to meet the criteria of the homophobic group he was joining. Cohen was the first to accept him, citing that the others had homosexual components.

Discussion of his rivalry with his father followed that of Cohen and another patient. He then started to reveal the violence underlying his pleasant ways. Reardon was discharged midway in his treatment.

The next patient, Forsyth, was another pivotal patient, this time in integration of the chronic and more acute patients. He was older, but inordinately muscular and physically able. His diagnosis could best be put as hebephrenic, but as he proceeded in treatment he displayed an underlying depression. He had a flair for dramatic and poetic expression, speaking in mock oratorical manner. He persevered in whatever he was doing, and fortunately yielded to the attendants, at times having to be separated from the group.

His clown, wise man, and poignant self revelation riveted the attention of the group. He revealed aspects of his family of origin in extremely perverse terms, by his devoted manner contradicting the material. He induced other chronic members to present their life data. In doing so, he began leaving the thrall of his hebephrenia, entering into a simple humanity, as an illustration of Harry Stack Sullivan's, "We are much more simply human than otherwise."

He started wearing appropriate clothing, and with Jefferson's help edged towards discussion of his wife. By the end of the work with him, under the stress of meeting Jefferson's challenge to relate to his wife, he retreated to the gadfly role, acting in a housekeeping manner re the window shades.

At the end of the work, this chronic patient was engaged in both the White Therapy Group and the Integrated Group in discussion of group concerns and his life problems. He assumed a leadership role in the latter group, mimicking the therapist, in managing the microphone, calling on members to join in, and in allocation of time for entertainment and discussion. This was done in a hebephrenic manner, as clown, devoted participant, and rebel. As he participated, he grew more serious, moving from poetry and word salad to the reality of the group.

It was apparent that the self he had been alienated from was one of an extremely hypersensitive man, of monumental sentiments and rages, who experienced his feelings with such immediacy that he could not allow himself to experience them in reality. In this way, he resembled the others in this presentation, especially Street, Cohen, and Rampa, the last of whom who initiated my search for the "had to" that stemmed from alienation. In the midst of having to rebel or play the clown he showed the sadness that came with reconciliation with current reality.

Foster, a sexual psychopath, was cooperative from the first, asking for help with his faults, then displaying them in a manner that was extremely resistive. He stated that he would crack without his defenses. They consisted of aggressive pestering of others, in part of homosexual nature, plus confabulation. In time, adopted by Jefferson, who extensively criticized his agitative ways, he opened up about his relationship with his family and the inception of his illness after his wife's death, resulting in a regressive turn to child molestation. The members accepted him as chair, and he became calmer and collaborative. He realized he had to be boss, run everything like he had in his family, did a certain amount of mourning for his wife, and turned from a paranoid orientation to a messianic one.

The next patient to appear on the record was in the hospital for study of a transient psychosis, leading to assault on his wife, a situation similar to that of Bostic. Dormer collaborated from the first, soon arriving at appreciation of his low estate, "lost soul... rat." He related the course of his illness, involving marital stress (his wife's miscarriage) and wartime Navy firefighting school.

He and the group cleared up a posttraumatic amnesia, and the occurrence of post traumatic hallucinations. Along the way, he was helpful to others, in what he called a "serving capacity," analogous to that with his wife, and which he realized left him vulnerable to his rages. At the end of the work, he was working through his problem with rage at loss of the ideal in self and others, also homosexual tendencies.

The next patient on the record was an early middle aged sex psychopath who had molested adult women. It soon became apparent that Hollister held himself superior in a manner that agitated the others in a manner that resulted in his humiliation. This was in part his attitude towards himself. The members noted that he was sexually obsessed, taking the form of molestation of "distressed women." In time he revealed what he held to be evil, also messianic aspects to his personality, accepting membership in the group, attainment of the position of chair, and abandonment of an exceptionalism that had defeated him in his career aspirations.

Murphy was pessimistic about ever leaving the Hall, despite his cooperativeness. At first appearing cooperative, the members found that as chair he was high handed. He reported having been beat by his father. A picture emerged of a strong conscience and alienated perverse identity. He acted with the therapist as a momma's special boy, serving the group through aping him in notetaking. By the end of the work he was a full fledged member of the sexual psychopaths group, working on his life course issues in relation to his perversity.

The next patient, Bolster, had been proselytized to join the group by Cohen, from one of the chronic wards in Howard Hall. He had been hospitalized for paranoia, after having murdered an attendant at a Veteran Administration hospital. A former Army officer, his commanding presence resulted in being called Captain Bolster. In time, he related his crime, crying afterwards. He then became enraged at an interruption, exemplifying his problem with himself. Jefferson supported him, and he gradually let go of his temper, discussing his omnipotent and defiant character.

Certa was an early adult Alaskan Indian who had a background of a physically abusive mother and absent father, and inception of his illness on her death. He had been an excellent student prior to the family's problems, and showed traces of that status early in the record, growing stronger as the group proceeded. Small in stature and boyish, he was patronized at first by the members of the group, becoming a full member towards the end of the work, sobering in the process.

The next patient, Forthright, had lived on a chronic ward for some years, volunteered for membership in the White Therapy Group towards the end of the work. He asserted his right to do as he had, had no remorse, and would answer his mother back. He provided another lead in an allusively worded statement about an escape attempt by means of a rope, that it was dead, and everybody might leave that way. He was on the way to further exposition of his murder, in alliance with Jefferson.

Holster, the next patient on the record, a black minister, had molested female parishioners and from the first was tearfully open about his crimes. He then reported that he was massively preoccupied with sexual impulses and thoughts, ascribed to evil spirits. The members accepted him in its work, and he was on the way to work on the dynamics of his current family and family of origin.

Like Forsyth and Bolster, the next chronic patient, Lopez, was drawn into the dynamic of the Integrated Group. He also assumed a leadership role, that of making representation of his case and that of Filipinos who had been wronged. Under the group's and my inquiry he revealed that he had no family, no job, was depressed and then that his wife had killed their son in 1926, and he had been reborn in America in 1929. Forsyth played a role in drawing out this man's story, and eventually the assertion that they were "ordinary people trying to get along." These unlikely partners gave evidence of moving into reality.

The next patient, a middle aged sex psychopath, Morton, had from the first stated he had given up on life and molested young girls. He became passionate, though, in claiming that he could not change. He later claimed he was impotent, then that he was afraid of women. His affability and confabulation led the group on a merry chase, and the members were not able to reach acceptance by him of his alienated state, beyond his initial statement that it would be impossible for him to change.

Frank Forster

This somewhat older, chronic, black hebephrenic patient gave eloquent evidence of early therapeutic alliance ("the day you came, and opened up, you were perfect . . . an open door, to grasp the opportunity . . ."). He impetuously broke into an account by Bostic, to cite having been beaten up by his mother, hinting at his murderousness. Subsequently, he went on to relate his lack of fulfillment as a member of an achieving family, to account for his compulsive orality.

He commanded the agenda of entire group sessions, revealing his mastery of English and his profession of teaching. He revealed data about his regressive spells, involving eating of feces and other experiments with self ("acting crazy in a crazy house"), down to nadir status. There he noted his homosexuality and sadness, and alienation from himself. At that point he induced empathy by members of the group, one of whom commented that he had "no voice of his own." In that nadir state, he absented himself for months, returning dramatically, enacting his issues, in the course of which he brandished a chair over a fellow homosexual's head, ostensibly to soften his obstinacy.

Like Street and Forsyth, Forster provided the members a window on their deepest sense of alienation, acting as weathervane for the winds blowing through the group, making initial progress towards reconciliation with self and resumption of human status.

The last patient in this commentary, Austin Thomas, was a black 37 year old, extensively educated; who claimed that had been a minister. He held himself to be superior, "somewhat of a psychiatrist." He announced that he had reached a near identity with God, also the depths in a low estate, also data pertaining to polymorphous perversity. Very much a leader, he once led the White Therapy Group into a useful discussion of alcoholism, then enactment of homosexual behavior. In the Black Therapy Group he went on to discuss his case, his problem with his family, in which his wife allegedly treated him like a child.

A COMPOSITE PICTURE OF DYNAMIC FACTORS

By the end of this work, I had come a distance in discernment and alteration for the better of the compulsions or "had to's" of the residents of Howard Hall. Yet I had no comprehensive picture of any one case, though a number no longer needed maximum security, and met criteria for release to the hospital and court. The most complete picture was of Wilfred Bostic, who started massively catatonic, and collaborated in his treatment until recovery, and beyond. We worked on a character he eventually recognized as vulnerable and dangerous in a relation with women. As with others in the work, my individual relationship with him developed in the group process, except for occasional short individual and family interviews. Yet he did undergo analytic regression, as himself, in the service of the therapy, first into a messianic transference, in which he trusted and believed in the therapy for deliverance from what I sensed was a subjective world of hell. Then he swerved from that transference, back to a lifelong orientation as with his mother, joining in a legal move towards a writ of habeas corpus.

Even were I to have engaged him in the individual psychoanalysis I had no time or training for, it is doubtful we would have penetrated to the internal factors leading to the driven state behind his vulnerability to his victim. In his case and that of a number of his fellows, the inquiry pointed to an early tie with a mother figure. In his illness, he was convinced his mother was dead. William Cohen had a similar delusion, combined with belief that she was an impostor. Jefferson gave evidence of severance of the tie with his mother, in favor of a black "mammy."

We have precious little data on the ties to a maternal figure of the others in the 23 in this presentation. Bostic, Jefferson, and James reported they were bewitched by women they also held to be domineering. Of the sex psychopaths, Hollister had a contrary, if suggestive, experience, one of compulsive ministration to women in straits. Another sex psychopath, Foster, massively regressed when his wife died. The presidential assassin, Smith, exhibited delusional material involving on the part of Mrs. Roosevelt of transmutation to a young girl.

The fathers of the patients were mostly absent from the story, or at best sketchy, certainly ambivalent. A strong strain of homosexual affiliation, present as a transference, is suggestive of a product of the alienation of father from the family. Importantly, Bostic, Jefferson, Cohen, Foster, and Certa went for a period through regression into homosexual phases in the treatment, then returned to reality. Lauton and Street did so, in a manner I believe they intended to be supportive, if bizarrely so.

Bostic was quite aware of ego defects, manifested first as difficulty in conceptualization, then expression that extended to simple phonation. His awareness then moved over to that of massive anxiety, admixed with rage and mourning, both occasioned by loss of ideal concepts and states. A number of others—Jefferson, Cohen, and Certa—arrived at awareness of such ideals, devastation at their loss, and their transformation into perversion.

Work with Bostic in his recovery led me to sensitivity to the altered state of consciousness he had traversed and the world(s) he had lived in during his catatonia. Lauton attempted communication with a dead sister. The matter of alternate worlds became of great moment in later work.

Correlate Data from the Author's Self Analysis and Practice

I had no formal training in psychiatry, much less psychoanalysis, when I began this experiment, though I had served as wartime psychiatrist for a Post Hospital, then a Rehabilitation Center. I now consider this lack to be largely advantageous, opening the way to engagement of aspects of my personality that the discipline of psychiatric, even psychoanalytic training, would have inhibited or obviated. My mentors at the Washington Psychoanalytic Institute insisted I discontinue my Howard Hall work, as a condition of further training.

I left the work at Howard Hall, to continue training in psychoanalysis, in a private practice context. I would be free to engage in intensive, disciplined inquiry, with the research record keeping I had been following in Howard Hall. Also, a seminal task was analysis of my own psychic correlate in the therapeutic equation, comparable to Rampa's "had to," hopefully less imperative. I can only infer that my two analysts inadvertently blocked the emergence of the sort of data in me and my private practice that my patients in Howard Hall had been approaching.

I was able to intellectually, but not emotionally comprehend the maternal tie at issue, having arrived at the formulation through work with a group of mothers and daughters elsewhere at St. Elizabeths. They were fixated in a state of concomitant alienation and affiliation. (*Maternal Dependency and Schizophrenia: Mothers and Daughters in an Analytic Group*, Abrahams, J.

and Varon, E. International Universities Press, 1953). They gave evidence of the idealization I had noted in the patients in Howard Hall.

Looking back, I would infer that an arrest in my psyche impeded the group dynamic from deeper penetration into their relationships. Later, in my practice, a series of patients, severely disordered but still functional in their lives, advanced my comprehension. One, like Bostic in Howard Hall, was paradigmatic. He was a pathologist who could not mourn a father who haunted him in the manner exemplified in Shakespeare's *Hamlet*. Insomniac and depressed, this man became addicted and suicidal. His operant ego was taken over by identification with both his parents, of incestuous import. Psychoanalytic intervention, potentiated by a range of analytic group therapies which amounted to total immersion, resulted in transferential yielding of a dream in which he separated himself from an introjected parental figure, his father's rotting corpse. This was attended by profound grief and release from his previous inner imperative, his "had to."

Not long after, during the inception of a mid-life crisis, I arrived at inklings of that drama in my psyche, in the form of a dream and associations. In the dream, I found myself in a coffin, dead, lid on, and would really die, were I to struggle. I was strangely acceptant, determined to study this conundrum. I sensed that my psychic death and nadirhood were somehow related to my mother's grieving her mother and inability to climb out of a depressive pit. I was able to go on in my life secondary to an inherent messianism I had derived from my mother. My third analyst avoided analysis of the messianism, and the analysis was to limited avail. However, another patient came along with a deeply delusional tie to a dead father, inability to mourn, and the capacity, within the modifications I had prior developed in my analytic practice, of analytic family therapy, intensive psychoanalysis, and therapeutic community, to confront her autistic ties, mourn, and like the pathologist, free herself from previously crippling inner imperatives.

In my further self analysis, I experienced further dreams concerning death and restoration, and a growing comprehension of the transference from my family's tragic course and its impact on my life and practice. In short, I inferred that the tie, in a three generation hypothesis, was messianic, in which the generations belonged to one another, saving each other and attended by excruciating guilt on autonomy and freedom from that tie.

I attempted replication of the work in Howard Hall in a contemporaneous setting, the Atascadero State Hospital, 1990–1996, to be published as *An Adventure in Self Transformation, Therapeutic Community at Atascadero State Hospital*. A review of my career in psychoanalysis is forthcoming, as *Terra Incognita: Exploring Psychoanalytic Frontiers*. Recently published: *Turning Lives Around: Wartime Treatment of Military Prisoners*, Author House, 2006; *A Passionate Psychoanalyst: Dreams and Poems*, Abrahams, J., Xlibris, 2007; *The Messianic Imperative: Scourge or Savior?* Abrahams, J., Xlibris, 2007.

Chapter Five

Summary and Inferences

By the end of the four years of this work, the Howard Hall community had changed significantly. We had replicated features of the Fort Knox program, its complexity and single minded mission of individual change to fit the person for a life in the reality outside the Hall. As at Knox, a certain general patterning emerged in the therapeutic encounters in the group and individually. I have noted the pregnant pause or hush that befell the groups, as they transitioned from the antisocial psychopathic position to the prosocial "normal" one. I have also noted the anxiety and perturbation that ensued in daily life, as the individuals missed their previous ways, suffered their loss, and lived into a life in current reality. This dilemma was clearest in Vince Jordan, in losing the companionship and direction of his voices.

The new found capacity of the group to identify with me and one another was clearly evident in the case of Ron Holden, followed by a capacity on the part of the members of the group to induce him to shed his superiorism. He worked his way through anxiety and depression, and was able to assume leadership in aiding others. He was discharged before we could assemble a natural history of his disorder, and develop insights into its genesis and effects.

A hebephrenic member, Street, paradoxically induced the members to drag him into experiencing the nightmare of a dementia praecox-like inception of his disorder late in adolescence. As he regressed, he hinted all the while about a deep depression. The group, especially Street rose to the occasion of the emergency situation presented by the advent of Bostic in catatonic crisis. There laid bare was the inception of disorder, and its dynamics. He was particularly susceptible via a close relation to his mother (whom in a delusion that spoke of some underlying truth, he thought dead), to investment in a relationship of deeply ambivalent nature that advanced to a crisis in which self esteem was pathologically manifested by murder of a denigrative romantic partner.

Aspects of this configuration were present in the stories that emerged, as the members in fragmentary fashion worked their way back to capacities and identities lost during their periods of alienation. Bostic, too late, unraveled the skein of circumstance his lover and he had been caught in, emerging shaken, much sadder, and wiser, and much more able to choose and court another. Jefferson turned out to have loved the wife he had murdered, who had denigrated him. Cohen believed his mother dead, and was impelled to kill a father figure. The sex psychopaths told stories of perversity that ensued after failure in their family relations. All, or near all, in time desired reconciliation with their families of origin or the ones they had initiated.

Study of the earlier work with psychopaths had taught the need for a deeper element of intimacy I called messianism. The alienated members readily demonstrated a negative identity, but also a dialectically opposite character vector, a wish to be saved and to save. Psychic attunement to these factors, within and without, enabled the group processes to open up to a reconciliative transaction. I was surprised that the dead-enders of Howard Hall yielded as readily as they did, to collaborate as did the young men at Fort Knox, building a considerable and sophisticated program.

This surprise extended to the collaboration of the hardened psychotic criminals and the new sexual psychopaths assigned to the program with the inception, post-War of the Miller Act, pertaining to sexual offenders. Personnel expected combat between the psychotic and sexually psychopathic members, perhaps mortal. But the program, operative for about a year and a half, took it in stride. After a certain amount of insult and opprobrium, the members agreed that they all suffered pathology, and that was already yielding to their work in the groups. They expected that these "queer ducks" would turn into simple and complex human beings like themselves, and make their way back to their families and society.

The therapeutic course of the sex psychopaths turned out to be analogous to that of the psychotics. First came their defensive ploy, as with Foster or Hollister, in which they arrogantly asserted their superiority. The psychotic members, having gone through that phase with Holden and Street, saw through it, responding with integrity and appropriateness, leaving the members to lose their bearings in their pathology, and begin the decompensation experienced prominently in the war-time work with psychopaths. In the meanwhile, they began yielding up their personal histories, understandable to the members. All were drawn into the manifold activities of the occupational therapy program, the reading groups, and the educational program mounted mostly with patient teachers.

The attendant staff in Howard Hall played an important part in the work. I attempted to orient them to the endeavor, mostly through example and transparency. I met briefly with them, after the sessions, explaining my motives and actions, and evoking discussion. Some lent themselves to the group dynamic, by simply sitting, even participating. Others boycotted, complaining through channels about the noise the patients made afterwards, and "difficulty settling them down." The initial conflict culminated in removal of the group from the Admitting Ward to one more chronic, ostensibly safer. The authoritarian style of leadership extant in the Hall was illustrated by a failure on the part of the Chief Nurse to consult with me on that move. Later, when patients improved sufficiently to be transferred to the main hospital, it was done so, independently of my input.

Establishment of the large Integrated Group, done after consultation with the Chief of Service, resulted in a crisis, marked by mounting racial hostility on the part of a clique of attendants. The black patients had become dominant in the sessions, through production of music and participation in problem solving. Attendants objected to their use of the bathroom and gathered during a session to vent their outrage towards me. I fended them off, later working it through with the Chief of Service and the Chief Nurse. A formal training program was later instituted as part of a Hospital-Wide Group Work Training Program.

Resolution of the battle with the attendants was a later development, leading to general recognition of the groups as valid in the eyes of personnel and patients. Before that came the recognition, as useful partners, by the Red Cross, the dietitian, and the occupational therapy department. All contributed to cultural normalization, followed by recognition by the press, consisting of the local newspaper and a national newsmagazine. By that time Howard Hall had achieved an aura, soon spread via *The Howard Hall Journal*, a newspaper established through the efforts of a patient William Cohen and Mrs. Janet Sheridan, the occupational therapist who mounted a sophisticated program in a trying setting. This in turn led to visits by psychiatrists from all over the globe, one, Yoshiko Ikeda, who came to be known by the patients as my "sidekick."

Unlike the work at Fort Knox, which came about through Army decree, this program was developed as we went along, and mutual confidence established, to counter an ever present sense of danger. That I had to prove myself is understandable, in light of prior reports of brief successes in the history of work with schizophrenics and the mortal danger of the work. The important variable appeared to be the sense of conviction of the intervener. Mine stemmed from my successful experience, identification with Colonel Miller and Lloyd McCorkle of Fort Knox, my messianism and a scientific attitude which called on me to test hypotheses.

A complete presentation of *This Way Out* has been handicapped by the inaccessibility of clinical records due to a decision by the Bureau of Records to destroy all but a fraction of the records, but for some rendered in a code, itself inaccessible to me. However, for scientific purposes the extraordinarily detailed and reliable session protocols I daily dictated are coherent and patterned enough from which to draw inferences. The mere fact that we were able to mount successful large groups, with up to 110 black and white patients is of significance, besides the detailed protocols. Then there were the coherent narratives of individuals and groups, their characteristic patterns of interaction, and discernable phases of development.

INFERENCES

Going in, there were a number of inferences, developed in the crucible of the wartime Army, pertinent to the work with the groups and individuals. The first related to the phenomenon of *alienation*, the break with self and others that resulted in severing of emotional and social ties. It appeared deeper and more difficult to alter than the usual Freudian mental mechanisms, repression, the most analogous. Alienation resulted in loss of human status, whereas the repressed individual remained essentially human.

We learned to infer the presence of alienation through behavior, history, and most important, intuition on the ego state of the alienated other. A corollary inference was that of *reconciliation*, the acceptance of the reality of self and the other. This process appeared to be accompanied by deep displays of emotion. I early learned to sense its advent through a subjective psychosomatic sense in my chest and head, my intuitometer, which I was able to teach to my personnel. Another important aspect of the alienation/reconciliation experience was the decompensation, noted earlier, psychopaths experienced in the course of loss of that defense, manifested by depression, confusion, insomnia, psychosomatic disorder, and brief psychosis. More on that later, plus its set of inferences.

A third phenomenon had to do with group process, including the diad of therapist and other. It is called *regression*, a state of psychic traversal from a previous state, to one of greater depth. Regression could be trusting and generative, or further alienating and destructive. At Knox we became practiced at discerning both, again through observation, external and internal. The trusting regression enabled the subjects to encounter with alienated aspects of self in the dialogic manner, intrapsychic and interpersonal, of psychoanalysis, through the transference of aspects of the past present in the ego. In Howard Hall, the Black Therapy Group displayed trusting therapeutic regression early, in the thirteen step analysis, plus, surprising appearance of the trans-ference. Again regression could be inferred through behavior, history, and intuition.

A fourth phenomenon noted at Knox was that of *the group as an entity*. We learned to sense when a group became its proper self, the roles members took in that process and its furtherance, and its specific patterns of behavior. We learned to detect the atmosphere it gave forth, and the different characteristics of its different sizes. The latter consideration was instrumental in the estab-lishment of the Integrated Group in Howard Hall, which paradoxically was more effective than the smaller groups. . Noted earlier, the establishment of the Black Therapy Group as an entity is examined in detail in a microanalysis. It became overt, with the capacity to negotiate with the dietitian and election of chairman.

A fifth phenomenon was the fact of *normalization* that ensued with the establishment in previous work in the Army, of cultural assets like a radio station, newspaper, the Colonel's music hour, and an orientation to the war program in which the prospective soldiers taught each other re the issues in the war and its progress. The lessons learned there were essential to the success at Howard Hall, preparing the patients for life in reality. Central in normalization was the education program, which existed formally at Knox, less so in Howard Hall. But the process of therapy was inherently educative, with the added massive task of debriefing from psychopathic and psychotic ways and their sets of knowledge.

Sixth and most important is the spectrum of phenomena, resultant from alienation from self and others, of *psychosis and psychopathy*. In extreme form, it was the subject of incipient research at Fort Knox, in the person of Rampa. My thesis was that understanding of that man, leader and charismatic figure for the rest, would yield the comprehension of how to reach our failures in the effort. His alienation appeared the ultimate of purposefulness, leading me to conceive that in the enactment of perverse ideals, he was following some inner core of his personality. I suspected that the core was a negative version of the Freudian ego ideal. But the literature of psychoanalysis said little about that phenomenon in the psychotic and psychopathic. In fact, Karpman, an advanced researcher on the psychopath, spoke of *anethnopaths,* completely without ideals. One can infer that Karpman's anethnopath had an ego ideal that denied having ideals.

At Knox we inferred the presence of that extreme of psychopathy by the, to us, distinctive appearance, mode of verbal and action representation, history, and our intuitions. As I noted in this volume, I set myself the task of further research, and was gratified with the opportunity presented by Howard Hall for work with multiple Rampas. Marking his perverse ingenuity and vigor, at

Knox we enclosed Rampa within a prison within the prison, behind double barbed wire, set on dig-proof large caliber rocks. Escape proof Howard Hall was surrounded by 35 foot concrete walls, reached through a tunnel, capped by a thick iron gate.

That immurement became part of the research design, because Jordan, Holden, Jefferson, and Cohen had incorporated it into their identities as psychopath and psychotic. It was a source of pride, despair, and apathy. And so, while subsumed under *psychosis and psychopathy*, it was an entity of its own, awaiting the change from "hell hole" status brought about by the break through action of the patients in meeting with the Red Cross, dietitian, and occupational therapist, and in time, graduating from the Hall. My terror filled encounter with Jordan at the inception was a break in the wall of rage encasing this man. In work with him, I learned a great deal about his alienated worlds, and how to enter those of his fellows.

Chapter Six

The Work as Therapy and Research

I have made much of the impetus for research evoked by the dramatic self sacrifice of Rampa, the leader of the failures at the Fort Knox Rehabilitation Center. Again, Howard Hall gave us the opportunity to work with people as indurated in their pathology. I have expounded on my approach to both Fort Knox and Howard Hall, formally in the text and through a running commentary. There I have emphasized the influence of the Chicago Area Project, itself stemming from the research projects and community intervention stratagems of the Department of Sociology of the University of Chicago. I was introduced to group and role theory and practice by Lloyd W. McCorkle, who had participated with Professor Clifford Shaw in the Chicago Area Project.

Specifically, we considered that we studied the sociologic dynamics of our Center in the manner that Professor Shaw did his Project. However, we looked more deeply, through psychoanalytic methods, at the instance of a psychoanalyst, Dr. Alexander Wolf, who was pioneering in psychoanalytic group therapy. This led us to look into the family dynamics of our subjects. We learned the value of systematic session protocols for mutual consultation and research. Above all, our treatment team, which included Colonel George Miller, our Commandant, developed hypotheses about the work, which we tested in our daily work and planned to test in future projects.

The first hypothesis related to the slogan we had developed, "From Gripe to Group." In the early phase of development, the groups would manifest antisocial griping, followed by a pregnant silence, then prosocial collaboration, discussing issues productively. In that, the atmosphere or feel of the group would change radically. This configuration would occur with almost clockwork regularity. We learned to predict its occurrence, a matter of scientific import. I had noted a coincident intuitively relevant substernal sensation that I later came to call, my "intuitometer."

We hypothesized that the pregnant pause was nexal to the process, involving social and personal crises in the participants. I adduced a notion I had developed of a spiritual nature to that pause I called messianic, that the rehabilitees had invested the therapists, and through us the entire institution with that messianism. We noted a strong emotional connection during their tenure at the Center, to us and to one another.

Another hypothesis pertained to the effect of this motivational dynamic on education, as explanatory of the ten point rise in educational achievement scores. Another related to the loyalty and adherence of the rehabilitees to the program after leaving it, as evidence of their voluntary involvement and adoption of a proselytizing stance.

Most telling, re research into the pathology of psychopathy, were the phenomena of depression, anxiety, and psychosomatic illness that ensued after loss by the rehabilitee of his psychopathic defenses. We hypothesized that in reconciliation with self, the rehabilitee was recovering from a state of alienation, and through psychopathy the person had transcended an intolerable internal state. We were struck by the fealty the psychopath had to his pathology, as a factor in the difficulty in its treatment.

We noted the importance of recognition of the sociologic concept of transaction, a unity of interacting entities, and its importance in recognition of our necessary involvement in the treatment. We were inherent parts of the prosocial gangs we formed in the course of treatment! We also noted the regression in the process that Freud had discovered, and the ascription of previous experience he had discovered as transference. Not only that, but we saw that we brought to it our previous experience and personality sets, something that came to be called countertransference. Then there were the cultural and historical transferences, as in the revolutionary and reactionary mobs of the past, reenacted before our eyes.

Stemming from the startling success of the large groups, we hypothesized that the larger size drew the natural leaders into compelling action, which regularly enabled us to significantly alter the leadership and the nature of the groups. They could not resist revelation of their antisocial stances. It was apparent that such large size called for specific leadership on our part, warranting deeper study.

Though the subjects of this volume were indurated psychotics (with psychopathic features), they surprised us by yielding to the therapy and forming a therapeutic community. This paradox was even more present in the large Integrated Group. The sex psychopaths also largely joined in and were initiating basic changes for the better.

The complex of hypotheses derived from the experience at Knox were largely applicable: (1) The groups in Howard Hall went through crises in the development of the therapeutic encounter, as in the "gripe to group" experience, but they were not as clear as at Knox. It was manifestly definitive in the large groups, which showed more of the perceptible pregnant pause; (2) The orientation of the members was altered in that they became invested in matters educational and cultural, developing institutions of literary and musical nature; (3) They reconciled with their premorbid selves, and also with their families; (4) Having breeched their alienation from self and others, they were opened to care for themselves, conceiving of self in their life courses, with a view to making choices in such. In doing so, they manifested the human transaction particular to psychoanalysis, with constructive regression and the appearance of transference; (5) They also went through the states of anxiety and confusion we had noted at Knox, on loss of their previous defenses. (6) Lastly, the dynamics of the members of the Integrated Group, 70+ in number, were closer to those at Knox, than the small therapy groups, in reaching through to alienated members, and establishment of mutual aid.

During the work in Howard Hall, I obtained glimpses of a process underlying the delusions and hallucinations of the members, the existence of myth. Vince Jordan appeared in a mythic thrall, with the array of autistic identities that distinguished him from his fellows. Jefferson enacted a mythic small town Southern leader. He and others had constructed what came in the psychoanalytic literature to be called personal myth, a screen for the underlying truth, full of distortion, concerning their families and lives. The groups became quite practiced in intuitive reaching through to underlying reality, by experience of their personal myth and otherwise mythic selves, through individually based and inter-member free association.

As a budding psychoanalyst, it became apparent to me that the group method, though not recognized in the psychoanalytic literature, enabled the patients to attain a state of transaction that put them in position for the analytic method proper. I also recognized that I needed further training in its application. I needed a theory of personal development, family dynamics, personality organization, and above all, the influence of the past on the present, psychoanalytic transference.

The reader will ask, how did this beginning psychiatrist develop the presumption to subject himself to patients with a known history of sudden, fatal violence, and expect to lead them into formation of a therapeutic community? The answer lies in prior experience that I cite here and in the volume, *Turning Lives Around*, of favorable kind with psychopaths. But more so, there were special aspects there of extraordinary sort that gave me special confidence in the work with severely alienated individuals.

I shall detail an important aspect of that work briefly. During the last of World War II, my treatment unit had been given the task of calming down a detachment of riotous Army prisoners. Shipped over from France, from the Loire Detention Training Center, they had been subjected to a punishing regimen of hard labor, denigration, sleep in slit trenches, eating out of garbage cans, and lack of change of clothes, resulting in lice. This regimen was supposed to punitively subject them to the hardships of soldiers in the field. By teaching them such a lesson, they would be sobered about their deviance and motivated to return to combat duty. That outcome was foreclosed by the end of the war in the European Theater. Their Commandant was court- martialed for his part, and they were on their way to Leavenworth Penitentiary, stopping enroute at Fort Knox for special processing.

The shipment numbered 500, heavily guarded. After being housed, fed, and clothed adequately, batches of 250 were provided aspects of our program, starting with group therapy. First came emotional ventilation, in a large group format. Their leaders opened up, wild, intending revenge by word and deed. However, the phenomenon we had encountered in the large groups prior, took hold. Their leadership fell in fits on the way to attacking me, or became incoherent to impotence. Cooler heads in the groups then proceeded to a thorough, at times poignant debriefing, and they went on their way. The potency of large groups with alienated individuals, in a structured program, became doubly apparent.

Following that, on VJ Day I had the experience that I have described earlier, with a thoroughly hardened psychopath, Rampa. There my inference was that, though we had failed to rehabilitate him, the program had reached him in his emotional core. There was an essential dialog going, encouraging me to go on in the exploration of the subject of alienation. Add to that the evidence we had accumulated on the facilitating effect of messianism, plus my own still untrammeled messianism, my motivation to take on the community of Howard Hall become understandable.

I was also encouraged by the experience of success in training of a corps of therapists taken from the ranks of soldiers judged grade C, unsuited for regular military duty. They ranged from former shoe salesman to orchestra leader, and were eager students. One of the rehabilitees became proficient as therapist. The success of the group method in our school at Knox led me to institute such early in the work in Howard Hall. Also at Knox, we found the rehabilitees proficient in establishing an orientation to the war program, leading their own discussion groups in their barracks.

So I had a model to replicate, though admittedly easier with the Fort Knox psychopaths. At Howard Hall we had psychotic individuals whose psychopathy was hardened in a manner comparable to Rampa's. I was highly motivated to resume work on their alienation and to develop a program as platform for that study.

I missed the close in support of Colonel Miller, but did have the benignly abstinent one of the Superintendent of St. Elizabeths, Dr. Wilfred Overholser, whom I kept closely advised of the progress. Then there was the support and collaboration of Dr. Bernard Cruvant, my Chief of Service, who had done group therapy during his wartime service, and in time began what we called administrative therapy groups.

Almost from the beginning, the Howard Hall patients took psychoeducational initiative, and sought recreational and cultural opening to the world. The hospital Red Cross eagerly met their needs, with ready supply of games, magazines, books, and musical instruments. The Food Service responded, again early, meeting with the patients, and changing the boiled to fried chicken, a major item. Then with the subsiding of danger, the Occupational Therapy Department met with the patients, sending Janet Sawyer, a courageous and talented young woman, who quickly formed positive relationships with the leaders of the patient groups, then developed a thoroughgoing program. It prominently featured a newspaper that was begun by one of the patients.

The entrepreneurial spirit of the patients, in building their own culture, reinforced their efforts in the therapy proper, and countered the powerful chronic mental hospital and prison cultures. It also enabled them to withstand the unfavorable climate generated by the attendants who adhered to their old ways of maintaining security.

I engaged with that entrepreneurial spirit in my first encounter with Vince Jordan, then with the initial group, plotting with them their release by self growth. Somewhere within their psyches, they must have sensed that I was joining with them as a fellow human being, and some sensed that I, too, had problems with alienation. Along with that, was a core messianic message. We formed a mutuality consisting of those three elements. The hope and support resident within enabled them to admit to their nadir-hood and alienation. The next step was resurrection of their human feelings. They could rejoin the world of reality they had left. From that platform they could renegotiate leaving their worlds of alienation and their affiliations.

Vince Jordan was vividly caught in that dilemma, arguing with the voices that had given him solace in the crisis through which he had left reality, while in solitary in prison. Subsequently, from his position as delusionary king, he had the obligation to be their enforcer. Failure there would engender guilt. Wilfred Bostic felt guilty towards his alienated ideals, for opening up in the group. The two fought physically for their honor and hegemony.

I sensed that, once in reality, both were vulnerable to haunts from the past, experienced as the transference. Lacking systematic individual therapy, I was not able to explore those ties, as I did in later work in a Maximum Security

Hospital. I obtained inklings of it in traversal of Bostic's onset of psychosis, and in work at St. Elizabeths with a group of schizophrenic women and their mothers (*Maternal Dependency and Schizophrenia*, International University Press, New York, 1953). I found both the Bostic couple and the mothers and daughters to be fixed in a transactional unity, with a role reversal and alienated tie. The mothers were abysmally dependent on their daughters, and caught in a deep ambivalence towards their husbands.

I did have a brief therapeutic encounter with the Bostic family, enlisting the aid of his sister in breaking away from the family's myth of denial of "trouble," enforced by his father and brother. Subsequent work along family analytic lines would have been helpful. Similarly, Cohen, Jordan, Jefferson, Reardon, James, Murphy, and Thomas all could have been helped analytically to reconcile with their families, or to make their way autonomously.

SUMMARY

The work at Howard Hall was built directly on that at Fort Knox. In both we achieved an institution that mobilized numbers of men, alienated from self and others, to seek reconciliation, and through that reintegration with society. In both, we learned the reliability of the therapeutic group formations, small and large, and to discern their phases of development. In Knox 40% of the rehabilitees had their dishonorable discharges remanded and made it back to the Army and combat. Rather than immured in chronicity, a steady stream of patients were discharged from Howard Hall to the courts and less secure hospital programs. Howard Hall was transmuted into a therapeutic community, with a sophisticated milieu therapy program. The success at Howard Hall emboldened personnel to develop a group work training program and extensive penetration of the formerly static services by therapy groups conducted by a broad range of professionals.

By the end of the work at both, we were well advanced in the capacity to discern when groups were formed as entities, role assumption in the process, and when they appeared to exist in our common reality. All of that proved testable, in our conferences. Along with that we developed hypotheses about alienation, group, interpersonal, and intrapsychic. We were on the way to discerning a relationship between alienation and the psychoanalytic transference, in which the transference was a step along the way to reconciliation with current reality. We sensed the crisis the psychopaths traversed in the process.

As important and integral to the success, was growing penetration to the conundrum posed at Knox, by the question of what impelled the psychopaths

in their self destructive courses, exemplified by Rampa. In his severe alienation Rampa could be considered as psychotic, in the manner that Cleckley
described as moral insanity. He was disabled in a core function, a thought
disorder pertaining to his conscience. On the way to his death, he gave evidence of inner conflict, eventuating in revelation of an inner imperative, an
alienated conscience that called for his death.

In the Howard Hall experiment, we were able to elicit and focus on that
alienated conscience, starting with core considerations of alienation from self
and other, of 23 individuals, as they participated in building its therapeutic
community. In itself, that community structure can be considered as a seminal
achievement. The struggles of Vince Jordan and Loren Jones with their alienated consciences, especially in the case of Jordan, provided leads to further
inquiry into the natural history of that core alienation.

Despite the interest of fellow residents and staff members in the work in
Howard Hall, we did not form a study group comparable to that at Fort Knox.
Recognition of the validity of positive institutional changes did result in formation by Dr. Overholser of a Hospital Wide Group Work Training Program,
which in turn developed training groups, but not research capabilities. I did
participate in the Veterans Administration Group Therapy Research Project,
and the publication of my findings in work with large groups, in *Group Psychotherapy*, Powdermaker and Frank, Harvard University Press, 1953, and a
research project at St. Elizabeths Hospital, *Maternal Dependency and Schizophrenia*, Abrahams and Varon, International Universities Press, 1953.

FURTHER RESEARCH

The work at both Fort Knox and Howard Hall led to an array of observations
to be confirmed, and hypotheses to be tested. For 40 years my arena of inquiry
was a psychoanalytic practice which encompassed the severe disorders and
also group consultation in a number of clinics, hospitals, and the National Institute of Mental Health. I early discerned that I sought to attain the poignant
connectedness of the hushed silence of the Fort Knox groups, manifested by
what I came to call my intuitometer. I had taught my therapists at Knox to
detect theirs, before I gave it a name, and extended that lesson to my group
consultation. Its absence on the part of the residents who substituted for me
in Howard Hall impaired their capacity to lead those groups.

In my private practice I developed combined group and individual therapy
in psychoanalytic work with a broad range of mental illnesses, teaching such
methodology with groups of mental health professionals, including encounter
groups. I adapted the detailed record keeping of my work at Howard Hall and

the work with mothers and daughters at St. Elizabeths to my private practice. The results of their analysis will be published as *Terra Incognita: Exploring Psychoanalytic Frontiers.*

I had the opportunity to test my methods and hypotheses institutionally at the Atascadero State Hospital, 1990-1996. There I applied therapeutic community lessons and hypotheses in individual therapy I had learned in four decades of analytic work with the severe disorders in private practice. At Atascadero my office on the ward was open to patients who in good faith wished to work on their problems. A number did so, meeting with me, from two minutes to an hour, and from one to five times weekly, complete with dream analysis. Despite initial trepidation of the staff, my trust was never abused. Half of the ward of 24 were members of a Living in Reality Group, making sense of their lives and empowering themselves. Administrative difficulty got in the way of systematic family therapy. The work will be published under the title of *An Adventure in Self Transformation: Therapeutic Community at Atascadero State Hospital.*

Chapter Seven

The Maximum Security
Mental Hospital of the Future

This is an opportunity to rethink the philosophy and practice of a maximum security mental hospital. First consideration is the element of security. The traditional way to maximum security was through construction of fortress-like structures, barriers to egress and ingress, with provision for internal sequestration. Howard Hall was a good example of that. The John Howard Pavilion that replaced it looks like any other mental hospital, and attains its security through a certain amount of structure, but mostly through its way of handling its prisoner patients, through the efficiency of its sally port, but more so through its therapeutic program.

At the inception of the illness of these severely disordered individuals there is certainly need for maximum security, for their protection and that of society. Should it be by means of a 35 foot concrete wall, or even a twelve foot double wire, electrified wall? Certainly not. Where should it be located? Certainly where it is needed, and readily accessible to the families of the patients and training facilities of forensic nature.

I envision that the maximum security mental hospital and its allied treatment prison of the future would have a "university behind walls" that would be a center for research and training in matters forensic (see *Turning Lives Around: Wartime Treatment of Military Prisoners*, Abrahams, Joseph, AuthorHouse, 2006). We are increasingly aware of the incidence of mental illness in prison populations, and the likelihood that psychopathy in its alienation is closely linked to mental illness. The maximum security mental hospital therefore would have an integral relationship with the treatment prison in the training of personnel, exchange of prisoner/patients, and above all in the academic core of the prison, its University Within Walls.

The architecture of this hospital would follow its function, but adapting heavily from resort hotels, even cruise ships, to reflect its many-sided therapeutic interventions. We note the grand architecture and grounds of the Dorothea Dix mental hospitals mean to bring out an aspiration towards culture, the dignity and enlargement of the individual.

Then there is the issue of architecture for the groups inherent to therapeutic community. A particular challenge is a living space for the large groups. At Knox, we found ourselves able to manage therapeutic groups of 225. The chapel in Howard Hall could manage 110. The large size of the groups was instrumental to their successful dynamics. The question left was, how much larger could they safely be? How to design ready access to a group, in emergencies? Another issue would be provision for intensive work with families, and multifamily assemblages. Then there is the issue of housing for overnight and more extensive stays of families and marathons.

Along with the emphasis on an integral part for academics and research, goes the normalization of the hospital culture. The full range of media, recreational, and athletics would be employed, in coordination with those of current society. Transparency would be sought, tempered by the need to protect privacy.

This progressive venture would be best begun and developed in the context of a progressive political administration, devoted to a progressive penal practice. In my book, *Turning Lives Around*, I advocate for an Institute, the California Institute for Research in Crime, which would have role of research, development, and advocacy.

Appendix A

Glossary of Terms

The terms in this glossary differ significantly, at times radically, from their definition in the psychiatric and psychoanalytic literature, and call for elaboration. They reflect the author's conceptual development as he traversed the experiences at Fort Knox, Howard Hall, private practice, and that at the Atascadero State Hospital.

Advent Phenomenon

Because of the importance of the concept of that which is impending in the human self, I have taken the liberty to adapt to it the term *advent.* It denotes an event of arrival, of special moment, personal and social. In religious experience it is the term for the coming of Christ, of profound salvationist meaning to his contemporaries and since. In the work at Knox I noted a significant phenomenon, a hushed, pregnant state, followed by evidence of conversion from alienation to reconciliation with common reality. Discussion in our therapeutic conference brought the realization of the momentousness of what had become a systematic occurrence, with overtones we increasingly recognized as messianic. Further evidence of the advent phenomenon is presented in this Glossary in a discussion of messianism. The advent phenomenon may be considered as a transitional state, bordering on the parapsychological, pertinent to issues in that aspect of the self denoted as soul. Also, see soul in this Glossary.

Alienation

Alienation at core refers to estrangement and the state of being a stranger; interpersonal withdrawal or separation, including the affects; and intrapsychic separation or splitting. Alienation from self is a central factor in my hypotheses of mental and emotional disorder. It results in rupture of relationships with others and regression to earlier developmental levels, also states of deficit, which in turn result in secondary phenomena of hallucinations and delusions.

In its massiveness and psychologically earlier occurrence, it is differentiated from repression, a Freudian mechanism of rendering thoughts and affects unavailable to consciousness, in the context of an already operative superego, or internally guiding and governing agency. I hypothesize that fundamentally alienation stems from injury to the developing psyche, extending to the nervous system, altering it towards functional blighting, then flight to higher and lower centers, and consequent alteration of essential functioning of the entire nervous apparatus. This blighting would be experienced as a temporary psychic death, followed by reestablishment of function, or resurrection. See resurrection in this Glossary, also death.

The original psychiatrists were termed alienists. Their hospitals were termed asylums, set apart geographically. From time immemorial, the mentally ill separated themselves from others, or pressed their alien theses forth, to the point where they were sequestrated as nuisances or potentially violent. Some were reflective of current dilemmas, becoming, through charisma, great religious and political leaders.

This alienation from self and others results in regression to earlier and lower levels of development, dehabituation, loss of mental and emotional faculties. Clinicians—Kraeplin, Bleuler, Meyer, Sullivan, Langfeld, and Schneider—noted different aspects of this phenomenologic elephant. The latter two are of note: Langfeld cited depersonalization, autism, emotional blunting, insidious onset, and feelings of derealization and unreality. Schneider cited symptoms of the first rank: audible thoughts, voices heard arguing, commenting on one's actions, influences playing on one's body, thought withdrawal or interference, diffusion of thought, delusional conception and perception, ascription to the other of impulses and volition.

That was the experience, along with manifest violence, of the members of the Howard Hall group, evidence whereby they were confined there until they changed sufficiently to live on one of the Hospital wards, or could live in the District Jail or Lorton Reformatory, or were fit for trial or execution. The criteria for such reconciliation emerged in the group life they mounted in treatment. There they recapitulated the experience of the rehabilitees at Fort Knox. In the work at Knox and Howard Hall we evoked the full force, the reality, of their state of alienation, in the context of an emerging therapeutic alliance. We offered them the choice of reconciliation to their and our reality. The therapeutic alliance had core messianic and human components. The members systematically went through an experience of communion, marked by a hushed, contemplative state, followed in the group by the emergence of pro-social leadership, as differentiated from the previous antisocial leaders.

With that pro-social cast to the rehabilitee group, the members gave evidence of initiative at normalization of the Center, development of media (newspaper, radio, recreation, an orientation to the war program), and an esprit de corps. A corollary feature was the treatment by the medical clinic of states of depression and confusion on the part of the rehabilitees as they lost the comfort and safety of their psychopathic defenses.

Similar phenomena appeared in Howard Hall, as the therapy progressed, and it became socialized. Recovery from disordered, alienated states led to inferences on the nature of alienation. Data on those inferences and the processes of their development permeate this work, chiefly in the running commentary, and the section on the courses of individuals.

Animistic

This would be an early stage in the development of religion, involving identification with and worship of aspects of nature. The surfer may be animistic, in worship of the God of the Curling Wave. My thesis is that we all experience mankind's religious past and its stages of development. This awareness is of moment in working with regressed schizophrenics and their strange gods. Vince Jordan identified with panthers, a feral animism. Bolster was a nature lover, seeing it and a farm as curative.

Autism

One of the pioneers in looking afresh at the human situation, this time at children, psychiatrist Kanner in 1943 described a state of aloneness or social detachment he called autism. It was marked by obsessive desire for preservation of sameness, a specific relationship to objects that contrasted with the child's inability to relate to people, an intelligent and responsive capacity, and either total mutism or variety of language not intended for interpersonal communication. Others have refined these observations and noted an enlarged prevalence in childhood, adolescent and adult populations. In a search for still earlier incidence there were noted additional absences, those of eye contact, anticipatory reaching, smiling, facial responsiveness. Further noted was apathetic indifference, and lack of reaction to affection and physical closeness. Violation of the state of sameness required by the autistic person results in panic, terror, and deeply disturbed behavior. Bizarre motions, emotional states and verbal behavior are present. While retreat in autism obviously occurs, a rich inner fantasy life has not been identified, but remarkable intellectual capacities are presented.

The patients in Howard Hall were beset by autism. They fought to preserve sameness, appeared detached or its opposite, related better to objects, went in and out of muteness, and exhibited underlying intelligence. Some acted bizarrely. Donald Street, a hebephrenic manifested a florid autism.

Autonomy

Each item in this glossary is central to conceptualizing the situation of the patients in the Howard Hall venture, but this one is most of all, With the exit from Howard Hall dependent on the attainment of the capacity of the patient's ego to live in his own and common reality, as differentiated from the thrall of psychosis and psychopathy, the members were called on to transact in a therapeutic alliance with treating authority. This was made possible by what I call messianic mutuality, in which there was conversion to an already present messianic aspect of self, versus the psychopathic and psychotic self. From that vantage point the individual could contemplate and examine his developmental past, to discern when he split away from his ego reality and resume transaction in that mode. Taking counsel with me and their peers, they learned to live again with one another and the world at large. In that exercise, they grew in autonomy and self confidence. Again, Of the 24 chosen to illustrate the courses of the patient population, Vince Jordan's internal struggle is the most documented and dramatic, engaged between autonomy in current reality, and autistic autonomy. In Dr. Powell's popular literature discussion group the members earnestly worked on what it meant to have a mind and options of one's own. Cohen learned to exercise his ego in counseling his fellows, becoming stronger in fighting off his demons.

Death

Death figured prominently in this work and that at Fort Knox. At Knox we prepared the rehabilitees to face mortal combat when, in the well documented Orientation to the War Program, we followed and reviewed the battles in the Pacific, North African, and European Theaters. Also in the Fort Knox experience, Rampa held that he "had to" die, and did so literally in my arms. In Howard Hall, in terror, I faced death at Vince Jordan's hands. Loren Jones fantasized bombing me to death. William Cohen was determined to kill the Commandant of his psychiatric hospital, and John Jefferson accomplished that act with seven blows of a hammer to his wife's skull. Cohen was convinced his mother was dead, and his live mother an impostor. Wilfred Bostic also was convinced his mother was dead, and later killed his fiancée, and believing he was dead, was surprised to be alive. Donald Street tried to murder his psychiatrist. Frank Certa became psychotic on the death of his mother. Dennis Smith came close to murdering a president.

Much of the death in those stories was intended, some experienced as present in others and self, and in still others, compulsively perpetrated. I considered all those versions to be equally worthy of study, from a dynamic point of view. Within the psychic realm, death appears to be spiritually coupled with resurrection. I link that to messianism, an inborn saving capacity, in turn capable of carrying the organism to other levels of organization and capacity.

It was apparent to me that Rampa professed a perverse ideal that resulted in his death. In exposing myself to Vince Jordan's imperative to kill me, I was enacting an imperative ideal of my own. Transcendent ideals can be identified in most of the cases cited here. As explanatory theory, Freud arrived at a transcendent myth, that of a basic death instinct. Yet there is also a myth, that of Narcissus, that allows us make sense of this core conundrum.

Narcissus knew that his death had been foretold by the sage Tiresias, who had stated that he would die, when he knew himself. It is a short step to posit that as he gazed at his glorious image in admiration, in time, remembering Tiresias, he looked in the water for data on who he really was. His lineage was that of son of a river god and a nymph. Stemming from the doubt incited by Tiresias, he disassociated himself from the glory of godhood, the water turned dark, and he died, disillusioned. His paramour Echo had already died, secondary to his absorption with Olympian glory.

Narcissus was one of the spring flowers of Greece, along with the hyacinth and anemone. In early Greek tribal history, children were reputed to have been sacrificed to ensure the crops. In later myth, the crimson Anemone sprung from the blood of Adonis, over whom Aphrodite and Persephone fought. The hyacinth was derived from Hyacinthus, who was killed by his elder and lover, Apollo. While Hyacinthus seemed to have some element of choice in associating with Apollo, Narcissus for the while fully gave himself over to the Olympian ideals of glory and beauty. Deviation from such fealty called for death and self sacrifice. This element of sacrifice, stemming from involvement in the toils of the Gods, was present in the great exercise of narcissism and turning point in world history, the enthusiastic flocking to the colors of French, German, and English at the inception of the First World War. That glory, attended by sacrifice, came to be seen as an illusion if not delusion, by the time of the battle of Verdun in 1916, and massive death on the part of the French. This resulted in a sense of reality and the death, pro tem, of the national ideal of glory as well as the death of God himself. Narcissus got to know himself as a dupe, and died.

I have inferred that Rampa sacrificed himself for a perverse, narcissistic ideal. Vince Jordan, beholden to his voices, was prepared to sacrifice me, was deterred by adherence to a parallel God-state, in which he was a messiah. Loren Jones transcended self into godhood, giving him the authority to bomb and kill. William Cohen was entirely willing to mete out such punishment to the Commandant of his military hospital, subsequent to the delusion of the death of his mother. Wilfred Bostic, likewise, was convinced his mother was dead, that his fiancée had killed something deep within him, and taking her with him to an actual death, was surprised that he was still alive.

I further infer that these individuals were caught in mythic thralls of various permutations and combinations, in which actual death was consequent to psychic death. The emotional ties would be deeply regressed, in which they belonged to one another and were swallowed up by one another in the manner of the Greek generations of God. These formulations were *in nuce* at the time of the work in Howard Hall, to be developed further in my private practice and at Atascadero State Hospital.

Ego ideal

In his ideal self concept, the initial protagonist in this piece, Vince Jordan, held to an apogee, as King, Nat King Cole, the President-General, and Christ. Later in the therapy he held that he was at the nadir of human identity. In both high and low estates, he exemplified an aspect of personality I hold to be central to this study, the ego ideal. The assumption is that there is an organizing function of the personality that Freudians call the ego. Its governing aspect is recognized as the super ego. The superordinate function as template and repository of ideal states, standards, and outcomes has been termed the ego ideal. As effecting monitoring of the relation to the whole and its parts, it would be the mediator of reality.

Its core significance to our study became apparent. The sessions at Knox manifested a series of crises, centering about ego ideal issues. I have cited the dramatic, systematic occurrence of a pregnant pause in the griping in the psychopathic groups at Knox, followed by civilized collaboration. We inferred a spiritual component, having to do with the ego ideal. The identity of the participants may be considered to have changed from criminal to normative. A similar but more complex version of this phenomenon occurred systematically in Howard Hall. William Cohen changed from exemplary bad actor, a likely assassin, to ideal proselytizer of therapy; his visage, mein, stance, and behavior changed accordingly.

I hold that the locus of organization of personality accords with the Freudian concept of ego ideal. That concept would be one aspect of a group of entities—

self, identity, superego, ego ideal, soul — all contained in each other like Russian dolls, subject to reversal of position. Notably, I have added soul to the formation, in recognition of the place of essence and essential functioning.

Freud had it that the ego ideal watched over the ego for how it measured up to its ideals, the self as the self would really like to be. The super ego became the enforcer, measurement left to the ego ideal. The ego ideal later was conceived to be the repository (through identification and introjection, of idealized parental figures, and aspired to careers and states). Freud held that the ego ideal was formed late in adolescence, when the individual forsakes childhood issues, turning to adult concerns, forming individual life aspirations and self guiding values and concepts. But throughout, he had the two, superego and ego ideal, bound together. He was graphic in denoting the ego ideal as central in the constitution of human groups, which would include the group of two. It would account for amorous fascination, subordination to a hypnotist, and submission to a leader, "put one and the same object in place of their ego ideal, and have consequently identified themselves with one another in their ego"

It would appear that the ego ideal, in its centrality is concerned with life aspirations and positioning in larger reality, would be the mediator on issues of reality itself. Otherwise stated, through it we ascertain our sense of reality and position in regard to it. The ego ideal would by that token be the repository and effector of the course of life and sense of destiny, of hope and doom. Vince Jordan, in his Hamlet-like peregrinations centered his thought and feelings about ego ideal issues.

The role of the ego ideal in group functioning, so vividly depicted by Freud in *Group Psychology and Analysis of the Ego* was centerpiece in the Howard Hall groups. That was evident most clearly in the Integrated Group, resulting in ready conversion of deeply regressed members, like Forsyth, Lopez, and Jones, to ready collaborators.

Generations of God

The evolution of the Godhead, personal and societal, is here conceived to be in a multigenerational manner, most clearly shown in the Greek theogony, starting with Chaos, then Chronos, Zeus, to Prometheus, who conceived of, and generated man. Chronos swallowed his children, and was caused to disgorge them. This happens to man, psychically, on a soul level. In the Semitic god system, Jehovah denied the existence of previous gods, such as Astarte, although the Old Testament has passing reference to Gods. The study of the generations of god, from animistic to the current version, is of great moment, in inquiry into the god experience and the transformations that Vince Jordan experienced in his psychosis. Jones early regressed into godhood, as did Thomas later in the work.

God

Starting with the experience and definition of God as the supreme or ultimate reality, one moves into conceptions and attributions that are personalistic, and the qualities of human existence (creation, sustenance, judgment, redemption, righeousnessness, etc.). Study of the anthropology of God reveals thousands of deities, as evidence of the plasticity of the experience, also its universality. The inference can be drawn that the experience of God is inherent to the human psyche, and is a man-made attribution to nature. That nature is evidently systematic, but we clearly impute purpose there.

The God experience is also inherent to the stories of the men in Howard Hall, to which they systematically regress, claiming they are God, or a representative.

Id

The work in Howard Hall was impelled by messianism and a scientific curiosity, effected through intuition that was related intimately to an awareness deep within the personality, which Freud termed the id. He derived that concept from Georg Groddeck, who called it the It, "a wondrous force which both directs what he himself does, and what happens to him. Man is lived by the It." In work with the psychopaths at Fort Knox and the criminal psychotic population in Howard Hall, I sensed that id force. That awareness led my hair to stand on end in the initial encounter with Vince Jordan, in response to a feral mobilization, as a panther-god. Along with that was the sacrificial myth, Christ and the criminals alongside, incident to the messianic career line. (See *The Messianic Imperative: Scourge or* Savior in the Annotated Bibliography).

Freud saw the id as a primary reservoir of instinctual drives, and repository of a primitive past, on which the ego was built. Groddeck attributed to it a deep intuitive, animal intelligence. That intelligence was exemplified in Howard Hall by the patient Street. In his hebephrenic self mobilization and id-awareness, he was a weathervane in the group, letting me know of deep currents of feelings I would otherwise miss.

The intelligence was configured in mythic fashion, in turn stemming from what Freud held were instinctual sources. However, in modification of his instinctual theory, he introduced a death instinct. Death played a large part in the lives of the members of the groups, and in my patients subsequently. My thought on the matter stems from what I term a death experience, coupled with resurrection. Both are best conceptualized in reference to the organization of a soul.

Identity

Much of the dialog of the members of the groups related to who they were, their identity on the human scene, with particular reference to the small society of Howard Hall. Erikson's schema re identity, is most useful, with its tracing of the issues humans traverse and resolve in maturation, from birth through senescence. As the members constructively regress in the therapeutic experience, they reencounter issues they have failed to work through in adolescence and early adulthood. Their resolution in the treatment prepares them for graduation from the Hall.

Intuitometer

I developed the concept of intuitometer as a manifestation of an inherent human, and to an extent animal capacity, to sense the existential situation of self and others. My thought is that in the exercise of intuition the personality mobilizes its entirety towards human connection, including the hypothesized id. We know of that connectedness intrapsychically, psychosomatically, and interpersonally. I discovered that gauge of interpersonal connection in my work at Fort Knox, with the appearance at critical junctures of substernal sensation. Later, I learned to correlate it with thoughts, affects, and meaning. See the article on "My Intuitometer."

Malevolent Transformation

This term was first used by Harry Stack Sullivan, to denote the onset of antisocial attitudes and behavior in youthful males as they made transition from family to street. Its transformative nature is of interest here, implying an inner systems approach. Indeed, Sullivan did employ the term self system. Jordan underwent a malevolent transformation later in his life, during nightly crises. I first noted a transformative process in the groups at Fort Knox, from malevolent to benevolent.

Mesmer

Mesmer was an Austrian physician of the latter 18th and early 19th Centuries, who had a profound effect on European and world medicine through the introduction of a phenomenon he called "animal magnetism" and a method of hypnotism, for the treatment of psychosomatic disorders. I take the anima of "animal" to be a phenomenon of the anima or soul. His healing groups or banques were marked by manic fits similar to those experienced in my work at Fort Knox, noted in the text. In the text, the patient named James reported that the group was under a hypnotic spell.

Messianism

This phenomenon is central to this work with the severely disordered. It provides a linkage of psychotic to reality. My observation is that messianism is inherent and ubiquitous, and becomes prominent when the individual is under extreme stress and disorder. I noticed it first when I inquired why groups of psychopaths manifested pregnant pauses in their usual disruptive behavior, followed by prosocial collaborative sort. I also noticed substernal sensation I later called my intuitometer. I related the two, and conceived that they were responding to a state of being in me and themselves I had long suspected as messianism.

Study of the phenomenon and reading of the experience of authors in the philosophical, religious, and psychiatric literature has resulted in the formulation that messianism, and its saving expectation in issues of the soul. is present in the personality of each human being (see *The Messianic Imperative: Scourge Or Savior*, Abrahams, Joseph, Xlibris, 2007). In prior history it was even more prominent, as witnessed by regularly occurring gathering in expectation of the momentary arrival of a messiah, ushering in a final outcome. My study of populations, in hospital and out, is that individuals experiencing themselves to be messiahs, are many, and more frequent in earlier ages.

The messianic experience and encounter is ushered in by what, to my mind, needs to be called an advent experience, described earlier in the Glossary. I have best studied the advent experience in my private practice, as premonitory to mourning a deep intrapsychic loss. Report on that practice awaits publication of *Terra Incognita: Exploring Psychoanalytic Frontiers*.

A few instances from that practice will have to suffice. The first is that of a woman suffering from a mid-life depression. Her narcissistic defenses could no longer sustain her. Dream analysis opened her to mourning the self sacrificing grandmother who had raised her, and guilt her rational mind rejected. The advent of mourning was marked by dreams, in which she encountered a hooded figure that turned out to be the ghost of her grandmother.

In the second, a depressed middle aged man had experienced, prior to the onset of the depression, an apparition of his father, on the way home from the funeral. Unable to mourn, he immolated himself in a depressive fugue, with multiple suicidal attempts, culminating in a dream of residence within him of his incorporated father's rotting corpse. He separated himself from it by convulsive flight. He then revisited it, to mourn him and a lost life, with recovery. In the third, a young schizophrenic adult experienced the advent of a delusionary savior figure who transported her to preserve the life of a father who had died. She transferred saviorhood to me, mourning her father. After a long, painful analysis in the context of a therapeutic community, she recovered from a schizophrenic state, to come into her premorbid reality.

Each of these patients may be inferred to have messianism as a strong component to their personality. They formed a messianic mutuality with me, and then the advent experience ushered in the transference enactment and mourning of losses in their lives. The messianic tie with me of the first two yielded to standard analysis; that of the third partially so.

Myth

The word stems from the Greek mythos, or tale, related to the Gothic *maud-jan*, to remind; Old Irish *smuainim*, I think; Old Slavic, *mysli*, or thought; Lithuanian *mausti*, to desire ardently. Involved is deeply emotional cogitation, pertaining to human aspiration or experience. Use of the concept myth has been bedeviled by attributions of non verifiability, a quality of uncritical acceptance and veiled allusiveness. But myth has been generally accepted as an underlying mode of psychic function which shapes social and personal reality.

It can be thought of as comparable to the genetic code for its capacity to organize and reflect human experience, in a nuclear manner enscripting it in the psyche. The Freudian id may be thought of as a repository of myth, down to its primeval beginnings.

In this work I take a comprehensive approach to myth. Especially applicable was religious mythology, and the Greek generations of God, from Chaos, through Chronos, who swallowed his children, then Zeus, Narcissus, Prometheus, culminating in man.

In his multiple identities, Vince Jordan reached back to myth and legend for meaning, following a solitary regressive epiphany while in prison. The members of the group, themselves caught in their mythic thrall, wrestled with him, as did the angels with Jacob in the Biblical myth.

Generally accepted as an underlying mode of psychic function which shapes psychic and social reality, myth has played a large part in the conceptualization of this work. I recognized from the first that Vince Jordan was in a mythic thrall, sucking me into one, where, as victim, I would be a sacrifice to his regressed hegemonic and deistic drives, also his regression on a feral level to the panther he simulated as he tread around me. Reflection on that set of phenomena gave me a clue to understanding the driven state of Rampa as reflective of mythic regression.

Mythopoesis

If immersion and tie to old myths is central to pathology, separation from them and creation of new myth is essential to therapy. When Jordan relinquished a Christ identity for that of minister, he created a new mythic identity, still intimately tied to the old, but surfacing as a contemporary individual. He did not have to sacrifice himself as Christ would, in the myth. In starting a radio repair shop, Jefferson embraced the freeing American entrepreneurial myth of Horatio Alger leaving behind his heroic Custer's Last Stand. Cohen likewise came into a new mythic identity when he started the Howard Hall Journal.

Central to this work is the challenge of creation of new myth. Scientific study stems from such creation in the form of hypotheses, which are then tested for their approximation to reality. The challenge of modern man is creation of new reality, through such mythopoesis. That birth is accompanied by the death of the old myth, as I discuss under the rubric of narcissism. When Narcissus got to know himself, he died psychically.

Narcissism

This is a central concept in this work. In my lexicon it denotes an altered state of existence, resultant from intrapsychic trauma early in life, in which the individual enacts the mythic figure Narcissus. I have noted the story of Narcissus in my discussion of death, earlier in this Glossary, but its centrality calls for amplification. The son of a river god and a nymph, Narcissus embodied the Olympian ideals, and was central to the life of his amour Echo, who was rendered mute but for the capacity to repeat the words of others. Their fate was tragic, in accordance with Tiresias's dictum that Narcissus would die when he learned who he was.

My take on the story is that Narcissus found out then that he had been a dupe of the Olympian Gods, glorying in their ways, and that he ascertained that insight whilst he gazed into the River Styx, which in its blackness stood for his depression on learning the truth.

So, Narcissus did not love and glory in himself, but in an illusion. Humankind learned this truth during the Great War, at Verdun, with the death and maiming of a million men. On the way to that titanic struggle, in reality an early holocaust, the young men of Europe joyfully marched to combat, heroes to instilled ideals of glory. There in Verdun they found only slaughter and despond. They had stormed, taken, and relinquished redoubts such as Fort Duamont a dozen times, culminating in intimate coupling with their squad's rotting corpses. The French turned from "Revanche" and "Pour La Gloire," then from a provident God, to mutiny and bleating like sheep, as they separated themselves from the ideals of glory of their forebears. Later, Sartre wrote his play, *No Exit*, concerning the ambiguity and agony of transition to a new reality for Europe.

My thesis is that the characters in Howard Hall, caught in their individual and joint tragedy, needed to analyze through their narcissism and their mythic thrall, to find their exit to reality. The title of this work, *This Way Out*, stems from that journey. The group experience was of inestimable value in stabilizing the individuals as they went through the inevitable mourning on loss of their narcissistic position and ideation. Again, Vince Jordan was the poignant example of that thrall and pain of loss.

Post Traumatic Disorder

As we become more aware of the rights of human beings, in the context of human history, we recognize the traumatic effect of the violation of those rights. Harry Stack Sullivan alluded to one of those rights in emphasis on the need of the human for interpersonal security, versus anxiety. Trauma is incident to disjunctive experience, experienced as disasters—natural, accidental, and the large category of man-made nature—assault, war, torture, etc. Early childhood trauma, disjunctive to intrapsychic and interpersonal security, has been implicated in the genesis of a wide range of mental disorder.

In this study, we have not penetrated to data pertinent to trauma in the early childhood of the participants, but one can infer severe disruption in the early life of many, Cohen and Jefferson as examples. Dormer certainly underwent what he experienced as trauma in firefighting school, followed by post traumatic re-experiencing, anxiety, nightmares, impaired concentration.

Parapsychological

The altered states involved in the messianic experience are marked by parapsychologic phenomena, such as telepathy, clairvoyance, visionary experience, and telekinesis. Jefferson edged towards a telepathic stance, and Jordan and Street, clairvoyance.

Psychoanalysis

Psychoanalysis provided me with an essential assist in my mission to explore the alienation of the patients in Howard Hall. The groups at the Fort Knox

Rehabilitation Center had operated much as Freud had described in his *Group Psychology and Analysis of the Ego* and his associate August Aichorn in his *Wayward Youth*. Aichorn held that errant or psychopathically inclined youths could be treated, but Freud held that psychoanalysis was for neurotic individuals. At Knox I had been able to discern his phenomena of free association, regression, resistance and transference, all present in groups larger than the dyad of psychoanalysis. In fact, the larger the numbers, the more overt the psychoanalytic phenomena! Though involved and active to the extreme, an overt modification of the method, I was able to practice professional neutrality and abstinence.

These experiences gave me the capacity to attempt similar work with psychotic individuals, people Freud held untreatable by his method. In the preceding paragraph I have related the phenomena of psychoanalysis, discovered by Freud in the course of his researches into human psychic pathology. I came to important aspects of the intellectual basis for my researches, before formal psychoanalytic training, through prior training in history, biology, physics, and medicine. Especially pertinent was extensive experience in attending women in birth, in those days without the assist of imaging techniques. One waited and watched for the signs of passage through the birth canal, aware of the dangers that called for active intervention. This exercise in activity and abstinence, marking the dramatic passage of the fetus and mother, from a unity, to separate entities, can be seen as analogous to the therapeutic experience of individuation.

Even rudimentary knowledge of the developmental crises of gangs, and of the revolutionary and reactionary ones of history gave me a beginning frame of inquiry. I had been intrigued by the birth of democracy from the *ancien regime* in France, royal rule in England, and colonial order in America, each attended by intellectual study circles, then insurrectionary mobs. I discerned both in the large groups at Knox. And I could correlate awareness of my inner alienation with that of my subjects.

All this provided a dramatic backdrop to the sessions. Then came the phenomena consequent to what I learned was messianism in the most unlikely of places, psychopaths, and also in myself, something I had long suspected. I have described this set of phenomena at length in the text of this work. Suffice it to say that what appeared on the surface as the least likely of scientific states, the pregnant pause in psychopaths, followed by deep cogitation by the members, then demonstration of capacity for reason, provided the platform for scientific study, for psychoanalytic inquiry into the lives of the members.

The aim of the work with the patients in Howard Hall was, through verbal and non verbal dialog, to bring them into their own and common reality. This involved application of Freud's mode of dialog, called psychoanalysis, modified appropriately, to inter-member free association, on the way to that on the intrapsychic level. I had learned to conduct dialog with psychopathic groups, and noted psychoanalytic mechanisms in the groups, then in work with individuals.

Why psychoanalysis? Why not attempt education, such as habit retraining, as is done in current boot camps? Fortunately, an educator, Col. George Miller had realized that the psychopath is deeply handicapped in character, alienated from self and others, to a degree that made education relatively fruitless. Miller's eyes were opened by the work of an associate of Freud's, August Aichorn, in the treatment of alienated youth, reported in the book, *Wayward Youth*. Aichorn successfully modified Freud's approach, to direct dialog with groups, combining it with educational methods.

Freud's approach may be defined as the art and science of ameliorative change of the human personality through collaborative transaction. The usual phases of development involved first establishment of trust leading to a therapeutic alliance, then free association, then constructive emotional regressions, with emergence, through analysis of psychic resistance, aspects of past reality that has distorted and obviated life in present reality. In the process, the analyst and the subject, called analysand, are intimately involved, related in what is called a transference-countertransference dyad.

In his study of consciousness, Freud was able to identify an aspect of it he denoted as the unconscious, variously kept from consciousness through a dis-associative process he called repression. Through the analytic process, one could study that consciousness, for its aberration. In the work with psychopaths, then schizophrenics, we learned that their consciousness had been significantly altered; they had escaped to other motivational worlds. Concomitantly, their value systems, or ego ideals, were altered drastically. Their superegos were present in the obverse, and even more severely.

To engage with groups larger than the dyad of psychoanalysis proper, we had to engage in what were called parameters, significant changes in approach and technique. However, the basic stance of psychoanalysis was sought and attained. At Knox, we obtained feedback, through submittal to each other's scrutiny and guidance, as well an ongoing therapeutic seminar. In Howard Hall, we had the collaboration of my fellow residents, as well as Dr. Cruvant. The views of visitors from abroad on what they had experienced were useful in rendering us perspective.

Reality

Reality has been arduously constructed by humanity over the millennia, and becomes what man is searching for and experiences contemporaneously.

Vince Jordan and his colleagues in Howard Hall had constructed an alternate reality, and were in fear, at times amounting to terror, of its relinquishment. He would be betraying the voices, which manifested his conscience, to which he was true, in part right up to the end. It was in conflict with a basic sense of reality, through which he was making a transition back to his family and life in Michigan. He expected to return to the reality status of automobile worker.

He had to let go of a personal myth of status as a lieutenant in the US Army, and of hero of a race riot, transmuted in his crisis at Fort Leavenworth into popular singing star and Army General. Central to his inner mythic struggle was a capacity to re-conceive of himself as a simple human being. This new conception called for mythopoetic capacity. All of these functions would take place in his ego ideal, the personality's instrument of the sense of reality, and positioning in the human and material universe. It would be a sign of humanity's tenuous hold on reality that it anchors its life in the expectation of an after life in a heavenly group assembled with God.

Regression

At Knox we had observed that the groups progressed to being civilized, on the way to becoming valid soldiers, but also regressed to their former psychopathic ways. Some of those who failed in the program and were headed to prison regressed in self care towards sloppiness. In one instance the group reached nadir, and only an armed guard stood between the psychiatrist and the group howling for his scalp.

We learned to recognize the earliest indications of progress and regress. So we were puzzled by the regression within themselves the members seemed to experience when they exhibited the full fledged phenomenon of advent, the hushed, contemplative state of transition between alienation and reconciliation with reality. I later learned of the concept regression within the ego, as a process on the way to the development of the transference that is central to psychoanalysis. That regression would be a trusting one, entered into by both parties to the diad. I was aware at Knox of regressing in trust as I conducted sessions, remarking to myself, "These are my people," as I remembered fondly my earlier experience with and wish for membership in a gang of Irish toughs on the lower East Side. It would appear that I was leading the group non-verbally through initiating and joining in such regression.

That regression brought the members and myself intrapsychically to earlier and past aspects of our selves, and awareness of resistance to their disclosure. But in the dialectic of therapy, described early in this volume in the micro-analysis of an early session, denial was superceded by affirmation, and the underlying reality, in the form of transference, emerged.

Resurrection

This is a key underlying concept in the development of my thought about narcissism. There, after the psychic death of the organism, there is resurrection in a new identity. My thesis is that Narcissus suffered a psychic death early, was reborn in identification with his parents' Olympian ideals, held them forth for his lifetime until he realized the truth about himself, as was foretold by Tiresias, and reverted to the original death. He then was in position to come back to his authentic life. By that token, Vince Jordan's delusional world was resurrective, needing to undergo death, for his salvation.

Role Theory

In our reality we enact a range and gamut of roles, each a patterned set of actions in the maintenance and furtherance of a social position in a social unit. Therein we develop careers, marked by developmental crises. Through empathy and intuition we are able to comprehend each other's roles and careers, and communicate gainfully in the process. Through study of role theory at Fort Knox, I had been sensitized to the range of roles in membership and leadership in the groups. This enabled me to actively relax and evoke such in the much more difficult groups in Howard Hall. Likewise, I was able to relate the members' problems at role assumption to their inner dynamics, and guide the process accordingly.

Schizophrenia

The first person we encounter in this work was profoundly schizophrenic, as well as psychopathic. I have described how he represented himself, as King, and the profound anxiety he induced in me, through the threat posed by his powerful regression, manifested by his stance, visage, and clenched fists. But I had been able to work my way through the challenge of riotous psychopaths, and learned to have confidence in the dialogic capacity of my professional and personal self, informed by a capacity to regress along with the group. I had learned that its messianism was able to win over those psychopaths, as well as earlier schizophrenics of my medical school training. I equated that to a positive transference on their part to me as a physician.

So why were these, as well as the schizophrenics and psychopaths of Howard Hall, able to attach themselves to me and other enterprising therapists, and later recover from their self alienation, to their premorbid selves, when Freud held that could not be done? My answer to that conundrum is that Freud abstained from the exercise of his, to me, obvious messianism. I infer that he tried to abstain, in the service of an identity as a scientist. Kaplan and Saddock (*Modern Synopsis of Psychiatry III*, Williams and Wilkins, p. 328) cite Rumke to the effect that the diagnostic criterion for schizophrenia is the praecox feeling on the part of the psychiatrist that enables intuitive contact with the schizophrenic individual. Emotional distance would preclude that contact, and it may be that Freud did not permit himself to engage his praecox feeling. The reference cites that in a study 1,000 European psychiatrists, 54% declared that the praecox feeling was a reliable criterion for diagnosis of schizophrenia.

Freud held that the schizophrenic individual is so narcissistically regressed within self as to be unable to cathect or relate to others in a manner he called transference. More on that essential concept later. Bleuler described the core aspects of that regression as the four A's: ambivalence, disturbance of association, disturbance of affect, and autism, with a preference for fantasy over reality. Meyer held that schizophrenia was a reaction disorder, in a unitary schema encompassing all of mental disorder, based on habitual patterns of maladaptive responses, in turn based on organic, psychologic and sociocultural factors. Sullivan emphasized deeply disturbed interpersonal relationships. He emphasized damage to a self system, related to security, self esteem, and fulfillment of psychological drives. Harperman emphasized the damage done to the development and adaptive function of the autonomous ego by uncontrolled aggression. He noted the vulnerability of dependent individuals, dreading separation and loss.

Menninger emphasized schizophrenia as a reaction to stress, carrying Meyer's unitary hypothesis from nervousness, to neurotic illness, overt aggression, dis-association from reality to psychotic disorganization, depression and death. Tracing a normative course, Mahler conceived of the child's maternal attachment in the first three years, identifying inordinate attachment to the mother. This renders the child emotionally dependent. Following this lead, analysts have focused on ego impairment, the inability to bear anxiety and depression (Zetzel, Segal), and family enmeshment (Lidz, Abrahams and Varon, Searles, Bateson, Wynne).

Treatment of individuals immersed in the schizophrenic dilemma has a long history, starting with man's emerging capacity for a mind of one's own, and its correlate, one's personhood. Through the Enlightenment, mankind woke from prior dogma and rote thought, in the 18th and 19th Centuries. Freud and his followers looked at man's mind and very soul afresh, as did Kraeplin and Bleuler. Sullivan paved the way for treating the schizophrenic as someone caught in unfavorable circumstance, undergoing an inner transformation, looking for freedom. Menninger waxed eloquent on that mission.

Semrad provided the most detailed guide to working with the schizophrenic as a human being and provision of personal and interpersonal experiences of ameliorative nature.

I published on my experience in the treatment of schizophrenics in 1946, 1953, 1957, and 1964. The unitary hypotheses of Meyer and Menninger made sense to me. However, from the first I have addressed the impact of alienation from self and others on an ego previously developmentally impaired. In that experience, psychic death and resurrection play a central role. Vince Jordan is illustrative of the altered and impaired ego, and its vicissitudes in the inception of illness and recovery. See my exposition on death, also alienation.

Soul

This work is a record of the soul-searching of a small society that at first knew no exit from its limbo. The member who made first representations, Vince Jordan, in his psyche had escaped from that reality, through life in other worlds, of kings, super-stars, Presidents, Generals, and Gods (in which he was Christ). Instead of killing me, as would his fellow assassins, it turned out he underwent an epiphany, in which he as Christ, communed with me as messianist, and joined with me as leaders of a helping community. I propose that those data and that to follow are best approached when we add the concept and percept of soul to the psychological analysis.

Jordan thereafter underwent an excruciating journey, struggling with the essence of his identity, its vector, quality of good and evil, relation to the deity, salvation of self and others, and depression at the loss of glory as he learned to accept reality's mundanity and ambiguities. Reading the text of that journey is an excruciating experience.

I had been prepared for the rigors and satisfactions of that journey by several years of struggle with more than a thousand alienated young men at Fort Knox on their core motivations. I had grown to realize that a spiritual component was in play, and had focused on what I recognized as my messianism, and an obsessed prisoner who had dramatically sacrificed himself for his cause of alienation. This man, Rampa, had formed a positive relationship with me that I sensed was messianic, when he stated that he could not be reached, then had urged me to help his more reachable fellows, and they to accept me.

My focus there was on what was he essentially about, when he stated he "had to" commit the act that brought on his death? That focus was still in operation when I sensed that Jordan meant to kill me, and also when I revealed to him my messianic intent. His sadness at that point had been manifest in Rampa's eyes when he stated he could not be reached. I had in mind the criminals' cross alongside that of Christ, and speculated whether he was masking an inner Christ at that point.

Rampa appeared to be in massive denial of any prosocial idealism, which nevertheless shone through perversely in messianic and satanic purposefulness, both evidence of soul. Jordan appeared to be the essence of soulfulness, in his manner and array of identities, especially that of Christ and his dialectic, satanic criminal, "the meanest, worst person in the world." This phenomenon of Jordan's personality was one of transcendence and essence: the height of national identity, president-general; the height of popular stars, Nat King Cole; and the height of transcendent religious identity, Christ.

I have noted his tendency to epiphanic experience, the malevolent transformation he underwent in solitary in prison, also in his encounter with me, plus his nightly crises. He devised religious costumes, and ritually recited re a materialist talisman, a Cadillac automobile. He was different from his fellows, in that he identified himself in ideal absolutes. Therein lies another aspect of the human soul, the highest and lowest essence of human identity.

I have noted another characteristic of the human soul, the advent phenomenon, whose most frequent occurrence is as a haunt. There, in the course of developmental crises, the person conceives of and perceives the advent of loss or gain in a parapsychological manner, as the appearance of Hamlet's father as an apparition, prior to a mourning of his death that never took place. Jefferson sensed his coming mourning of his wife through some telepathic experience. Street held that he anticipated one's thoughts.

So we have assembled the phenomena of soul, which I define as the core organizing principle and factor of the human personality and identity. It incorporates the representation of the entire personality in its essential, on a different order of existence, perhaps explicable through complexity theory. It is sensed intuitively, sensate in the chest, head, eyes, and hearing apparatus, leading to an altered state of consciousness. Psychoanalytic and religious regression are pathways to such sensation. I conceive of the work in Howard Hall as essentially a struggle for the souls of its population.

At humanity's current level of comprehension, we conceive and perceive the existence of entity in the world and its essential meaning as soul. Death follows departure of that animation, that soul. As living creatures we tend to experience that life as present in the future, and therefore immortalize the soul. We conceive of a career for that soul, postulating in myth stories of genesis and ultimate outcomes.

It would appear that religionists and philosophers first conceived of the essential and the ideal aspects of its governance of self as soul. However, there are *anlage* in myth of that development elsewhere in society, such as the career in Greek mythology of Prometheus, who broke with the Gods, and the development of democratic ways on the part of northern European tribes, eventuating in democracy in England, France, and America. That would lead one to think that humanity would have come to the conception and perception of the essential self and other were Abraham not to have heard the voice of an ultimately personal God setting him on a mission in selfhood for his tribe. Along the way, God's design for the entity and dignity of the human being was revealed in abstinence from human sacrifice, then in the cultivations of the prophets, and the evolution of the soul of Israel as an example for the world.

My thinking about the soul is an extension of Erikson's formulation on identity. He had it both as a process and product. Through that combined function and psychic structure, the manifold aspects of the ideals and aspirations, linkages and affiliations to others and their ways, how the individual enduringly identified self in time, space, personal and social reality.

The soul would be such on both a higher and deeper order. The soul would have wings as well as heart, indicating representation of psyche and soma in an essential way. The soul would be reflected in the dream life of the individual at critical times in the life course, as with Jefferson's contentious tie to his father, and Jordan's dream experience of having been bitten by a rat. Hamlet's soul was racked by his tie to his father, who doomed him to a mission of revenge, on the parapet. We experience the souls of the living and the dead as presences in our daily life, and especially in crises. Our lives pass before our eyes in severe crises.

We experience evidence of our soul-connectedness with others in our chests and heads, as in my *intuitometer*. We experience essence of self in our chests and heads as internal or external auras. Then there is the *terra incognita* of parapsychology, where we have the task of separating fact from fancy, but where "there are more things in heaven and earth than are dreamt in your philosophy."

Therapeutic Alliance

I did not know it at the time, but Vince Jordan formed a therapeutic alliance with me in our initial encounter, harrowing as it was. His alienated ways turned affiliative, and he became my chief ally. He sought to sit next to me, become the group scribe, helped his fellow patients present their problems. I inferred that it occurred when, hair standing on end, I averred that I was there to help. I think he was somehow aware that I meant business, though frightened, and that the business was that of the other side of his psychopathy, messianism.

Therapeutic Community

Therapeutic community may be defined as the practice, of systematic assemblage of the participants in a therapeutic venture, to make sense of, guide, and further its mission. At its heart is the therapeutic alliance. The practice of therapeutic community formally appeared late on the human scene, during and immediately following World War II. (Maxwell Jones, Tom Main). In the early 1920's August Aichorn conducted a group home for delinquent youth that can be thought of as presage to therapeutic community.

It made sense to me, early in my career as a psychiatrist at a regional Army Hospital, to meet with my patients to orient them to the task of recovery, debrief them from their wartime experience, and mobilize their assets in the process. Earlier, preparing for combat on the part of a medical detachment of a tank destroyer battalion, I assembled them systematically for emotional orientation to combat, and contingency problem solving.

Similarly, during the war, Howard Hall's Chief of Service, Dr. Bernard Cruvant, had met in large groups with neurotic soldiers who would currently be diagnosed as post-traumatic. The idea was simple, get everybody together in a town hall style group meeting, to identify current concerns and their solutions. Such convocation has a long history in America, in New England town hall meeting, Chautauqua religious and educational convocations. In the 18th Century, Mesmer in Europe held his *banques*, imbued with animal magnetism, with deep emotional exhibitions, including the fits I noticed at Fort Knox. Mesmer's charismatic venture had a salvationist, authoritarian cast.

The work of Maxwell Jones and most therapeutic communities involved simultaneous meeting of the entire staff and patients in large groups structured to evoke the experiences and sentiments of the members, including personnel, towards problem solving. At the Fort Knox Rehabilitation Center for Military Prisoners, we employed extremely large groups of deeply disordered psychopaths to stabilize them, for further treatment. That experience demonstrated to me and my colleagues the feasibility of working with groups afflicted with the severest disorders, indeed, as an avenue to research at reaching them therapeutically.

That experience led me to attempt the assemblage of almost the entire population of Howard Hall, despite its dangerous potential. In time, we included the Chief of Service, several nurses, a number of attendants, myself and a few other residents. We took up housekeeping and administrative issues, plus the issues that emerge in therapy. Dr. Cruvant, who had previous experience with group therapy in his Army service, ran the administrative meetings. However, he mostly held his administrative group therapy with the much smaller ward groups, to which patients from adjacent ward were brought.

The groups reported in this text were in the category of group psychotherapy, with therapeutic community overtones, as when we conferred with the Red Cross for games and educational material, the Occupational Therapist re conceiving of and constructing a program, or with the dietitian re coming off war-time boiled chicken. We did some of the psychoeducational work of therapeutic community, such as projection of the slides devised for the psychopaths in the Army, or book discussion groups. But the sessions were generally structured to evoke the issues of the members: "What does the group want to talk about. Let's figure it out." At times my fellow residents conducted the sessions, yielding to a chairman elected by the members. I have gone into the experience in some depth in an ongoing commentary. Suffice it to say here that psychoanalytic phenomena, appropriate to group life systematically surfaced, once the members communed in the simply human manner described by Harry Stack Sullivan.

Transaction

Psychoanalyst Eric Berne identified this aspect of human interaction, its formation of a unity, a gestalt, of interacting entities. Unity is the keynote here, denoting a new psychological entity, governed by the ways appropriate to its numbers, as diad, triad, quadrad, etc. We behave differently embedded in each level. Psychoanalysis up to now is a science of the diad, analyst and analysand, and is on the verge of expanding its horizons outward, to encompass specific study of larger units of humanity. The gestalt aspect of transaction is hardly noted by social psychologists, nor is the transactional nature of the gestalt by gestaltists.

Berne entered the realm of the individual within the transactional unit through conceiving it as possessing and enacting both the child and adult within the operative self. He also conceived of the encrypting of scenarios of action-sequences, which he induced his subjects to play our through recitation. J. L. Moreno, through psychodrama, staged those sequences, adding the element of spontaneity. The psychopaths at Fort Knox who fell in Mesmerian fits were regressing in transaction with me. We fell short of the fits in the Integrated Group, but the unity of our interaction became evident.

Transcendence

It occurred to me early that the psychopath and schizophrenic transcended reality, to live in other worlds. At the same time, protected by what I learned was messianism, I experienced my analogous other worlds, and gained a degree of access to those of my subjects. The messianism itself involved transcendence of self. When, through analysis, I was able to relinquish a preponderant messianism, I gained access to a depressed earlier ego state, escaped through an inherent transcendence. Lessened reliance of this transcendence has followed. The members of the Howard Hall groups grew adept at noting this lessened reliance in their fellows. I expect that neuroscience will depict all this through imaging.

I invoke this concept to explain the other worldly nature of the messianic experience. It occurred to me early in the work with psychopaths that they lived in different worlds, a state evident in the case of schizophrenics, especially with paranoid and hebephrenic individuals. Conceptualizing what was being transcended and the role of alienation came later, as did the complexity theory.

It appears that humanity has less and less need for transcendence into other worlds, as reality becomes more bearable, in the womb and afterwards.

Transference

This psychoanalytic concept was developed by Freud in an attempt to investigate the penetration and obviation of current reality by that of the past. He enlisted the analysand in comprehension of the current situation via a dialog in which free association figured prominently. Resistance blocks full consciousness, first towards the act of free association, then to specific problems arising in its course.

In the initial phase of the work the members would both discern and impute to me a messianic identity which past authors would call positive transference. While past affects would be so transferred, and the path in therapy laid for trusting regression as fellow human beings, that in turn set the stage for the emergence of experience from which the individual was disassociated, through what Freud called repression. As such, transference would be a late arrival on the therapeutic scene. Freud held that the schizophrenic was incapable of transference. Jefferson arrived at a transference experience when he opened up about his colored mammy.

Eliciting the phenomenon of transference is central to this work. Its appearance is marked by enactment in the present, on the way to their mastery, of life situations to which the subject is tied emotionally. I never did discern what ties to the past Rampa, of my work in Fort Knox, suffered, that led him to his sacrificial course. However, Jordan and Jefferson gave me glimpses of the relationship with their mothers and fathers that bent their psychic twigs into the psychotic and psychopathic characters they became. The transference appeared late in the work, after establishment of the messianic mutuality, human-to-human transaction, establishment of trust sufficient for regressive easing into revelation to the self of the individual and others.

Unconscious

The work in Howard Hall centered about altering the consciousness of the groups and individuals, to reconciliation with aspects of self and others from which they had been cut off or alienated. In that consciousness, death played a central part. Like the consciousness of our reality, that consciousness had its executive function, its censor and suasive power. A messianic transaction with the representative leaders, Jordan and Jefferson, was pivotal in that conversion. Their original state of mind appeared to have the characteristics of the Freud's theoretic unconscious—closeness to the instincts, primary process, childlike wishes and thinking. Forsyth, in poetry and Jefferson in his Mayoral rages, both regressed, were figures out of the system Unconscious. Jordan was regressed into a world of myth resident in the unconscious.

Freud later termed that elementary primitiveness the Id, derived from the at once primitive and sophisticated inner intelligence Groddeck called The It. Freud held that the Id had no internal organization, was a chaos of primitive instincts. I found that the regressed patient, from Forsyth to Jefferson, acting as operant Ids, could "read" the unconscious of his fellows and communicate such to me. Analogously regressed in my therapeutic role, I was enabled to reach their fellows and bring them into the therapeutic transaction. LaPlanche and Pontalis (*The Language of Psychoanalysis*, Norton, New York, 1973) claimed that Freud in practice transferred through this operant id his original unconscious, with its primary process, complexes, genetic layering of the instincts, and organized opposition of life and death instincts. Max Schur, in *Freud: Living and Dying*, International Universities Press, 1972, posited that Freud, in his superstition, experienced an inner demonic nature, wishing a death which would give him peace, from the "cross" he bore. Schur speculated that Freud elevated his experience of a demonic and uncanny wish for death into an instinct. (See extension of this, in the topic, Death, in this Glossary)

Appendix B

Occupational Therapy, the Parallel Program

The Occupational Therapy Program can be traced back to the earliest sessions presented in the text, when the original group responded to my question on what they wanted. They wanted better food, reading material, and recreational games. I had the members meet with representatives of the Red Cross, who furnished magazines and games, then material for construction of model ships and planes.

The members assumed responsibility for the possession and distribution of those items, in effect a partnership in an occupational therapy program. Musical instruments and mentorship followed, as well as literacy classes, conducted by the patients. Mrs. Merrill, the Chief of the Occupational Therapy Department of the Hospital, appointed an occupational therapy worker, Miss Janet Sawyer, to take charge of these developments, into a full fledged venture. Prior, the Hall had been off limits to women, because of dangerousness. Now, the patients did their own mutual discipline of unruly members, such as Vince Jordan. As an example of the change, Jordan, by this time, had graduated from feral enforcer of alienation, and been acting as recorder for the Black Therapy Group, receiving supplies from Mrs. Merrill, also a guitar for instruction of patients.

Also, another violent patient, William Cohen, had turned a talent for poison pen letters to the Superintendent of Mason General Hospital, to a request that he start a patient newspaper. Miss Sawyer nursed his talent into a successful editorship, and the birth of the *Howard Hall Journal*, which drew reporters from black and white populations, into the close collaboration called for in such an enterprise. The *Journal* achieved wide readership in mental hospitals across the nation and internationally.

EDITORIAL PAGE

In the first edition of the *Journal*, its purpose was also printed on its first and opening page. It read as follows "Published by the men of Howard Hall, St. Elizabeths Hospital, for mutual encouragement and rehabilitation. It is hoped that many will avail themselves of this educational opportunity for self-expression and exchange of ideas, and that our readers may be enlightened and inspired."

Mrs. Sheridan believed that the *Journal* would serve as a medium in which the patients would be able to express their thoughts and beliefs. This the patients have done, and by exchanging ideas they halve helped in many ways to rehabilitate themselves.

We here in the *Journal* are dedicated to the unfinished work which the men on the *Journal* staff before have so nobly advanced. The Journal has carried on, and still carries on the struggle to obtain and better things for the men of Howard Hall, now John Howard Pavilion. We are fighting a never ending battle to secure more and better treatment methods and programs, recreational facilities, and social outlets, all of which, in an effort to secure for all patients, regardless of status, an equal opportunity to gain an understanding of the mental illness that resulted in their hospitalization, to help them adjust to their new environment , to ease the daily tensions that grow where groups of men are continually housed together, and a means of preparing the patient to his return to the outside world and again take his rightful place in today's modern society. The JOURNAL has a voice that many patients are not aware of, and it is these patients that we try to reach.

I am both thankful and proud for this opportunity to relay to you, our readers, of this twentieth anniversary of the *Journal*, some of the progress that our publication has been instrumental in obtaining.

The *Journal* is no longer a nine page issue, printed on a hand operated mimeograph machine. The *Journal* is no longer a scared dolorous infant trembling at the mere sound of typewriter keys, and neither is there a fear of not being accepted. It has not fear of lack of accomplishment, or how important a role it can play in rehabilitating patients in and out of John Howard.

Its print is now large and bold; its voice can be heard near and far. The *Journal* now circulates throughout the fifty states and several foreign countries. Its growth from one to two hundred copies to well over eleven hundred is proof of its popularity and success and erases the rear of rejection. It is an assurance that the *Journal* is a permanent part of John Howard Pavilion and the Occupational Therapy Shop, out of which it functions. Howard Hall and now Howard Pavilion have accomplished much through the voice of the *Journal*. It has obtained recognition to the patients active in securing self-government, a list of social activities are to the *Journal's* merit, plus establishing in itself a true therapeutic outlet for all patients.

Recently, through the efforts of the Editorial Board, the Journal received two Awards, in recognition of its achievements in journalism. This is an added and constructive incentive cemented in the files of the *Journal*, for those who come after us.

Appendix C

Photographs of Howard Hall

Photos are from the archives of St. Elizabeth's Hospital.

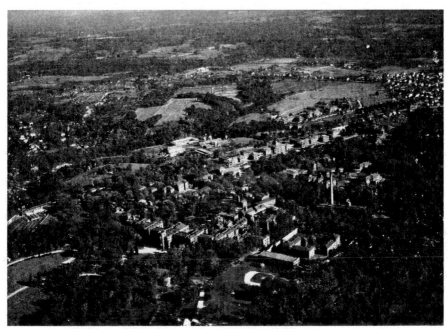

Aerial View of Howard Hall 1922.

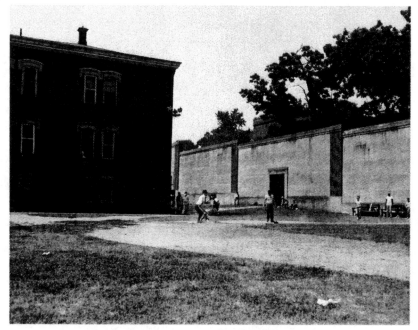

Baseball Game at Howard Hall (date unknown).

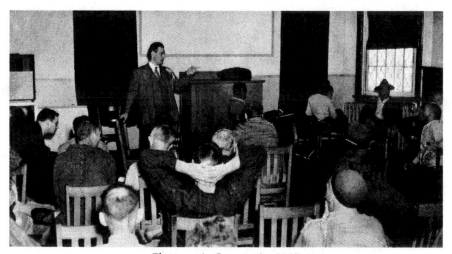

Therapeutic Community 1947.

THE JOHN HOWARD JOURNAL

A MEMBER OF THE INTERNATIONAL INSTITUTIONAL PRESS ASSOCIATION, INCORPORATED

VOLUME XX, Nos. 4 & 5   APRIL-MAY 1968

AN ANTHOLOGY COMMEMORATING
THE JOURNAL'S 20th ANNIVERSARY

1948 — 1968

Howard Hall Journal.

Annotated Bibliography

Abrahams, J. and McCorkle, L.W. 1946. Group Psychotherapy of Military Offenders, *Am. J. Sociol.* 51:455.

Abrahams, J. and McCorkle, L.W. 1947. Group Psychotherapy at an Army Rehabilitation Center, *Dis. Nerv. Sys.* 8:3.

Abrahams, J. and McCorkle, L.W. 1947. Analysis of a Prison Disturbance, *Jour. Abn. and Soc. Psych.* 42:330.

My associate, the sociologist Lloyd W. McCorkle, and I here report our adventure in treating psychopathically inclined youth during the momentous days of World War II. Narrative in form, these accounts were intended to set the stage for further research and development. He went on to initiate Highfields, a halfway house for delinquent youth; then became Principal Keeper of the New Jersey State Prison; Commissioner of the New Jersey Department of Institutions and Agencies; Professor, John Jay College; and author, with David Korn, of *Modern Penology.* The advances we report on, and continued for a decade were lost subsequently.

Abrahams, J. 1947. Group Psychotherapy: Remarks on its Basis and Application. *Med. Annals of D.C.* 16:612.

———. 1948. Preliminary Report of an Experience in the Group Psychotherapy of Schizophrenics. *Am. J. Psychiatry.* 104:613.

This is a preliminary report of the work in Howard Hall, leading in time to the establishment of a training program in group work at St. Elizabeths Hospital.

———. 1948. Group Psychotherapy: Preliminary Remarks on its Use in Correctional Institutions. *Bull. Correctional Service Assoc.* 1:12.

This Bulletin of the Correctional Service Associates marks the high water mark in a movement within the Federal Prison Service towards establishment of rehabilitation there on the Fort Knox model, also a National Institute for Research in Crime.

———. Group Psychotherapy: Implications for Direction and Supervision of Mentally Ill Patients, in Theresa Muller's *Mental Health in Nursing.* Washington, Catholic Univ. Press, 1950, pp. 77–83.

———. 1953 The Large Group, Chapter in: Powdermaker, Dr. Florence, and Frank, Jerome D., *Group Psychotherapy*, Cambridge: The Harvard Press.

Jerome Frank and Florence Powdermaker, along with Daniel Blain, Chief of Psychiatry of the Veterans Administration early post war initiated a research group, which in turn organized a group treatment project at the Perry Point Veterans Administration Hospital. Following the evident feasibility of extremely large groups, later called therapeutic community groups, we established a group of 87 patients, therapists and personnel.

The Chapter reports on that rewarding experience.

Abrahams, J. with Varon, Edith. 1953. *Maternal Dependency and Schizophrenia, A Group Analytic Study*. New York, International Univ. Press. Foulkes, Rev. S. H., Intl. J. Psa, 1955. 36:358; Jordan, A. M. Q., 1955, 24:300–302.

This group on a chronic ward at St. Elizabeths Hospital consisted of 6 mother-daughter pairs, a social worker recorder, and myself, meeting weekly for 2 years. The alienated tie of mother and daughter was subjected to analytic scrutiny, and yielded to cycles of reconciliation.

Abrahams, J. 1956. Some Views on Group Psychotherapy in the Mental Hospital. *J. Neurophsychiat.*, 4:39.

Abrahams, J. and Stanton, Alfred H. 1958. (Report) A comparison of individual and group psychology. (Panel: Am. Psychoanal. Assoc., Chicago, May 1956), *J. Am. Psa. Assn.* 6:121–130.

This paper is a report of combined individual and group psychoanalysis of a group of 10 private patients, their courses towards recovery, and my inferences. Alfred Stanton summarizes the work, which is still unpublished. The character analysis initiated in the group was a mainstay in the members' individual analyses. A remarkable feature was the insight afforded by delineating the role of myth in the life courses of the women.

Abrahams, J. 1960. (Ed.) Group Methods in the Treatment of Schizophrenic Outpatients, Scher, Sam C. and Davis, Howard R, (Eds.), *The Outpatient Treatment of Schizophrenia*, New York, Grune and Stratton.

This is a broad gauged essay into the theory and practice of group methods in the treatment of schizophrenic outpatients, occasioned by the initial efforts towards their treatment in community clinics.

———. 1962. (Ed.) *Group Work in the Mental Hospital: A Manual*, The St. Elizabeths Hospital Group Work Training Program, Washington, D.C.

The work in Howard Hall, Perry Point VA, and elsewhere at St. Elizabeths led to a Hospital-Wide Group Work Training Program. The faculty, consisting of the chairs or representative of the departments of the hospital—nursing, psychology, psychiatry, pastoral, educational, dance, occupational therapy, and psychodrama—learned to be members of and to lead groups, through training groups. Eventually, a large faculty (35) was established, along with 200 groups, hospital wide.

———. 2006. *Turning Lives Around: Wartime Treatment of Military Prisoners*, AuthorHouse, Bloomington.

The illustrative cartoons in this volume were a psychoeducational feature of the large groups in the rehabilitation program at Fort Knox, Kentucky, during World

War II. Drawn by a rehabilitee who understood psychopathy, they deepened the reach of the groups into the character disorders of the rehabilitees. There are narrative accounts of sessions, and presentation of a theory of alienation.

Abse, D. Wilfred. 1974. *Clinical Notes on Group-Analytic P*sychotherapy, Charlottesville: The University Press of Virginia.

This rich and masterful presentation of group analysis and therapeutic community, product of an original mind, is a far cry from Slavson's early work on the subject. Abse has coined a designation for the activity of interpretation in group therapy, *learning alliance*, in which the preconscious of the leader is joined with that of the group, to monitor consciousness, guiding the members in a state of derepression. He also comes out with condenser phenomena, in which associated ideas are pooled, to result in sudden discharge of deep and primitive feelings and ideas. He suspects that the group judgment engaged in problem solving at this primitive level. He notes the advantages offered in analytic groups of character analysis, and mobilization of *"totemistic" transference*. Elsewhere he mentions *motive analysis*, in the context of a profound discussion of anomie, suicide, and social integration and disintegration.

Berne, E. 1963. *The Structure and Dynamics of Organizations and Groups*, Philadelphia: Lippincott.

The ambitious title stems from a wide consultancy and practice of transactional analysis, a variant of psychoanalysis. Berne applied the valuable social psychological concept of transaction—a unity of interacting entities—to the unit of psychoanalysis, which in time created that of intersubjectivity. His ego psychological role analysis, done in parent and child terms, and ego defense analysis of "the games people play", plus their inherent scripts proved interesting in popularizing psychoanalysis, but of limited usefulness.

Bion, W.R. 1959. *Experiences In Groups*, New York: Basic Books.

Wilfred Bion and Maxwell Jones developed their group approaches under wartime emergency, and their work warrants closer and comparative inquiry. We gain greatly through their candor. Along the way they both underwent psychoanalytic training, and inevitably and uniquely let us into their situation. It turns out that Bion resists being a member of the group, while Jones glories in the experience. In this presentation we shall extensively inquire into Bion's experience.

Citing group work performed wartime with neurotic soldiers at London's Tavistock Clinic, psychoanalyst Bion lays the groundwork for operational statement of his experience post-war with large and small groups, and his inferences. Like Freud early in his *Group Psychology*, he regards the phenomena, group and individual, to be the same, regarded from different standpoints. Early in *Experiences*, he cites psychoanalysis to be a pairing, or dyadic group, centered on the Oedipal situation, and when examined as a group per se, centered on the myth of the Sphinx, related to problems of knowledge and the scientific method. The relation to the Sphinx is as enigmatic as the Sphinx itself. But such enigmas stud *Experiences,* midst largely pellucid language.

This work, published early in the development of analytic group therapy, is classic. In it Bion cites what he and the group members said and did, and gives a running account of his feelings, with essays into his intrapsychic workings, as illustrative of what may be going on in the members. Such an effort calls for reciprocation by others, for equally frank sharing of parallel experiences.

The session report referred to is rendered in Chapters 1 and 2, in which he presents specific behavioral sequences, apparently from a vivid memory. In succeeding chapters he goes on to build a group science with postulates of group mentality, group culture, basic assumption group, and work group.

Following the thesis that the Devil is in the details, I would like to review his report on a group, in the manner I cite as *microanalysis* earlier in *This Way Out*. To lend perspective, I shall insert in the account a running commentary similar to the one employed throughout *This Way Out*.

Microanalysis of Bion's Experiences in Groups, Chapters 1 and 2

1) Bion begins the account with how he got to "take on" the group in question. He had been asked by the Professional Committee of the Tavistock Committee to "take" therapeutic groups, utilizing his technique, which apparently had become famous, by this time.

2) He then cites his *discomfort* with the request, not knowing what they had in mind. He had persuaded the groups he led in the military to *study their tensions*. He could do that again, but he had found out that *the Committee expected cure*, something different from Bion's expectation.

3) He then reports that he expected the groups to *cure him of a symptom*, his "belief that groups might take kindly to my efforts."

This mordant statement was of great importance, to my mind. I would infer that the symptom is of a malady, related to an analogous belief prominent at that stage in my career, of messianic nature. In subsequent extensive efforts at self analysis, I attempted to cure myself of it. It plays a critical role in this account.

4) Then Bion prefaces description of a session itself by noting that a run of them had both patients and personnel, leading to a "peculiar quandary."

Implicit here was that the patients and personnel would have different expectations, significantly regarding the issue of cure, in the case of the patients.

5) Then he presents a session with mixed patients and others: Members gradually gather at the appointed time, engaging in desultory conversation, interrupted by *silence*, recommencing, then *silence*.

I make much of pregnant silences in my groups at Fort Knox and Howard Hall. Pragmatically, they were followed, as with Bion's group, by something other than desultory conversation, but deep, cogent emotion. In the Howard Hall and Fort Knox groups the group atmosphere changed markedly, in the manner described by Bion. But I am getting ahead of the story. In anxiety Bion interrupted the silence, confiding his sentiments.

6) Bion next reports that he "confided" his anxiety to the members concerning meeting the group's expectations.

He later reveals that he "blurted" this confidence.

I got to know Bion later in his life, during his residence in the United States in Brentwood, as a man who kept himself and his privacy under great control. He appeared to be in personality elevated above others. Blurting would be out of character, and I would infer that, under the anxiety of this new situation in the group, he had regressed inwardly at this point in an experience, of great consequence to his career as a psychoanalyst and the new discipline of group therapy. He has already revealed that he was conflicted by an impulse to "cure." By my token, were he to assume that stance, and the groups take kindly to it, he would be in the messianic position.

One of my therapists at Knox made a practice of disclosure of his discomfiture *per se*, in a manner so engaging that the members reassured him, without pursuing him further. Dr. Whitaker, a psychologist group therapist, and noted pioneer, as an initiatory act at this stage of the development of his group, lay himself down on the floor in front of the group, as if in a swoon, presenting himself as the subject for discussion. Monitoring the interaction, he later related to them what they had said and did, affirming their capacity for autonomous interaction. Both my therapist and Whitaker maintained their leadership role and position, engaging the group in the counseling stage of therapy.

I had found such maneuvers not necessary, waiting out the silence, while attuned to my and the members' phenomena. I became aware of how cogent and full of content the silences were. An associate, McCorkle, described a 40 minute silence with a group of young psychopaths, who responded to his strong authoritarian leadership by "staying with him" in communion.

7) Bion reports that his self revelation was met by mixed "indignation" and "friendliness."

He had not abandoned the leadership position, perhaps maintaining hope through previous success with his Army groups, when the inherent group dynamic led to polarization of those with and those against collaboration. Remember his previous mention of groups that "might take kindly" to his efforts.

8) Bion then averred that he sensed that the indignant members were expressing an underlying sense of entitlement.

He has regained his intuitive capacity, and is recovering from the anxiety that led him to blurt.

9) Allied with the "friendly" members who, trusting, gave him credit for knowing what he was doing, Bion engaged the group as a whole in free association to what they sensed as his motivations and presence. He wondered what their expectations were and what aroused them. They informed him: most were told he would "take" the group; some that he had a reputation of knowing a lot about groups; some that he would lecture.

That enactment was later termed brainstorming in the group dynamics movement, a guided evocation of data. It is apparent from his report that he volunteered as a democratic participant in the group, while maintaining his authority and position as psychoanalyst. He thereby provided leadership to the members in taking counsel with self and others on the role and capacity of leader and members.

10) He replies that their positions re him are based on "hearsay," and senses that the members feel he was denying his "eminence as a 'taker' of groups."

He is here saying that the members got his mission wrong, hearing what they wanted to hear, coupled in the same sentence with Bion's attribution to the group that he was denying whatever he means by eminence, and again, he brings up the phrase "taker of group" attributed first to the Committee. He earlier equates it with cure.

11) Bion cites the arrival of the vocal members to the position that the good expectations about him are disappointingly not true, and that his behavior is provocative, and that he chooses to be spiteful.

The realization that the members are disappointed in him is sinking in, moreover, that he is alienated to the point of being spiteful. I get the impression here that he is using this transaction to study this quirk of his personality.

12) He points out that it is hard for the group to accept that this is his way of taking groups, or that he should be allowed to, in such a way.

He would not let himself get away with it!

13) Bion goes on to discuss with us his rationale for his now admittedly provocative and evocative behavior, *whether he or the group was forced*, then brings up the issue of psychoanalytic processes, through mention of group transference and interpretation. He now admits that he was subjected to anxiety sufficient to cause him to blurt earlier. Moreover, he suspects he did so, somehow feeling persecuted.

I would infer that the issue of being forced had to do with compulsiveness of this personality trait. Also, the inference that, believing in Melanie Klein's theories of regression to depressive and paranoid positions, he was regressing to the paranoid, under the stress of assumption of the role of group leader with the new task of "cure," with all the ambiguity he describes.

14) Returning to the group account, he notes for the reader an improvement in the atmosphere of the group.

Certainly his introspection at this point would be accompanied by a lessening of the assertiveness with which he criticized them as subject to hearsay. He had then "taken" their criticism. It had traversed the initial formative stage he had experienced in his work with the Army groups, and he could possibly relax and guide its further development.

But this civilian group would not let him hide behind the position of authority he had held successfully in the Army. The members instinctively searched more deeply. In my Army experience at the Fort Knox Rehabilitation Center, my therapists and I had noted this expectation to be one of saviorist nature. When resisted, the group lost meaning to the members. It did not need acknowledgement in words, but in readiness to receive communication on that level and in that mode. I sensed it to be messianic, and they agreed to that formulation. I came up with the formula, "Scratch a psychopath, and find a messianist!"

15) Bion digresses, to admit in part that he provoked the focus on his personality, and purposive as interpretation of psychoanalytic transference, arrived at spontaneously.

Remember that he blurted out in the context of the deeply evocative silence at the inception of the group. I would estimate that he was engaged there in resistance to the act of transference, on the way to analysis of that quirk of his character. He indirectly admits at this point to feeling paranoid.

16) A leader of a subgroup, Mr. X, takes "helpful" initiative for the group, focusing on "elements in the group destructive of morale and good fellowship," identifies Bion's leadership as the problem. From the "eminence" of leadership of the subgroup

he interviews Bion as to his internal difficulty, which Bion cites as his object, why Bion cannot give a straightforward explanation of his motives. In reply, Bion apologizes, and offers the group testimony as to the motivation he had in prior work in the Army, "to study group tensions."

He either dissembles here, or has disassociated from awareness of the issue of cure and his state of inadequacy, either in individual psychoanalysis (involving the Oedipus myth), or group analysis (involving the Sphinx myth, both momentous and novel courses of inquiry.

17) The leader of the subgroup, Mr. X, queries others on their ideas re Bion's difficulty. He runs into resistance, and Bion picks up that they lean towards acceptance of the thesis that the Committee "must have some purpose in saying that I was to take the group," also that the group was of value per se. Members give testimony re their origins and possible value to a group which studies itself scientifically.

Bion is evidently monitoring this phase of self propelled group activity.

18) Another subgroup forms, vaguely discontented with the position arrived at so far. Bion senses this, interpreting that it is dissatisfied with his revelation re his motives and presence. The members reject this and enter a state he states he has experienced in every group. He cites that his "fitness for the role I am expected to fill is in question." The group *enters a deep existential crisis, with threatened dissolution of the group situation.* He anticipates reporting such to the Committee, and attributes such gloom to the members. He reports an inner transaction of memories of being excluded from other groups because of his personality.

Were he to relinquish what I take to be the self justified aspect, if not arrogance, of that personality, he would also experience the gloom he attributes to the members and be on the way to analysis of his character.

19) Another group leader emerges, Mr. Q, spokesman for the group's autonomy. He stated that logical argument would not get the data sought, and *it was up to the group to experience the nature of its phenomena for itself, and I must have good reason to take my line.*

There were three elements extant and accomplished here, the issue of logic versus its opposite, affirmation of Bion's reason, and the group's capacity to identify and explore its nature.

20) Bion notes a change of course in the group, a change he also notes as an improvement in "atmosphere."

It is accompanied by Bion's second thoughts on his resistive personality.

I would infer that he notices a lifting of the sense of silent challenge he reported at the inception of the account. In the emergent acceptant setting, he begins to work in private on the resistance that has caused him so much trouble in the past, in his work with groups.

21) Bion reports awareness of a former lower opinion of the group, and a personal bias against self revelation, which he reconsiders.

This would call for inner self scrutiny of analytic nature, and my growing thesis here is that he is resisting awareness of his arrogance and messianism.

22) Almost simultaneously, the members return to the former position of wanting him to lead in the manner he had resisted. Bion intrapsychically allows as how the

members are with justice annoyed at him for his resistance. Paradoxically his mind alights on the issue of a past sense of gain groups have experienced at this point, his attempts on his own to discern why that was so, and also to ask others, in vain. He finishes this introspection with the determination "to present a broader view of the situation."

I would infer here that he is determined to be more open, "broadly," to data about his personality.

23) Bion intrapsychically speculates, through ascribing such to the members of the group, that his internal resistances are also present in the transactions in the mental life of the group. He alludes to the mobilization of resistances going on in the group, to the possibility that the members are coming to the conclusion "that the label on the box is a good description of its contents." Realizing such, they logically would become alienated, and leave, as members have in past groups. He states then to the reader that the group is in crisis.

He senses that the members are making ready to infer that his internal mental contents match his resistive position, further that the group is in a real crisis and ready to break up.

24) He then reviews past history in a most peculiar manner, employing double negatives: that at first the group was unwilling to think it had not satisfied itself re hearsay about Bion.

One would infer that he pictured the group as satisfied re the hearsay, but with the profusion of negatives, simultaneously not so.

25) Bion alleges to the reader that he is but another member of the group, with specialized knowledge. He goes on to state that the Clinic has "given the seal of authority to a myth of unknown dimensions." Next he states that the group's tensions call for a God "fully responsible for all that takes place."

We are next door in awareness to a possible messianic identity for Bion, arrived at after the assertion he was just another member of the group, with specialized knowledge.

26) Members then assert that Bion had knowledge of what he was about, which Bion interprets as its insistence on its will. He later alludes to members speaking different languages.

If my hypothesis is correct that Bion was edging up on awareness of his messianic identity, although sensed as god-like, rather than messianic per se, the cognizance by the members that he knows what he was about would be the match of his internal cognitive process. Otherwise, he was ascribing to the members his own willfulness. He previously alluded to spitefulness, a state allied to willfulness. Denying his "eminence," he cites "the objective fact that he is only a member of the group possessing specialized knowledge". But it does bring up the question of the leader as a member of the group, and subject to the powerful forces he notes at this point. The metaphor of different languages refers to states of alienation.

27) The members turn to a self effacing member for leadership.
Bion senses that the members chose a leader representative of a self effacing mood.

28) Bion communicates the "bright idea" that the members are searching for a leader to give them orders, or for survival, or to deal with emergencies. He goes on to

speculate on such wish to be an archaism, stemming from what would seem as inappropriate fear of emotional, or some other emotional situation.

This swing is consonant with the dialectic established in the group, of swinging from one ego position to the other. In his speculation about archaism and threat in the group, he is edging into conceiving the transference. However, he is out of touch with those considerations, through his transcendent intellectual defenses.

He does not go further in report of this group, but it is apparent that he is the chief obstacle to inquiry, by himself and others, into what the members suffer from, and its correlate, himself as a healing agent. He has alluded to this conundrum in stating they wish him to be God, his approach to the subject of messianism.

29) He then reports further work with groups, and a pattern in which he discerns how members give away an aspect of their internal psychology by their seeking or aversive behavior in the group.

Discernment of this aspect of their internal psychology, by projective identification, is a great contribution by Bion to group psychoanalysis, linking it with Klein's work with individuals.

30) He then cites how the curiosity of the group in his personality slackens after two or three sessions, to be transferred to other members.

I would infer that he here intuits that there is cogency in that interest, a cogency my group therapists and I at Fort Knox noted in the silences, and identified as related to messianic expectations. We noted that traversal of this phase of the group development resulted in change from psychopathic behavior to that consonant with reality, or normal. In regard to this potentially momentous change, Bion earlier noted that "the group atmosphere changed for the better."

31) He reports that he interprets the interest in others besides himself is related ultimately to him. He gathers evidence of this he thinks will convince the group, and presents it as such. He terms it evidence of "transition."

Again, he intuits that the members are still after him to enact an aspect of his role and responsibility (I take to be messianic) before they will unburden themselves of the information about themselves he is seeking.

32) Bion brings up the issue of wisdom versus doubts.

I relate this reference to doubt and wisdom to the issue of the members' doubts regarding his wisdom as leader.

Throughout his assiduous and detailed exposition, Bion reiterates appreciation of the powerful emotional currents traversing the group and himself. His lucid and at times baffling prose has made him a touchstone in the treatment of the severe disorders, illuminating patients and self as persons in life dilemmas, momentous in nature, in a struggle for freedom hampered by their personality limitations.

An exposition, not as detailed, is found in the group report of another psychoanalyst, August Aichorn, in his seminal work, *Wayward Youth*, found in this Annotated Bibliography. While I am at it, I would like to cite the report of psychoanalytic experience, similarly conversational in tone, rendered by George Groddeck, in his *Book Of The It*, reported elsewhere in this Bibliography.

Brabender, V. and Fallon, A. 1993. *Models of Inpatient Group Psychotherapy*, Washington, D.C. American Psychological Association.

Early in this massive work, the authors seek to make explicit the assumptions about psychopathology and the processes effecting its alteration, goals and interventions that purportedly accomplish them. They pose delineation of models as the context of events and systematic intervention. They quote Yalom on the advisability of the consequent cognitive framework. They describe seven models.

The first is educative (Maxmen), in which the subject, using information furnished by the leader and the analysis of the situation in the group, learns to think clinically and behave therapeutically towards others. Meetings are held without staff.

The second is the interpersonal model, using Sullivan's principles of social learning, Yalom's relatively unstructured version, and use of data from the here-and-now for interpersonal learning, the go-around potentiation of group process, and agenda-setting for ego potentiation. Yalom also advocated focus groups for lower functioning members.

The third is the object relations/systems model, reflective of the organization of the patients' inner lives. Residency on the unit is advisable. Attention is paid to the relationship to inner schemata, or images, treated as objects, and their generation in experience with the external objects or family members. Attention is paid to early ego formation, and the phenomenon of splitting. The course in treatment of Vince Jordan is an example of the object relations approach.

The fourth model is the developmental, based on the developmental stages of psychotherapy groups. The group is conceived of as a social system, developing its unique structure. The development of the large group in the Powdermaker and Frank's *Group Psychotherapy* is a case in point. A great deal of attention is paid to development of the groups in This Way Out.

The fourth model is the cognitive-behavioral. While the patient's cognition is a primary concern in many of the psychodynamic therapies, the cognitive-behavior approach is a systematic therapy of its own. The patient is turned into a behavioral scientist, ferreting out data from the personal environment leading to incorrect, distorting, and self defeating theories about self, dysfunctional schemas. The therapist is a co-scientist and instructor, and the patient instructs self. The groups here are small, 4–12. The authors provide session protocols and examples of cognitive distortions.

The fifth is the problem solving model. Its centerpiece is skills training, taught by the leader. S/he poses the method, and modes of reframing of the problems presented in the sessions. Aids such as posters, slides, and films are employed, as in the work in Howard Hall.

The sixth is the behavioral/ social skills model. Empiric in basis, and begun in opposition to introspection, it sought phenomena that were subject to consensual validation, that which was observable. In practice, it centers on correction of untoward or defective behavior, phenomena present in inpatient settings. The empiric validity of an intervention with dilapidated patients was their change towards more normal and acceptable behavior patterns. It emphasized action and was ahistorical. Goal setting, skills training, and exercises are features of the practice.

The seventh model is social skills training per se. Base on stimulus-stimulus connection, or classical conditioning, or stimulus-response, and particular outcome, or operant conditioning. In addition there are vicarious or observational experiences, or reciprocal interactions, or "reciprocal determinism."

The authors discuss the increasing commonalities among the models, developed pragmatically in inpatient group psychotherapy, as the realities and complexity of the treatment situation evolve. "One true path does not exist" (Lazarus, Beutler, and Norcross 1992). That was the experience of *This Way Out*, though based on psychoanalysis.

Cleckley, H. 1976. *The Mask of Sanity*, St. Louis: Mosby.

In this pioneering study of psychopathy, still pertinent, Cleckley, in anecdotal fashion lays out his experience with psychopaths, leading to the inference that they suffered a deep alteration in their capacity to live in their and our reality sufficient to be described as psychotic.

Durkin, H. E. 1954. *Group Therapy for Mothers of Disturbed Children*, Springfield: Charles C Thomas.

Utilizing relationship therapy, an application of psychoanalysis, Durkin set to inquiring into the unconscious needs and emotions of mothers and the behavior of their children. Over a period of 15 years and 100 groups of meetings of mothers, once weekly, she found that the interference of the mothers in the treatment of their children was eliminated. Moreover, the neurotic pressure of the children in the family removed, and character change in the mothers effected. This was done through collaboration of the mothers in analysis of the transferences they brought to the group.

Eissler, K.R. 1949. *Searchlights on Delinquency: New Psychoanalytic Studies*, New York: International Universities Press.

This is a commemorative volume dedicated to Professor August Aichorn, a teacher and psychoanalytic pioneer, on his 70th birthday. His work in rehabilitation apparently started with an interest in the causes and treatment of delinquency, then a ten year crusade, as educator, against a military settlement for boys, in Vienna. With the fall of the monarchy at the end of World War I, he was given the opportunity to organize a new school, at Oberhallanbrun, adapting a psychoanalytic approach to treatment.

In a Biographical Outline, Eissler informs us at some length of Aichorn's personality, seminal to his success. He lauds his non egoistic passion, intuition, capacity for life in the other, alienated countries of crime and schizophrenia. It would appear that Aichorn provides us with the complementary side of Freud that, if pursued systematically, would open psychopathy and schizophrenia to psychoanalysis.

Oscar Pfister, the pioneer pastoral psychoanalyst, has a chapter on Aichorn's therapeutic approach and his ethics. He addresses the locus and core of idealism he and Aichorn term love. Failures in the arena of parent-child love result in waywardness. He personifies "noble and sublimated love," which Pfister equates with Christian. Pfister describes the mission of the therapist as like that of the Son of Man, "come to seek and save that which is lost, "a pivotal mechanism of his corrective education." This love transference is cultivated, acknowledged, and employed as reward to the delinquent in compensation for the rigors experienced in the process of self change. Aichorn expects his charges to lead useful lives, and expects to take pride in them, in a transference that does not end. Relapses are dealt with in a manner similar to that of Jesus.

Pfister calls for the creation of a new ego ideal. He cites that Aichorn permitted wild boys to abreact their rage, letting them subsequently to find, through his super-ordinative care, that they were heaping "coals of fire on their own heads." (Proverbs, 25, 22.) This was followed by tears of rage, emotional instability, then acceptable behavior. An essential element in the "cure" was Aichorn's ready engagement with his charges in discussion of daily life in which they poured out their troubles. There they discovered his strength. This became the core element in their new ego ideal.

In a footnote at the end of his piece, Pfister introduces the word messianic, in reference to a misguided aspect of science, independent of ethics. It does not offer "the faintest protection against the diabolical destruction of the highest human values, but rather it constitutes the most terrible danger unless the development of human, social-ethical attitudes keep pace with it." One can infer that in his Jesus-like approach, to Pfister, Aichorn was messianic.

Eissler and Pfister laud and analyze Aichorn in *Searchlights on Delinquency*, but the volume is a treasure trove of work done by Melitta Schmideberg, Edward Glover, Anna Freud, and Margaret Mahler. The last presents a report of work done with children of analysts, whom she calls, *enfants terrible*, for their arrogance and alienation.
Grotjahn, Martin. 1993. *The Art and Technique of Analytic Group The*rapy, North-
    vale: Aronson.

Another analyst who worked with large groups in the crucible of creativity that was World War II, Grotjahn in simple language attempts here to tell how he and his groups work. He defines his approach as analysis by the group, as differentiated from Alexander Wolf's analysis of the individual in the group, or J. L. Moreno's analysis of the group. He holds that all psychoanalysis is group therapy, but faults individual therapy for inducing regression into a transference neurosis that "swallow(s) the analyst." The group is a "theater in the round" for the projection of the entire mind. Grotjahn gives a vivid picture of not only his work with groups, but of his internal life therein.
Chasseguet-Smirgel, Janine. 1985. *The Ego Ideal: A Psychoanalytic Essay of the
    Malady of the Ideal,* New York: W.W. Norton.

Chasseguet-Smirgel reviews the literature on the ego ideal, especially Freud's contribution. However, she first details her own theses. She holds for the existence of an agency within the ego, its conscience, that has its origin in the earliest developmental period. She conceives the infant as precociously driven by inordinate ambitions that stem from an illusion of symbiosis with the mothering one. The infant seeks to reify the consequent ideal ego.

The issues inherent to this conundrum are central to the self analyses of the patients in *This Way Out*. They begin under the thrall of ideal, delusional states that are matched with their opposites, as with Vince Jordan and John Jefferson. These turn out to have developed during epiphanic states in their illnesses, that followed dementia praecox-like crises. Prior, it appeared that they were in narcissistic states, derivative of illusions of symbioses with parental figures, principally the mother. From later work, I have inferred that there was a sacrifice of identity in favor of the maternal object, accompanied by a state of psychic death. Freud identified that ubiquitous death as an instinctual state.

Freud, S. 1900. *The Interpretation of Dreams*, S.E. IV and V, London: The Hogarth Press

The patients in Howard Hall reported that they experienced their psychoses as dreamlike states. Their references in the record to their dreams were sparse, compared to those in patients in my later practice, extra-institutional and institutional. I infer that further training and experience made the difference. However, Freud's instruction in dream analysis was central in the transaction with the patients in Howard Hall, involving suspension of disbelief, acceptance of the emergent material within and without the therapist, while maintaining one's capacity to correlate and estimate it. This did not induce further regression into psychosis of the patients, as was feared, because of its grounding in the capacity to "figure it out" emphasized in the therapeutic enterprise.

———. 1921. *Group Psychology and the Analysis of the Ego*, S.E., XVIII, London: The Hogarth Press.

In this seminal work Freud intimately relates the character of the group and the individual, through the concept of ego ideal. In the formation of the group, members invest both the leader and members with their ego ideal, regressing in the process. Freud also correlates this process with the intrapsychic process that occurs in mania, where he holds that there the ego and ego ideal become as one. Vince Jordan and William Cohen in *This Way Out* traversed manic episodes, regressing into megalomanic states. Recovery involved relinquishment of that delusion, experiencing antecedent narcissism, which in turn yielded to analysis, with data pointing to psychic symbiosis with the maternal object.

Gibbard, Graham S., Harperman, John J., and Mann, Richard D. Eds. 1974. *Analysis of Groups: Contributions to Theory, Research, and Practice*, San Francisco: Bossey-Bass.

This classic has material on observation of groups, group process and development, the individual and the group, collective fantasy and myth in group formation, and authority and leadership. Much attention is given to data collection and analysis, integrating psychoanalytic (Bion, French, Foulkes) and social science approaches (Bales, Murray). Of particular note is the detailed presentation of training group protocols.

Glover, E. 1960. *The Roots of Crime*, New York: International Universities Press.

In this large work, Dr. Glover, a pioneer psychoanalyst, centers his inquiry about a superego defect. He cites the normal infant as "completely egocentric, greedy, dirty, violent in temper, destructive in habit, profoundly sexual in purpose, aggrandizing in attitude, devoid of all but the most primitive reality sense, without conscience or moral feeling, whose attitudes towards society (as represented by the family) is opportunistic, inconsiderate, domineering, and sadistic." He quotes a lady magistrate's remark, "But, doctor, the dear babies! How could you say such awful things about them?" Perhaps the answer to that conundrum is that she saw the messianic and he the satanic side of the baby, itself in an earliest state of alienation from self. The closest Glover comes to the phenomenon of alienation from self is in a mention of Franz Alexander's concept of the Neurotic Character as driven by demonic compulsion, with overpowering of the ego by an Id that produces tendencies alien to the ego. The inference is that the Id tendency would be alien in itself, locating the seat of alienation in the Id. Glover goes on to cite Wilhelm Reich's '*triebhafter*' character, taken over by instincts. Glover goes on to cite his 'neurotic characters' and there a change in the libidinal milieu, repetitive in nature. He goes further to cite that the "psychotic character' might be more appropriate.

Glover has the personality of the psychopath as within normal bounds, overcome by abreactive periods of psychopathic tension, revealing an underlying mental abnormality "almost as grave as that of an insane person, and absence of reality feeling or judgment, and frequent senselessness and peculiarity of behavior." A strong lead in research is the concept of unconscious guilt, in which the individual induces punishment due to repressed infantile wishes. Certainly the patients in Howard Hall had strong moral tendencies early, chiefly as requirements for the adults in their family.

Greenblatt, M., Levinson, D., and Williams, R. Eds. 1957. *The Patient and the Mental Hospital: Contributions of Research in the Science of Human Behavior*, The Free Press.

This important study reports on the papers and discussion of the Conference on Socio-environmental Aspects of Patient Treatment in Mental Hospitals. The Conference was rendered immediate by the deterioration of care in the state hospitals of the period, and the need for establishment of the therapeutic milieu, or community newly emerging on the medical scene. Participants were the leading lights in the state hospital, NIMH, and university (Harvard and Michigan) scenes. Added in this volume to the professions extant in the mental hospitals of the day (nurse, social worker, recreationist, occupational therapist, clinical psychologist, and chaplain) were the sociologist, social psychologist, and social anthropologist, to study the institution itself, in an ongoing manner. The Conference on Socio-environmental Aspects followed a Symposium on the Mental Hospital as a Small Society, with social science playing a central part.

The Patient and the Mental Hospital is the distillation of 60 investigators, of diverse theoretical and empirical approaches. That distillation is of seminal importance to the understanding of *This Way Out*, and is embodied in Dr. Harry Solomon's concluding chapter, entitled The Mental Hospital as a Research Setting: A Critical Approach. There he cites the critical ideas raised by the investigators: "social structure, formal and informal organization, culture, social position and role, transactional processes, group dynamics, ideology, identity, the social patterning of authority and the individual's relation to authority, unconscious conflict and ego defense." They are of moment sufficient for inclusion in the *This Way Out*'s Glossary.

Dr. Solomon goes on to cite the value of the naturalistic approach to research, for its "initial exploration of complex social and psychological processes and in the search for significant concepts and hypotheses." He goes on further to cite its limitation, as a single case study, insufficient formulation of variables, deficiencies in research design. These considerations were very much in mind in *This Way Out*, and reflected in its initial approach, running commentary, and inferences. In a section, entitled Role Dilemmas of the Mental Hospital Investigator, Dr. Solomon examines the issue of choice of problem, achieving a tenable position and role within the hospital, and interpreting, writing and publishing the research. All of these deeply cogent considerations were encountered in the text of *This Way Out*. Finally, Dr. Solomon argues for a field research role for the social scientist. This of course applies even more so to the psychiatrist and psychoanalyst.

Greenblatt, M., Sharaf, M. R., and Stone, E. M. 1971. *Dynamics of Institutional Change*, Pittsburgh: University of Pittsburgh Press.

This volume is of great importance to *This Way Out* for its problem in bringing about basic institutional change, as a platform of the therapeutic community. Greenblatt cites at length how he came to the concept of unitization, or decentralization. What he had in mind was in advance of the work in industry of centering organization about tasks. He re-created Boston State Hospital into four units, serving different localities, emphasizing autonomy and local responsibility, in a larger unity that was responsible to them, and of course, the community. He worked to re-orient the personnel, administrative and professional. All this is what happened in Howard Hall, started from the grassroots.

Groddeck, Georg 1935, *The Book of the It*. London: C.W. Daniel Company

In this seminal work, Groddeck spells out what psychoanalysis was about in its early years, through letters to an imaginary woman. This is the Groddeck who had established a psychiatric retreat in Bad-Baden, Germany, which Ferenczi and Freud visited. At the same time, Groddeck communed with trolls in a lair he constructed up the hill, nearby. He has one of them, Patrick Troll, sign his letter/chapters. One can conjecture a personality configuration similar to that of Wilhelm Reich, who contributed greatly to psychoanalysis, regressing later in life to experiencing reality in a religious manner. All this is in turn relevant to the issue of messianism in their makeup. Goddeck's spiritual side is reflected in his conception of the unconscious, which he called the It. Freud importantly changed the designation to Id.

A Morris Robb provides the Introduction. He employs lyrical language, seeing Groddeck as reverential, feeling from the heart, contemplating the mystery of life, its wonder and paradox. Complexity is reduced by symbolism, dealing with the soul and its cycles. Reduced are high/low, narrow/broad, discord/harmony, confusion/clarity. He saw Groddeck as sharing, fellow friend, genius, with strange ideas that somehow became part of one's life, breaking from terror, awakening that which has been asleep, outgrowing one's traditions and former sexual ways.

The inference I would draw from this introduction is that Robb senses that Goddeck addresses what we now would consider issues in the ego ideal, as would a dream analyst. The text of the book calls for translation from that of an informal letter to a friend. He starts with a confession I believe Groddeck cites that he was raised like Joseph above his brothers, by his father's offer of a profession, based on his capacity for empathy. He had sensed that his sister would be smothering her doll with excessive clothing, Along with that existed murder, based on envy of her. He goes on to examine the components and dynamics of his professional identity, eschewing, in identification with her gentleness, the blood of the surgeon and poisons of the physician, for massage and mental treatment.

He goes on to inquire into his relationship to science as a discipline. He starts by citing how his identity as a researcher stemmed from a fixation on his sister's cardiac condition. He attests to impatience with the acute, versus chronic. That impatience would interfere with looking at the affection systematically, a hallmark of science. He cites his father's heretical and doubting attitude towards science, his scoffing at the theory that bacteria as causative of disease, and autistic esteem for the curative value of bouillon. He also had an aversion towards science, because both his sister's friend and school were associated with Alma and Mater. He goes on to his experience with this mother, her need for a nursemaid because of atrophied breasts, and a hypothesized deprivation when he was a sucking babe.

He then went on to cite a woman who had been deprived early in the suckling stage, and developed a life long enmity to her mother: "As thou to me, so I to thee." This woman's gait is that of a pregnant woman, her breasts swell when she sees a suckling babe, and abdomen enlarges when her friends conceive. A yearning cry for the unattainable. He goes on to posit the truth of another child symbiosis, sealed in the nursing experience. From that truth, one escapes into the kingdom of fantasy, a fantasy similar to that of science.

This amalgam of science and fantasy, tied together through intuition, marks the rest of the book. In the second chapter he goes on to assert that man is governed by an unknown force, an It. It is present as the underlay of life, and we are cut away from it by our infantile amnesia. Yet we revert to it, and to manifestation of our parents, and of the It they bequeath. He attributes his strange ideas to Professor Freud. He goes on to speak of the ubiquity of ambivalence, mother love and mother hate, and its manifold assaults on the expected child and numerous psychosomatic abdominal disorders. "It only disappears when one succeeds in tracking down and purifying the filthy swarm in the recesses of the soul, the poisonous swarm which corrupts the unconscious."

Thus Groddeck paints a picture of a sentient self at the core of the personality of the individual, which he terms the soul. It is an intelligence that operates on mythic terms, not a region of unknowing chaotic forces. Suitably situated in a constructive stance through their messianism, the patients of Howard Hall were able to read and translate their Its in a manner similar to that of Groddeck and his trolls.

Jones, M. 1953. *The Therapeutic Community*. New York: Basic Books.

Describing the social structure of an industrial unit in a hospital, itself integrated closely with the surrounding community, Jones goes on to cite how local industries were employed in the treatment of the patients, plus the use of a large group conference to deal with emerging problems. The fortuitous designation, therapeutic community came into wide usage, as well as its underlying logic, of the answerability of the parts to the whole, and vice versa.

————. 1968. *Beyond the Therapeutic Community: Social Learning and Social Psychiatry*, New Haven: Yale

In addition to advocating leveling of hierarchy in the organization of the mental hospital, Jones espouses what he calls multiple leadership, or the assumption of leadership initiative on the part of its components. He acknowledges the pioneering work done by Laing and associates at Kingsley Hall. There they had "ordinary" people living with schizophrenics, who were allowed to regress to infantile levels, followed by reintegration. Howard Hall had regression, of controlled sort, modulated by both patients and personnel, in the context of therapeutic problem solving, as illustrated with William Bostic and Vince Jordan. Jones forsees a great future for therapeutic community and social psychiatry.

————. 1991. The Therapeutic Community: Dialogues With Maxwell Jones, M.D. Interviewed by Dennie Briggs. *Special Collections, The Library, University of California San Francisco.*

In this important volume Dennie Briggs, a long time associate, if not informal partner with Maxwell Jones in the development of therapeutic community, interviews Jones over a period of 21 years, most of it at Jones' instance. This is the distillation of notes and recordings, aiming to render understandable the phenomena attending therapeutic community in the groups and its leadership. Briggs cites that Jones created democracy within autocracy. Both Jones and Briggs underwent psychoanalysis in the course of their careers, Jones with Melanie Klein. He refers to his three years on the couch as ultimately burdensome, devoted to biography, reductive to earlier memories.

It is my inference that the messianism, the God, mystical, and spiritual experience he reports at the end of his career was present as an underlayment earlier. Wilhelm Reich, a psychoanalytic pioneer was similarly motivated towards social change, and displayed his spiritual side floridly towards the end. Maxwell Jones may have fled the couch when his messianism brought him into rivalry and conflict with his analyst, Melanie Klein. In his account of his career, Jones first cites the atmosphere he was able to establish (in his groups), then the failure of psychoanalysis to deal with his problematic emotions, the immense relief he experiences in his group work, but at the end of his career, still the drive towards what he calls transformation. He associates to that as spiritual or transpersonal. He retrospectively recognizes that he sensed the presence of God during prolonged silences in groups. He realizes that he needed to inquire further into what was going on there.

In my work, the groups at Fort Knox and Howard Hall developed the atmosphere Jones refers to, and a core component was messianic, saving. For the rest, the members related to one another on the simple human level described by Harry Stack Sullivan. They formed an existential unity, a transaction in the present, marked by the dialectic—thesis, antithesis, synthesis—described by Jones and Briggs. It proved be as powerful and pervasive, producing change in the individuals, the personal learning that was at the same time social.

In this review of Briggs's interviews, I shall traverse the notes I took of the fascinating dialogue. Dennie and Max talked, over the decades, in England, the Continent, America, and Canada. Briggs began by citing a remark by Jones that *therapeutic community happens when the total resources of patient and the institution are pooled.* Jones developed the original concept in work occasioned by the social dislocation of post-War London. He noted that, during the War, there was a common enemy, plenty of work, outstanding leadership, and high morale. Then, with peace, the problem subjects exhibited low intelligence, unemployment, alcohol, drugs, vague illness, deliberate idleness, hard core unemployment. Society transcended mental hospital and prison, through development of experimental rehabilitation centers, versus mental hospital and prison.

I would infer that Jones came upon the practice of therapeutic community when the groups of 100 he conducted as classes on effort syndrome during the war developed a life and initiative of their own. He then applied that group initiative to work with the ex-POW's who were alienated from themselves and others, then conceiving and enunciating the concept of therapeutic community.

Then Jones segued to his training in organic psychiatry in America prior to WW II, moving over to Maudsley in England, and a team with insulin and shock therapy. Then came the crucial war work with effort syndrome at Mill Hill, for 5 years. The teams found effort syndrome to be psychosomatic. The team decided to educate the soldiers re their condition as functional, not organic, through classes, in large groups. Attractive young women conscriptees were involved then, participating in classes of 100, with the appearance of curiosity on the part of the soldiers, evocation of contributing factors, future concerns, and then family concerns.

The therapeutic method evolved of its own momentum, according to Jones.

Smaller groups were conducted by the nurses, and discussions on a human level evolved. A Nervy Ned manikin appeared, also skits devised by personnel and patients. Prior patients educated later ones. The staff pulled back as the groups took over, on their own.

Jones and associates engaged in theorizing and notation of systematic patterns in the groups. They noted self-love versus self-hate, the binding of opposites, oscillations in the groups, with peaks, destructive periods followed by constructive ones. A soldier created and published a journal of the lecture-discussion, and addressed the issue of causes, functional versus organic. The skits evolved into systematic psychodramas, with dramatization of the core histories of members, and appearance of the voice of conscience.

This use of dramatic material was an inherent part of the work at Fort Knox and Howard Hall, though not through organized skits. We used media more, as well as audio-visual material illustrative of life courses.

Mill Hill went through behavioral crises, occasioned when the soldiers received pay, went off to drink, came back rowdy. Jones referred them to the groups to work through their issues, and got into "hot water" with the hierarchical nurses, by letting the offenders "get away with it." He was backed by his superiors, though. The theme became "Don't destroy Poor Max!" Unexpected positive leadership emerged in the groups and personnel. His fame spread, occasioning supportive visits by outside leaders.

In Howard Hall we went through similar crises with the nursing personnel.

Then came the work with returning Prisoners of War, who lost their sense of identity, suffered from alienation from self, family, and friends. Jones assembled a staff of 59, for a unit of 300. The course was 6–8 weeks, of community meetings. The ex-prisoners expected authoritarian rule, but were engaged in psychodrama, intuitive connectedness, part time employment, making their own destiny, and emergence of their latent abilities.

Then came the publication of a newspaper, *The Grapevine*, and improvement of the food. It was a democracy within basically a military situation, with emphasis on co-equality. Jones gave an example of a disturbed member who hid the Thorazine that staff believed had dispelled his symptoms, as evidence of the deeply curative value of the group process.

He and Briggs formulated it as a result of a dialectical process, social and intra-psychic: thesis-antithesis-synthesis. They had learned to depend on it in the group process to bring about changes in the individual.

They described the 8:30 Group. It met at that time in the morning, composed of 100 patients. It was followed by staff post-mortems. Doctors held groups then. Then lunch. Then a ½ hour meeting on the ward, conducted by the nurse, followed by work groups. There was a departure group, family groups. Though successful, Jones and Briggs held that the authorities, including the Anglican Church were opposed to its deviant ways, and they ended, leaving "prophets without honor."

Designation of themselves as prophets who expected some special honor is signifi-cant, attended by depression cyclically in their careers. Despite their notoriety and fame, they were acutely conscious of their minority status in the professions, and of its missionary character.

Jones then segued again to his career development. He cited himself as a life long rebel. His father, himself a mercenary soldier during the Boer Uprising died soon after it, when Jones was 5. Mother was an idealist and moralist. Maxwell, slight of stature, excelled at team sports, convinced life-long of the transcendent centrality of morale in effecting victory. He dreamt of becoming a coffee planter, choosing a medi-cal career instead because of political factors. He was enthralled by James' *Varieties of Religious Experience*. He cited John Kennedy on looking into one's own soul for courage.

He continued with exposition of work he did in education, in the introduction of peer counseling. But first he engaged in an exposition of what he calls social learning, the transformative acquisition of new ways of thought and behavior, and ostensibly unlearning of old. This occurred in the dialectical transaction in the group. He cited the hope induced in the process, and how children would not let lessons stop. One taught oneself, and Jones extended it to peer teaching. He quoted Shakespeare on "learning what sadness is made of."

In a telling exchange he confronted Briggs on the charismatic quality of Briggs' leadership, and they went into Briggs' work in prisons and his charismatic leader-ship. Briggs freed guards to advance to counselor status, shedding their uniforms. The leader's role diminished as the therapeutic community matured. They evoked the innate therapeutic capacity and sense of integrity of their social therapists. They then arrived at the term *affective integrity* that was formulated by Harry Wilmer, who pioneered therapeutic community in the US Navy. Relative to affect integrity, they hinted that they were exercising such when they left their respective analysts, "Leav-ing the couch is when the learning began."

In the work at Fort Knox and Howard Hall the members systematically arrived at the past which interfered with capacity to live in the present, the history that was the psychoanalytic transference. Dealing with it was transformative. Briggs and Jones, denying psychoanalysis as useful, encountered this phenomenon and designated it as social learning.

As an example of such learning, Jones described a situation when Diggs called on him to consult in an emergency with a potentially violent psychotic patient at Dingle-ton Hospital. He cited as background that he had in mind his initial encounter at San

Francisco State University and the formation of a lifelong partnership with Briggs. He noted Briggs' idealism, then his depression following defeats and losses in his initial mission to change the educational establishment. Jones induced Briggs to work with him at Dingleton, and he did so, after rousing and "strengthening" experiences with idealistic left wing students in Europe and England. Briggs was given his own ward, and took to eating with the patients. Briggs had identified with their plight in the work detail, the dirty cutlery, and the iniquity of being subject to foul cleaning fluid, also of being relegated to separate recreational space. Representations about the dirty silverware went nowhere, and the final straw was the fact that the patients had less rashers or sausages for breakfast. He then sat with the patients at meals.

He sensed a fellow prophet, willing to be martyred for the cause, the "truth." In the dialog with Jones, Briggs equated that act of rebellion with standing for the "whole truth," alleging that " therapeutic community was being used there to control "spontaneity and freedom." Jones sadly acknowledged he had been living there in an "illusionary world," to the effect that what was of moment on the level Briggs occupied had not reached his executive level. Had it done so, Jones would have subjected it to "social learning." It would overcome the "errors of family, school, and other formative influences that tend to produce a stereotype, the so-called normal person."

At the end of their careers, they were ready for analysis of its messianic components. Jones mentions the social learning he would have undergone, if he had descended from his illusionary height, at Briggs' instance. He would have associated to, in psychoanalytic manner, the lifelong mission he had pursued in addressing the morale of his athletic groups towards winning. The compulsive rebellion against authority and unfinished rivalry with authority, father figures would have come into view, etc. He might have encountered the contents of a recurrent depression which he managed to transcend by plunging himself into new challenges.

Jones went on to cite the problem with administering discipline, the problem Briggs experienced on his ward with the potentially violent patient. Jones advocated spontaneity and taking risks, and in the social dialectic, the surfacing of parts of the personality previously hidden. He went on to trace the development of the group identity formed at Mill Hill, to that in the ex-POW center, then Henderson. He had abandoned his training in psychotherapy, to admission to the patients that "we don't know how to treat you." He described the new method as "eye-ball to eye-ball" in a circle, one speaking at a time, not too long, group setting its rules, and each patient a participant in decision making.

I would infer here that the free interpersonal association and the formation of a transactional unity resulted in a new unity and separation from the past one.

Briggs and Jones agreed that faith, trust in the process, objectivity of the facilitator, representation of all, in equity, were essential. Result: new learning, new decisions.

Next in the dialog was a letter from Jones to Briggs from Nova Scotia, July 25, 1987, in which to Jones the foggy countryside was experienced as "a transcendental infinity, construed as an invisible reality." He went on to cite that he was "enveloped in the mystery of life if (one) cease to exist separately." He maybe "understands the meaning of pantheism and the divinity of the whole." God is not present in his conscious mind, but still part of the universe. Jones is "all or nothing." "Dialogue is creativity."

I would infer that the unity, the cessation of separate existence, was accomplished through merging with the divine.

In their dialog, Jones and Briggs then bemoaned the regression into stereotypy in the worlds of therapeutic community. Jones immersed himself in work at Stanford University and the San Mateo Program in 1959, also work with character disorders in prison work with Doug Grant at Chino. Briggs had initiated New Careers for the Helping Professions and the forestry camps in Southern California. Jones then went on to work in the Virgin Islands, which ended with disillusionment with the hierarchic white and black cultures, and the rigidity of the National Institutes of Mental Health. Both Jones and Briggs lauded Thomas Szasz for his opposition to medical domination and advocacy of life as that what was meant to be lived.

They now came to sum up. Jones cited the paradigm of open systems, but found that they were inherently self reifying. Jones stated that he has been accused as manipulative. But Briggs and Jones knew that multiple leadership was valuable and self correcting, leading to superordinate freedom of thought. There was transcendence and realization of inner self, and one became in touch with a higher being. Jung's universal unconscious was applicable.

Jones then noted that he was in a crisis, after 50 years in the minority, after attack by the medical profession, itself pathetic. It was a test of the integrity of the group approach as a whole, and in his case an instance of *metanoia* (fundamental transformation of the mind). Jones cited that he respected women more than men, despite their dominance. Children learn from each other. One needs to submit to learning about oneself. Myths do outlive one. There was a change from war to peace, on a condition of soul, Christ-like. The enemy was oneself. He has been a leader of the transformative movements.

He cited his despondence, and his "pain, for the while." There was always the inspiration of taking up another task, for the while. There was the inspiration, between waking and sleeping, awake dreaming, becoming and awakener. Krishnamurti dissolved the barriers of time and space.

Dennie then cited Max's life changes, from charismatic leader, to awakener, and guru. Jones did not like the thought of being charismatic. Dennie noted the shift to power involved. They discussed Robert Bly, who Jones found exhilarating. They took satisfaction with the creation of hundreds of drug recovery communities, stemming from Jones' "hope." They lauded women's liberation, and groups of all kinds. There was a contemporary discontent with bigness, concern for integrity. A new society was being born, and education prominent there. Here was peace through peer action, and learning the inherent order in things. Learning was through social process, and feedback, listening responsibly, getting to know the person and the group.

One recycled oneself, stepped back to move forward, into a new wholeness, new identity, insecurity giving way to challenge, learning from becoming. Jones then again revealed that he terminated analysis after three years on the couch, finding the process burdensome. He had lived life in the company of deviants. He noted that creative psychopaths have been contributive, citing Gandhi and Jesus. There was psychological contagion, intuition, linking with the supernatural and metaphysical, networking. There were 15 million in futurist, citizens movements, enveloping them, revolutionary. The human brain has been fully developed for 15,000 years; the Savage Man was present, in evolution and revolution.

With early problem solving by children, one could expect the disappearance of mental illness. Jones quoted Buber on the determination to engage in dedicated listening and dialog, following giving up on religion per se, after the suicide of a student he had ignored because of Buber's immersion in religious experience. Jones cited that major problems can be, not solved, but outgrown, through an ego-less, spiritual phase. He and Briggs went into the phenomenon of silence in the group, "a living silence in the group, that attended deep change. Jones went on to equate psychoanalytic with obsessive attention to biography, reducing the process to restoration of memories.

This ego-less, spiritual phase would be central to the social learning itself central to their group process.

Jones addressed the attainment of a state of grace in human experience, and the presence of God. Briggs returned to the role of silence in the treatment of prisoners, sailors, and psychiatric patients, linking it with assembling in a circle. Jones and Briggs agree that therapeutic community goes only as far as the staff allows.

Finally, Jones returned to his growing experience of spiritual, mystic growth. He has struggled to overcome his psychoanalytic training, through transformation and spirituality. Both Jones and Briggs stated that the passion for democracy was contagious, spreading all over the world.

Briggs included at the end of his volume a transcript of a large group, described by Jones as "ghastly," of student and teacher participants in a peer teaching experiment, led by Jones, that struggled to establish its separate identity, but never quite accomplished it.

This failure was ostensibly because it needed guidance at its agreed on task, a critique of a film on peer teaching, and was waylaid by Jones, himself, into self scrutiny, resisted stoutly by the members, except for one of the peer teachers, Alice.

Recurrently, Briggs and Jones brought up the failures of the Jonestown religious community and that of Synanon, an at first promising drug treatment community. They noted their authoritarian character as contributive, but did not go into it further. Throughout the volume they took satisfaction with the spread of the democratic ethos and practice in society, and Jones designated himself as a social ecologist, abandoning the designation of psychiatrist, especially psychoanalyst. But then he returned to his conflict with his analyst and his quitting of the couch, and the "social learning" he developed instead. My thesis is that psychoanalysis did not have within itself the instrumentality or theory of religion to enable his analyst, Melanie Klein, to analyze that transference resistance, of his rivalry with her of transcendent messianic nature. The reader is referred to the author's experience with that problem, in (2007) *The Messianic Imperative*, Philadelphia, Xlibris.

Klapman, J. W. 1946. *Group Psychotherapy: Theory and Practice*, New York: Grune and Stratton.

An early exposition on the value of group psychotherapy, with valuable discussion of its origins, also the place of psychodrama, this volume advocates it for its value in "affective reeducation."

Kanas, N. 1996. *Group Therapy for Schizophrenic Patients*, Washington, D.C.: American Psychiatric Press.

Kanas espouses what he calls an integrative group therapy model. He initiated an insight fostering one in 1975, in a military teaching hospital. He had found it to worsen psychotic patients, and in 1977 in a Veterans Administration Hospital developed a supportive, homogeneous model that focused on ways to cope with psychotic symptoms and improve interpersonal relationships.

Liff, Zanvel A, Ed. 1975. *The Leader in the Group*, New York: Jason Aronson.

A celebration of 35 years of leadership in analytic group psychotherapy by Alexander Wolf, this engaging work has chapters by Wolf, Schwartz, Liff, Foulkes, Glatzer, Aronson, Mendell, and Kosseff. Wolf inveighs against authoritarian leadership, emphasizing informality. In his practice he had his groups meet in alternate sessions without a therapist. It is of note that Wolf started the group therapy at Ft. Knox, and was transferred overseas because a problem arose over an insurrection on the part of the rehabilitees related to his lack of control. Of particular note in this volume is a presentation by Harriett Strachem of couples and family group therapy.

MacNamara, E.J. and McCorkle, L. Eds. 1982. *Crime, Criminals, and Corrections*, New York: John Jay Press.

The chief contribution of note in this work is its chapter on Contemporary Trends in Corrections, and within that, a detailed presentation of the Highfields Experiment conducted by Lloyd McCorkle. Within that is an absorbing account of sessions of its centerpiece, guided group interaction. The aim there was to support the adolescent, 16 years of age, in traversal of his difficulties with the law, his normalization, and alteration of his untoward behavior. Within that frame was a certain amount of character change and attainment of insight, but the theme and thesis of treatment in depth of the work at Fort Knox and Howard Hall was eschewed.

Nevertheless, Highfields claimed to cut the recidivism rate by half, over a comparable population that chose a roughly similar institution, but for its guided group interaction.

McCorkle, L. W., Elias, A., and Bixby, F. L. 1958. *The Highfields Story: A Unique Experiment in the Treatment of Juvenile Delinquents*, New York: Henry Holt.

Credit for this experiment goes to Lowell Bixby, a criminologist in the State of New Jersey, who conceived of a home for 16 year olds, with minimal personnel, and a short term, intensive stay centered about group counseling, led by a responsible professional, here, Lloyd W. McCorkle. An equal cohort was assigned to a regular reformatory. Built into the design was study of the sessions, termed guided group interaction, and the outcomes. The residents learned to achieve self control, through identification with the program, the director, and the group. There was improvement of relationship with a probation officer (67%); relationship with family (72%); attitude towards self (73%); work adjustment (57%); overall adjustment (59%). There was no in depth inquiry, as in Howard Hall.

McKay, M. and Paleg, K. Eds. 1992. *Focal Group Psychotherapy*, Oakland: New Harbinger Press.

This relatively recent work is indicative of the widespread employment of group therapy for specific areas of concern, ranging from shyness, through agoraphobia, anger, eating disorders, rape survivor, domestic violence, incest offenders, to addiction.

The language is clear and the protocols are useful in setting up psychoeducational groups in institutions.

Meloy, J. Reid. 1988. *The Psychopathic Mind: Origins, Dynamic, and Treatment*, Northvale CT: Aronson.

This serious and significant work on psychopathy, from a psychoanalytic point of view is of special moment when it comes to treatment. This becomes even more important in a forensic hospital or prison, where individuals with varying degrees of psychopathy are incarcerated. Meloy starts his section on treatment by noting the "heart and soul" it takes to undertake such a venture. I would infer that he is edging there into the messianism that is entailed and that I consider an initial essential to the therapeutic alliance with the severe disorders. Meloy further emphasizes that he assumes initially that the subject will deceive him. It is possible and necessary to hold both ego positions.

In the chapter on treatment Meloy goes into the internal operations of the psychopath inquired into by the psychoanalysts Edith Jacobson and Otto Kernberg. Search for the role of messianism as an avenue to treatment is fruitless. Yochelson spoke of conversion of the psychopath as an essential step in treatment. In the work at Ft. Knox and also Howard Hall, abandonment of psychopathy was attended by transient psychosis and neurosis, an indication of a psychotic base to character disorder. Meloy does arrive at that position in a chapter on structure and dynamics.

Powell, John Walker. 1950. Group Reading in Mental Hospitals, *Psychiatry: Journal for the Study of Interpersonal Processes*, 13:2, May.

Dr. Powell extended his practice of reading discussion groups from libraries in San Francisco to Chestnut Lodge Sanitarium and Howard Hall. It was an extension of the adult education movement (late 1940 to 1960) of Professor Alexander Meikeljohn, of the University of Wisconsin. Meiklejohn held that a great task of democracy was the further education of adults. Powell applied his theory and practice through reaching alienated populations. In Howard Hall, utilizing group leadership similar to mine, he was able to engage with the members, white and black, in discussion of America's founding tracts, such as the Declaration of Independence. Trained in critical thought, members further contributed to the *Howard Hall Journal* and to their recovery.

Rachman, A. W. 1975. *Identity Group Therapy With Adolescents*, Springfield: Charles C Thomas.

Based on Erik Ericson's concept of identity formation and development, Rachman's group sees group therapy as the treatment of choice with adolescents. The crises inherent in development are gone into in detail and related to group phenomena. This work is of moment for its similarity to the Fort Knox and Howard Hall experiences, whose sessions were marked by traversal of developmental crises. Rachman describes marathon sessions that in essence resemble the experience reported with Wilfred Bostic.

Rosenbaum, M. and Snadowsky, A. 1957. *The Intensive Group Experience*, New York: The Free Press.

The authors and contributors cast a wide net, encompassing group dynamics, group encounter, institutional group work, psychodrama, Alcoholics Anonymous, intentional communities, millennial communities, etc. attempting to identify that which is "intensive" and effective in accomplishing change. The review of work in prisons is valuable, for its exposition of difficulties presented by the prison situation.

Rubenfeld, S. 1965. *Family of Outcasts: A New Theory of Delinquency*, New York: The Free Press.

Rubenfeld centers his theory on oppressive ideals imposed by 'sure' parents, resulting in massive reaction formation on the part of youth who are pursuing deviant personal values of their own that amount to a culture of their own. Alienation from self and other is systemic, fixating developed patterns. The way out of that dilemma lies in negotiation of new values and redefinition of selves. Rubenfeld inquires into the economically and other culturally advantaged groups, identifying enthrallment to celebrating the ego, personal power, individual competence in work, play, and sex games. All of this analysis is done in eloquent, vivid style, in a chapter entitled, National values, Neurosis, and Delinquency.

Rubenfeld's begins exposition of his theory of delinquency with the proposition of *eunomie*, or normative collaboration, itself a reciprocal relation within a culture between end state attainment and social synergy. Integrative failure there results in "outness," self destructive roles, and "hardening." He cites opportunity theory and role preparation in a career in crime. These constructs underlay the work at Knox and Howard Hall, in search for causes and courses in recovery. They were prominent in the methodology at Fort Knox, taught pre-war to McCorkle by the sociologist Clifford Shaw at the Chicago Area Project, a successful counter-delinquency venture.

Slavson, S. R. Ed. 1956. *The Fields of Group Psychotherapy*, New York: International Universities Press.

Slavson's authors cover the fields of mental hospitals, psychosomatic disorders, addiction, alcoholism, stuttering , allergies, geriatrics, mothering, delinquents, child guidance, family services, private practice, community mental health, industry, training and research- all indicative of how rapidly and widespread group therapy had become.

———. 1964. *A Textbook in Analytic Group Psychotherapy*, New York: International Universities Press.

This is a massive compilation of half a century of work by Slavson, a social worker who was one of the initiators of group psychotherapy. Done in a forthright manner, he starts by citing how he discovered the process, in searching why he and his colleagues were successful in a recreational project, finding that the group per se was the operant variable. He later discerned Freudian mechanisms. He has concluded that limitation of group size to eight is necessary for results, a notion at odds with the work at Knox and Howard Hall.

Spotnitz, Hyman. 1961. *The Couch and the Circle*, New York: Alfred Knopf.

Spotnitz was an analyst, Consultant to Slavson's domain, the Jewish Board of Guardians, who started a group with "untreatable" patients whose treatment in turn seemed to be at a standstill. At first surprised at the ease they experienced in adjusting to one another, he came to rely on their capacity to bring out latent capacity for problem solving and expansion of each other's horizons. He called analytic group therapy the third psychiatric revolution, and espoused small groups as the modality of intervention.

Stanton, Alfred H. and Schwartz, Morris S. 1954. *The Mental Hospital: A Study of Institutional Participation in Psychiatric Illness and Treatment*, New York: Basic Books.

This seminal work, a socio-psychiatric report of a 3 year study of Chestnut Lodge, a psychoanalytic mental hospital, is of moment in understanding the structure and functioning of Howard Hall. Stanton and Schwartz, "living on the wards" found that there were too many people making decisions, they were emotionally skewed, and there was insufficient feedback. Their reports resulted in concomitant centralization, federalization, systematic conferences, and separation of administration from therapy. Applying those theses to Howard Hall, one may cite that the attendants "in the line of fire" decided too much, there was deficient consensual upper and mid-level authority, no systematic feedback by conferences. Emotional skewing by attendants was rife. Both institutions in time worked towards the therapeutic community model, with differences in individual therapy in Chestnut Lodge and group therapy in Howard Hall. Both called for increased competency on the part of patients, and answerability on the part of therapists.

Sullivan, Harry Stack. 1953. *The Collected Works of Harry Stack Sullivan*, New York: W. W. Norton and Company.

Sullivan held that "we are all much more human than otherwise" and evidenced capability of talking with his patients in a simply human fashion, empathically reaching them. He is widely accounted as a pioneer in the treatment of the severe disorders.

In this volume he sets forth his interpersonal theory and practice. His prior experience was at St. Elizabeths, Sheppard and Enoch Pratt Hospital, and Chestnut Lodge, where he adapted psychoanalysis through his focused interview technique. He also evolved an ego psychology based on a self system that was altered through anxiety and what he called "parapraxis." Anxiety was central to the disturbance of maternal-infant relationship in early childhood. Another contribution was in the concept of malevolent transformation, a process in mid-childhood of transformation of the self towards the malevolence of psychopathy.

Thorpe, J. J. and Smith, B. 1952. Operational Sequences in Group Therapy with Young Offenders, in *The International Journal of Group Psychotherapy*, Vol. II, (p. 24–33).

Thorpe and Smith describe operational sequences in interaction with young offenders at the National Training School for Boys, in the course of development of the program there. Thorpe and Smith cite the need to integrate the group therapy into the program. They go on to pose the problems related to security and the need to "sell" the program. Certainly, that issue was made clear by the attendants in Howard Hall, in the course of the Integrated Group.

Weeks, H. A. 1958. *Youthful Offenders at Highfields: An Evaluation of Effects of Short-Term Treatment of Delinquent Boys*, Ann Arbor: University of Michigan Press.

A group of authorities, academic and forensic, examine an application by McCorkle of the work done at Fort Knox. It came about as response to judges who balked from assignment of adolescents to reformatories and training schools for youth they held redeemable. It was held on the former estate of Colonel Lindberg, and the youth stayed generally for three months, working in a nearby state hospital, attending the hour-long group sessions five days per week. It was designed to have a generalized constructive impact rather than an individualized treatment result, differing significantly from the work at Knox and Howard Hall.

Weiner, M. F. 1984. *Techniques of Group Psychotherapy*, Washington, D.C.: American Psychiatric Press.

Dr. Weiner here presents a pragmatic approach to group therapy, ranging from advice and counseling, to evocative, insight oriented treatment. A chapter is devoted to a history and overview of a wide range of the group therapies, that includes Recovery, Inc., Synanon, also teaching and training aids.

Whitaker, Dorothy S. and Lieberman, Morton A. 1964. *Psychotherapy through the Group Process*, New York: Atherton Press.

In this valuable work Whitaker and Lieberman, starting with the psychoanalyst Thomas French's focal conflict theory, approach group process in the microanalytic mode featured in *This Way Out*. Like Powdermaker and Frank they identify basic themes, "under progressively expanding cultural conditions." They fail to identify the crises and resolution inherent to the cultural change. An important feature of this work, in its effort to arrive at a way of inquiring into group process, is a comprehensive and critical review of others, such as Bion, Ezriel, Powdermaker and Frank, Foulkes, Corsini, and a host of others.

Wilmer, H. A. 1958. *Social Psychiatry In Action: A Therapeutic Community*, Springfield: Charles C Thomas.

Wilmer patterned his meetings with the admission ward community at the Psychiatric Treatment Center at the Oakland Naval Hospital on those of Maxwell Jones, T. P. Rees, and T. F. Main, in England. The experiment went on for 10 months (July 1955 to April 1956). He cites its humanitarian utility, as well as usefulness to the staff, in the betterment of the patients. The patients were in flux, varied in number and capacity for collaboration. Personnel were trained by attendance at the meetings, which are described as humanizing. Wilmer cites his motives as stemming from a rescue situation in a mental hospital, and determination to counter the brutality of its personnel. His meetings were attended by large numbers of personnel, also visitors by naval officers, including Admiral Nimitz himself. Dr. Wilmer had larger aims to "humanize" Navy personnel practices, to alter the toll of psychiatric illness. He was assiduous in the study of his experience, dictating a note after each session, recording a number of them by film and tape, and devoting time to their study.

Wolf, A. and Schwartz, E. K. 1962. *Psychoanalysis in Groups*, New York: Grune and Stratton.

Alexander Wolf was the initiator of the group psychotherapy at Knox, its large and small groups, and its psychoanalytic bent. Under his leadership, the groups worked through its issues, leading to inquiry into the deeper issues of the individual, leading to character changes. But insufficient authoritarian aspects of his character led to difficulty with the prisoners leading to impasses, near riot, then his replacement. Lloyd McCorkle, who followed him in charge initiated what he termed guided group interaction, in which he exerted what he held was the necessary authority, in guiding the members to conform to the norms of group therapy, including issuing military commands. Somehow, the members found my interventions appropriately authoritative, engaging in the dynamics initiated by Wolf, down to working through to the individual dynamic mechanisms.

Psychoanalysis in Groups is an exposition of Wolf's theory and practice in treatment of individuals in his practice prior to and after his military service. First, he emphases the equality between therapist and person afforded by the group. Then he notes its advantage in reality testing. Not only that, but the group stimulates interpersonal communication as well as the intra-communication of psychoanalysis. Moreover, he has his groups meet without him, for testing, exploring, and consolidating. It is cited as a specific for isolation and socialization. He sees the psychoanalyst of the future as giving up his isolation, eschewing the intrapsychic as "mystical abstractions," and embracing the group dynamic in his practice.

Yalom, I.D. 1983. *Inpatient Group Psychotherapy*, New York: Basic Books; (1985) *The Theory and Practice of Group Psychotherapy*, New York: Basic Books.

This psychiatrist has contributed seminally to the field of group psychotherapy in inpatient and outpatient settings. His approach is active and interpersonal, with emphasis on guided inquiry into the here-and-now as demonstrated in the group dynamic, also carefully structured feedback. Lower functioning patients are placed in groups of non-exploratory or supportive nature. He generally also structures groups towards support and problem solving, avoiding psychoanalytic regression and decompensation.

Yochelson, Samuel, and Samenow, Stanton. 1976. *The Criminal Personality: Profile for Change*, New York: Aronson.

Yochelson and Samenow report on 15 years of research in the criminal personality at St. Elizabeths Hospital. They arrive at the thesis that inquiry on the part of the criminal into cause results in perpetuation of the disorder. Instead they focus on inducing the abandonment of the personality traits that lead to crime. This reeducation occurred in a conversion process "reluctant converts," proceeding to systematic reeducation. The last was done outside the hospital, because of administrative problems with personnel. This is reminiscent of the problems with the attendants in the work in Howard Hall reported in *This Way Out*.

In their groups the criminal presented his 24 hour phenomenologic report, and the inquiry extended to his thoughts as well as actions, in "microscopic attention," leading to the person's view of life. They cite the view of life as abstract, but it was an abstraction that was at the core of the individual's problem with alienation. They assured the criminal that following their method would lead to the building of a meaningful life. This sounds similar to the implicit contract made in *This Way Out*. "Impeccable functioning" differed from later emphasis on responsible arrival at decisions more than the decision itself. Families were separately consulted for data, as privileged communication.

It becomes apparent that this work grew to resemble that reported in *This Way Out*, also differed markedly. Both strove to arrive at conceiving of the person's life purposes, collaboratively, engaged through mutually arrived at idealism and state of mutual responsibility. The context of the work in time was separated from the hospital, because of failure to arrive at a state of mutual confidence. Eschewing insight led to handicap in the long term. And, despite for the need of a certain degree of authoritarianism in a security bound situation, there appeared to be an excess here. That criminality is exposed and destroyed by rationality and logic appears to be a delusion and snare. Unacknowledged messianism would more rationally be behind the project's changes.

Index

Abrahams, J., xv, xvii, xxxiv, 348, 758, 759, 797, 798
Abse, Wilfred D., 799
abuse: childhood, 227–28, 393, 408, 424–25, 428, 430, 701, 741, 742; by father, 742; by mother, 429–30, 431, 701; substance, 224, 259, 260, 295, 296. *See also* women
Acheson, Dr., 330
actualization, 657
addiction, 224
administration, 174–75, 492, 493
administrative theory, xxxi–xxxii
Admission Conference, 138–39
advent phenomenon, 763, 772–73, 778
affect: in schizophrenia, 16; transference of, 29
affection, 32
aggression: response to, 19, 57–58; towards women, 216, 226, 233–34, 240, 247, 253, 276, 741
Aichorn, August, xxv, 784, 807; messianism of, 808; *Wayward Youth* by, xiv, 776, 777
airplane kits, 91, 92
alcohol, 296, 433, 435–36, 720
alcoholism, 224
Alexander, Franz, 809–10

alienation, xii, 734–35, 736; of Bolster, 399; of Certa, 449, 703; cycles of, xvii; definition of, 763–64; from despondency, 257, 258; from doctors, 343, 344; of Forster, 215, 725, 743, 744; genesis of, xxxiv; Glover on, 809–10; of Hollister, 393, 682; inference of, 750; of James, 501; of Jefferson, 393, 394; of leadership, 2–3; letting go of, 10; racial identity, 121, 132, 133, 405, 449, 682, 703; regression from, 764; with schizophrenia, 781; from therapist, 328; from women, 463
alienists, 764
Allen, Frank, 75, 80
ambivalence, 194, 214
amnesia, 296. *See also* Bostic, Wilfred
Anacostia River, 22–23
anal sex, 356, 357
Analysis of a Prison Disturbance (Abrahams and McCorkle), 797
Analysis of Groups: Contributions to Theory, Research, and Practice (Gibbard, Harperman, and Mann), 809
Anemone, 767
anethnopaths, 751

680, 697; criticism by, 390; denial
by, 682; family of, 407, 676, 680,
682; Foster and, 666; history of,
377, 384, 393, 397, 678, 679, 680;
homosexuality of, 387, 402, 484,
676, 677, 678; individual analysis,
676–83; James and, 642–43, 679;
Jefferson and, 387, 617, 676, 679;
leadership by, 678, 680, 683; low
self esteem of, 380, 384, 385, 678;
messianism of, 742; as outsider,
402; on Poe, 404; racial attitudes
of, 682; rehabilitation of, 389, 481,
483; on relationships, 379, 380,
384, 385, 387, 677, 678, 744–45; on
religion, 376, 767; resentment by,
481; superiorism of, 742; therapeutic
alliance with, 683; as underachiever,
680, 681, 683
Holster, 246; anger of, 710; crying
by, 264, 743; delusions of, 254; on
Forster, 248; history of, 253–54, 708;
individual analysis, 708–11; Jordan
and, 253; masculinity of, 253–54;
relationship of, 213, 216, 264, 267,
283, 709, 710, 711; on religion, 709
homosexuality, 48, 101–2; acceptance
of, 318–19, 328; assault with, 356,
357, 743; of Bostic, 210, 591; of
Certa, 510, 700, 702; of Cohen, 327,
630; of Dormer, 263, 304, 305, 673,
742; father and, 484–85, 654, 745;
from fear of women, 265; Forster
and, 214, 215, 498, 724, 725, 743;
Foster and, 659, 660, 741; of Harvey,
417; of Hollister, 387, 402, 484, 676,
677, 678; James on, 483–84, 642; of
Jefferson, 375, 426, 439, 601, 604,
612, 615, 616, 619, 620, 623, 676,
700, 740; of Jordan, 271, 538, 737;
of Lauton, 487, 576, 739; of new
member, 211; in prison, 263, 265,
269, 483; as problem, 270–71; of
Reardon, 327, 332, 335, 336, 646,
648, 649, 650, 740; regression into,

744–45; resistance to, 367; of Street,
149, 487, 576, 738, 739; White
Therapy Group on, 446
Hospital-Wide Group Work Training
Program, 759, 798
Howard, John, xiii
Howard Hall, xi, xiii, xxiv, *793, 794*;
1, 4–5; 2, 172; 3, 67, 96–97; 5,
xxix; 6, 121; attendants at, 36–37,
38, 63, 64, 193, 194, 214, 215,
244, 355, 373, 409, 463, 468–69,
470, 476, 492, 550, 555–56, 749,
822; fear of leaving, 414; Fort
Knox Rehabilitation Center for
Military Prisoners and, 758; group
size at, 453, 754, 762; location of,
xxv, 752; normalization at, 735;
recordings from, 122, 123–24;
regression at, 812–13; rehabilitation
at, 754–55, 758; reputation of,
xv; segregation at, xv–xvi, xxxii,
313–14, 443–44; sexual offenders
at, xxx–xxxi; therapeutic support at,
22, 23; transaction in, 813; women
in, 789
The Howard Hall Journal, xvii, xxviii,
32, *795*; board of, 403, 408, 412,
667, 681, 718; editorial page of,
790–91; founding of, 314, 399, 447,
626, 735, 749, 774, 789; leadership
of, 292–93; Sheridan and, 790
Hyacinthus, 767
hypochondria: of other patients, 131; of
Street, 88, 93, 97, 98, 100, 109, 110,
111, 120, 134, 136–37, 146, 155,
566, 567, 570, 571, 572, 738
hypomania, 233, 234

Id, 770–71, 773, 809–10
ideals, 4, 338
identity: Cohen's, 774; Erikson on,
783; Forsyth's, 474; gender, 474;
Harvey's, 510, 511; Jefferson's, 774;
Jones, L.'s, 15; Jordan's, xxxiv, 774,
778; lone wolf, 348; racial, 121, 132,